Also by Timothy S. Hall

Surgical Systems: Structure and Function

Surgical Systems: Quality Management

Cover Design by Elizabeth C. Hall

SURGICAL

SYSTEMS

GENERAL SURGICAL RESIDENCY CURRICULUM

Timothy S. Hall, MD

Two Golden Rules Publishing

http://twogoldenrules.wix.com/info

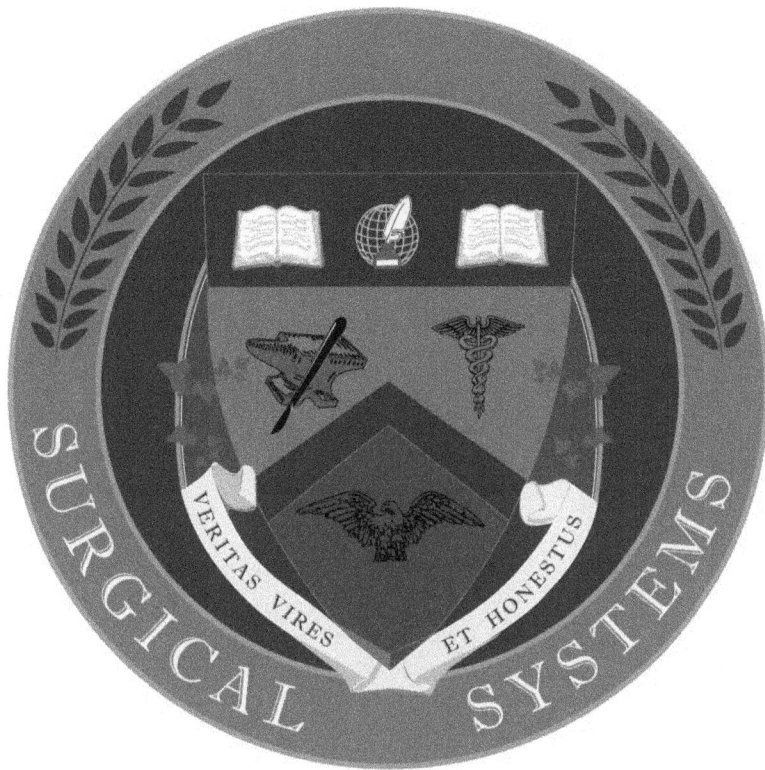

Published by Two Golden Rules Publishing, Connecticut

ISBN   978-0-9885542-6-9

Preface

This surgical curriculum draws heavily from the Intercollegiate Surgical Curriculum Project from the UK, prior recommendations from the Association of Program Directors in Surgery and original curriculum materials. It has been modified to meet the ACGME curriculum recommendations and regulations. The companion volume, Surgical Systems: General Surgical Residency Assessment provides the program structure and details of the applied tools to verify the success of using this curriculum. An outline of that material is presented in this volume, but that content was too extensive to include in this text.

> *"When you don't know where you are going, any road will take you there"*
> Talmudic sayin

The quote above is noted to be of several origins but it is historically referenced to the Talmud. It is also popularly known by its use in "Alice in Wonderland", a story that may seem to parallel life for surgical trainees. The objective of this curriculum is twofold. First, it is to provide a "road map" that sets goals and objectives for the residents to direct their studies. The second goal is to provide the baseline material to meet ACGME requirements. The construction of the curriculum represents a combination of both purposes. It has been modified at least quarterly to continue to meet the needs of residents and the ACGME and will most likely require the same schedule of change in the future.

> "All you need is the plan, the road map, and the courage to press
> on to   your destination."
> Earl Nightingail

As surgeons, we spend many hours directing residents or demonstrating to residents how to conduct the practice of surgery. It is easy to forget that there is a difference between training and educating. To consider educating learners in the discipline of Surgery, the curriculum provides the focus of the educational program. The curriculum is where the residents start; by reviewing the required competencies and goals it puts their educational efforts in context. As they are training; regular reviews of the curriculum will help trainees identify their strengths and weaknesses. As residents prepare for their final proof of competency, the curriculum will serve to measure their preparation. For the surgical faculty, the curriculum will serve to focus their teaching efforts; both in extent and detail and assist in future improvement in their teaching efforts.

TABLE OF CONTENTS

CHAPTER 1

PRE-REQUISITE CURRICULUM

*P*rogram overview

STRUCTURE

The overall program consists of 3 parts. First, structure from reading of a basic text in surgery, such as the "ESSENTIALS OF GENERAL SURGERY" by LAWERENCE. The aim is to create a common based of knowledge and language prior to starting the clinical work. Second, each new intern should be assessed on their medical knowledge, basic science knowledge and clinical skills. This requires testing on the first 2 days of orientation. Recently we have included examinations on non-medical areas such as Emotional Intelligence as well. Typical assessment subjects are listed below.

ASSESSMENT

       HISTORY TAKING

       PHYSICAL EXAMINATION

       TREATMENT PLANNING

       CUMMUNICATION SKILLS

COORDINATION OF MEDICAL SERVICES

ANATOMY

PHYSIOLOGY

CHEMISTRY

PHARMACOLOGY

PATHOLOGY

HOSPITAL SYSTEMS

The final section that is part of the pre-requisite training program is a Summer Training Course. This consists of a combination of education on medical knowledge, logistical requirements and skills training to enhance the transition from medical student to intern. This program is best conducted and run by the Chief and Senior Residents. As a "resident run" program, it offers an opportunity for resident bonding and program solidification. Common topics incorporated into the training include:

RESIDENT ORIENTATION

SIMULATION PROGRAM INTRODUCTION

ULTRASOUND TRAINING

PATHOLOGY COORDINATION

ASEPTIC TECHNIQUE AND PROPHYLAXIS

SURGICAL EMERGENCIES

LIBRARY SERVICES

An important part of the Pre-Requisite Curriculum is the new intern or resident assessment, through the testing of medical knowledge, skills review and personal interactions. From this process, a formal assessment is created to emphasize the new intern's or resident's strengths and weaknesses and a plan for improvement. This plan encompasses the "assignment" of a senior resident or chief to each new intern or resident to guide their progress and as a future resource for the next most difficult years of their lives.

CHAPTER 2

EXTRA CURRICULAR PROGRAMS

Courses and Take Home Exams

TAKE HOME EXAMINATIONS

With the hours restrictions, Program directors need to be creative in forming educational activities. One approach is to look to new types of educational approaches and for educational opportunities in the residents busy schedules. A solution to the difficult scheduling of educational events are take home examinations. The subjects may include important topics that could be performed in the resident's free time, usually on a quarterly basis and then reinforced through the ABSITE practice testing. The performance on the Take Home examinations are weighted and included in the Assessment Grid. The full explanation of the Take Home examinations content will be included in the Volume on Resident Assessment. A listing of the commonly used topics includes:

Take Home Exams-(Cycled over 2 year period)

1.   Interpersonal Communication

2.   Informed Consent

3.   Professionalism

4.   System Based Practice

5.   Evidence Based Medicine

6.   Practice Based Learning

7.   Peri-operative Risk Assessment

8.   Cross Cultural Training.

COURSES AND SUBJECT REVIEWS

Another supplement to the training of the standard medical subjects is to provide limited courses and reviews with specific training aims. These are subjects that require more time than the typical hour or two related to most educational sessions and can be supplemented with offsite reading and preparation. Many of these subjects are about process and culture, the "tacit knowledge" component of successful surgical intelligence. Similar to the Take Home Exams, these courses are often quarterly; in addition they can be varied by level. The full content of these courses will be incorporated in the volume on Assessment; several examples are provided.

Courses or Reviews

9.   Management and Leadership

10.   Critical Thinking

11.   Self-Assessment Program

12.   Sleep and Fatigue Training

13.   Surgical Culture-History,

14.   "Commander's Intent"

15.   Training Pyramid

16.   IRB Certification

17.   Resident Teaching

Management and leadership Course

Each PGY level will be introduced to basic management and leadership training which will be level specific. Using the provided materials, a take home exam will be completed and the material reviewed during the mentoring program meetings and at the biannual review.

OBJECTIVES

To educate and develop the skills and tools for team and system management and leadership using the management introductory series from McGraw Hill. This series; in an uncomplicated manner, uses checklists, special tips/tactics and focused exercises to inform and educate surgical residents for management and leadership roles.

STRUCTURE

Starting in May of the Intern year, residents will be expected to complete the assigned reading and complete the associated take home exam. Management and leadership Meetings with groups of residents will then review and focus on the management or leadership issues that are typically encountered for that level of surgical practice.

Level Specific Goals and Objectives will be incorporated into the curriculum

RESOURCES

PGY 1 The New Manager's Handbook. Morey Stettner McGraw Hill 2006

PGY 2 Managing Multiple Projects Michael Tobis, Irene Tobis Mc Graw Hill 2002
      Read Chapters 1 to 10, 12

PGY 3 Skills for New Managers Morey Stettner, Mc Graw Hill 2000
      Read Chapters 1 to 10

PGY 4 Leadership Skills for Managers Marlene Caroselli Mc Graw Hill 2000. Focus on
      Chapters 1-6, 8
      Read Chapters 1 to 6, 8 and 10

Critical Thinking Course

As outlined below, a course of critical thinking will be incorporated into case presentations and assessed as part of the communication competency.

> *"Not everything that can be counted counts,*
>> *and not everything that counts can be counted."*
>> *--- Albert Einstein*

> *"If a man will begin with certainties, he shall end in doubts.*
>> *But if he will be content to begin with doubts he shall end in certainties."*
>> *--- Francis Bacon*

We all engage in clinical decision making and problem solving every day. It is a reasonable question to ask "what is the value of reviewing a skill we already have". Unfortunately the practice of surgery is a "bounded rationality" in which reasonable decisions can degenerate to irrational results due to clinical constraints. Our conference on Excellence in Surgical Education (ESE) each week provides case presentations that illustrate inappropriate assumptions, false dichotomies, logical fallacies and demonstrates why a more formalized approach can improve patient outcomes and surgeon performance.

Our goals are:
1. Teach the foundations of critical thinking to create an acquirable skill
2. Create an environment for critical thinking application with reasoned debate, not dissent, as a foundation for surgical education.

Using this review material we will apply a context-dependent model for critical thinking which will be the cases presented at ESE. Our methods will apply the Paul and Elder Model which uses a multidisciplinary perspective under the purview of a facilitator in an environment that encourages reflective skepticism and open discussion. We will encourage the identification of "automatic thinking" (no stop and think) the clarification of data (How do we know what we know), the clarification of how success can lead to narrow mindedness (Egocentric memory and blindness). We will try to emphasize the role of clinical based guidelines and best practice (heuristics) in both aiding and creating errors in decision making. We also try to emphasize the value of multiple perspectives and input to aid decision making. We will try to identify incidences of confirmational traps, overconfidence, attribution errors, self-serving bias, logical fallacies, false dichotomies, and weak analogies (Glossary of Terms attached).

Assessment

Surgical Residents will be assessed for critical thinking during case presentation during the ESE conference.

Extracurricular AV Study in Surgical Techniques

The extracurricular study in surgical techniques include Audiovisual Materials for you to review as an initial form of training, The Course material will be signed out or scheduled on a regular basis and must be completed and returned by the end of the academic year. A short examination on the material will be incorporated into your biannual meeting with the program director.

Simulation Curriculum-open and Laparoscopic, Robotic

PICC line-PGY 1

AV Fistula-PGY 2

School of Breast Oncology training -PGY3

FLS Certification -PGY 4

Limb Ischemia –PGY 4

Laparoscopic Colon Course -PGY 5

Resident Teaching Program

As a surgeon, part of the requirements to maintain an excellent practice is to be able to educate your staff related to your practice and specific patient needs. Additionally, educating students from all fields enhances and improves a surgeon's expertise in the subject area involved. Previously, resident teaching was modeled based on prior residents and faculty behaviors, often missing the important educational concepts that form the basis of effective teaching. A course of study has been designed to develop or improve the educational abilities of residents for their teaching of students, each other and faculty. The course content is included in the Assessment Volume; the subject list is included below.

1. Resident Teaching needs Assessment
2. Teaching to Teach-Micro skills
3. Principles of Adult Learning
4. Providing Constructive Criticism
5. Teaching Psychomotor Skills
6. Chief Resident Leadership Teaching

Complex Surgical Case Management/Surgical Case Series

The historic Mortality and Morbidity Conference is often resident presentations of complications and mortalities aimed at education regarding preventing poor patient outcomes. As was reviewed in the Quality Management Volume, the value of this approach is often limited and it neglects the potential learning from complex cases that were well managed or that represent unusual clinical situations which can provide an enhanced learning opportunity. To address these limitations of the M and M, a supplemental educational program on Tuesday mornings will incorporate a 1 hour presentation of recent complex case management or a specified topic related to patient management using a problem presentation and evidenced based review.

Cases will be presented by the involved resident and attending with their Clinical Documentation and Imaging in a step by step process focusing on decision making and management.

Chapter 3

ASSESSMENT PROGRAM

*T*he general surgical residency Assessment program is presented in its own volume; "General

Surgery Residency Assessment Program". What will be presented in this volume will be an

outline of the approach.

OUTLINE OF APPROACH

1.   OVERVIEW
2.   ASSESSMENT TOOLS DESCRIPTION
     A.   EVALUATIONS-ATTENDING AND RESIDENTS, 360
     B.   CONFERENCE ATTENDANCE
     C.   SELF ASSESSMENT
     D.   ABSITE PERFORMANCE
     E.   ABSITE ANNUAL REVIEW
     F.   ANNUAL BASIC SCIENCE EXAM
     G.   JOURNAL CLUB PRESENTATIONS
     H.   MORK ORAL BOARDS (SENIOR RESIDENTS

I.   OPEN SKILLS ASSESSMENT

J.   SIMULATION COMPENCTIES

K.   LAPROSCOPIC SKILLS ASSESSMENT

L.   CASE LISTS

M.   ATLS/BLS COURSE COMPLETION

N.   CASE BASED DISCUSSION CBD

O.   SURCIAL SKILLS OBSERVATION SSO

P.   PRACTICE BASED EXAM

     I.   EVIDENCED MEDICINE EXAM

     II.   MEDICAL DECISION MAKING

     III.   RESIDENT RESEARCH

Q.   INTERPERSONAL SKILLS AND COMMUNICATION ASSESSMENT

     I.   COMMUNICATIONS/INTERPERSONAL SKILLS EXAM

     II.   RESIDENT PRESENTATIONS

     III.   CHIEF RESIDENT PRESENTATIONS

R.   PROFESSIONALISM ASSESSMENT

     I.   PROFESSIONALISM EXAM

     II.   INFORMED CONSENT EXAM

S.   SYSTEM BASED ASESSMENT

     I.   JOURNAL CLUB

     II.   SYSTEM BASED TAKE HOME EXAM

     III.   PATIENT SAFETY EXAM

3.   PROGRAM RELATED ASSESSMENT AND IMPROVEMENT PROGRAM

4.   RESIDENT MENTORING PROGRAM

OVERVIEW

A requirement of the ACGME is to implement an assessment program of the surgical curriculum and to institute an improvement program based on the assessments results. Enclosed is an outline of a Surgery Assessment Program, the full version is provided in the Assessment Volume of this series. That volume provides the assessment tools and how they are applied to resident evaluation. Many of these assessment tools have been adapted from ACGME related workshop recommendations and from the Intercollegiate Surgical Curriculum Pilot from the United Kingdom. The assessment tools are meant to complement the standard resident evaluations and case logs to improve the breath of training consistent with the ACGME competencies. The new assessment tools are applied to enhance simulation training and the applications of information technologies. On an annual basis, an overall assessment score is created for each resident based on the cumulative results of the assessment tools to help guide decisions regarding promotion in the program.

Another required assessment is an annual overall program evaluation and improvement plan. The program assessment tools descriptions follow the resident assessment program. A cumulative score for the program can be generated from the program assessment tools to assess the success of the program and to focus on areas of improvement.

RESIDENT RELATED ASSESSMENT TOOLS

EVALUATIONS

Residents will be evaluated by rotation or quarterly by the surgical faculty using the evalue system, which includes the ACGME competencies assessments. Additionally, a year-end review will be included to confirm the appropriateness of promotion to the next level. The resident's rating will be compared to their peers and tracked during the residency for progress, improvement and for sited deficiencies.

CONFERENCE ATTENDANCE

Attendance at Journal club, Weekly Case Review, Surgical Mortality and Morbidity Conference, Surgical Grand Rounds, Basic Science Course, Trauma service review and Service related Tumor Board is required. Resident attendance will be recorded and monitored. Video recorded lectures for those not able to attend related to hours restrictions will be recorded from the library sign out.

SELF-ASSESSMENT

Resident self-assessment will be appraised by review of their professional journals for completeness related to case activity, patient related outcomes, self-assessment notes on performance, evidence of self-improvement objectives. It will be part of the biannual review with the program director.

ABSITE PERFORMANCE

Resident performance on the ABSITE examination will continue to be a primary assessment tool for resident medical knowledge. Residents with total ABSITE scores below the 20th percentile for 2 years sequentially will be placed on probation. A third year below the 20th percentile will be grounds for removal from the program. The sited ABSITE deficiencies will be reviewed with an improvement program annually.

ABSITE ANNUAL REVIEW

Resident performance on the ABSITE examination will be used as an assessment tool and review program for resident medical knowledge. Residents will be required to review their sited errors on the ABSITE exam and prepare a short review related to the question of concern. The sited ABSITE deficiencies will be reviewed with an improvement program biannually as part of the directors meeting.

BASIC SCIENCE TEST

An examination for each subject reviewed will be completed on a weekly basis and a comprehensive exam will be given annually. The examination results will be reviewed with the resident and a study plan implemented to address deficiencies.

OPEN SKILLS ASSESSMENT

Surgical skills will be assessed for open procedures by performing basic surgical skills related to level of training. Skill sets will be assessed for time and quality, tracked for progress and with improvement programs instituted for remedial performance.

SIMULATION COMPENTENCIES

Using the surgical simulation laboratory basic skill sets will be completed successfully as part of the procedural competencies. Completion of required competencies will be necessary for progression to the next training level.

LAPROSCOPIC SKILLS ASSESSMENT

Surgical skills will be assessed for laparoscopic procedures by performing basic surgical skills related to level of training. Skill sets will be assessed for time and quality, tracked for progress and with improvement programs instituted for remedial performance.

ATLS/ACLS COURSE COMPLETION

ATLS/ACLS courses will be completed as part of the resident training program with residents maintaining currency in BLS.

CASE BASED DISCUSSIONS-MOCK ORALS

Each senior resident will participate in a mock oral program with an assessment reviewed during the semiannual review with a study plan developed for deficiencies.

CASE BASED DISCUSSIONS-CBD

Case based discussions are focused case reviews similar to mock oral boards using the ICSP template assessment program. When possible, these will be cases drawn from the resident's case records to allow for complete assessment. Case categories will be selected based on curriculum objectives for each level.

"Answer to Operate" Program

To help increase the motivation of the residents to increase their learning activities, we are using the "Answer to Operate" Program. For residents to be allowed a significant role in an operation they will be required to answer at least 3 questions about the pathophysiology of the patients disease, the operative technique and the clinical outcomes.

Residents that cannot answer the question will only be allowed to assist during the case. This is a department standard.

SURGICAL SKILLS OBSERVATION

Direct Observation procedural skills assessments are focused assessments. Residents will arrange assessments with the staff surgeon for selected cases. The case categories will be based on curriculum objectives by level of training. Performances will be reviewed using the SSO review document and returned to the program director. When appropriate, improvement plans for the residents will be developed.

PRACTICE BASED EXAMS

The section on practice-based medicine will focus on the use of evidence-based medicine and its incorporation into clinical practice as demonstrated by examination. Medical decision-making will be included in this course of study as a separate evaluation.

Practice based-EBM exam

Medical Decision Making exam

INTERPERSONAL SKILLS AND COMMUNICATION ASSESSMENT

A course related to interpersonal skills and communications will be included annually with an examination. Residents will also be expected to present a topic annually for evaluation. The Chief residents will present a Surgical Grand Rounds each spring that will be incorporated in their final evaluation. These skills will also be assessed in the general evaluations during rotations.

Communication-orientation-

Resident presentations

Chief Grand Rounds presentations

PROFESSIONALISM ASSESSMENT

Professionalism will be assessed through an educational program and an examination focusing on ethics. Part of this course of study will include a course and examination on informed consent. These skills will also be assessed in the general rotation evaluations.

Profession-take home ethics

Informed Consent-take home exam

SYSTEM BASED ASSESSMENT

System based issues will be addressed by a course and examination on health care access and with review of the residents evaluation of the scientific literature as part of their participation in the weekly Journal Club. These skills will also be assessed in the general rotation evaluations.

System based- take home exam

Journal Club Presentations

Mentoring program

Although the mentoring program is designed as a support system for the residents, it also functions as part of the overall assessment program. Because these interactions occur outside of the clinical arena, it provides the faculty with additional insights into the resident's activities and personality, and thereby can improve the overall resident assessment.

Resident mentoring programs have been cited as a method to improve faculty and resident communication and enhance role modeling. Although the resident and faculty interaction in the program has always been good, it has been sporadic for the interns and second years. To address this issue, we will have a formal mentoring program for all the residents.

Interns will be assigned mentors at the beginning of their careers with the expectations that they may change when they determine their specialty interest.

Residents will meet with the Mentors at least quarterly, but preferably monthly for at least 30 minutes to discuss their careers in a setting of their own choosing.

Mentors will be available for advice and support on an ad-hoc basis.

Biannual Program Director review

This meeting should be an overall review of resident related progress including case activities, completed educational goals, performance measures and evaluations. The review should also be "open ended" and "quiet enough" to allow the resident the opportunity to reflect on progress, successes and failures, goals and plans.

PROGRAM RELATED ASSESSMENT

The overall program review is meant to encompass more than just assessing the residents involved in the program and their progress. This assessment should try to engender the review and criticism of the entire spectrum of the training program from orientation to certification of chief competency, include resident, and faculty research and scholarship and the program's commitment to humanitarian goals. The best approach to creating the appropriate atmosphere for contemplation of perspective and content is a faculty retreat. Some of the basic data sources for preparation for the event include:

GRADUATION REVIEW

Graduation Assessment

Board Certification Percentage

Staff privileging success

Survey Assessment- alumni

Noted accomplishments

ABSITE REVIEW

The overall resident performance on the ABSITE will be reviewed for program related deficiencies and form the basis for educational modification of the curriculum presentation.

ANNUAL FACULTY REVIEW

Annually the residents and faculty will be surveyed regarding the strength and weaknesses of the program. These results will be tabulated and reviewed in the surgical education committee and subsequently presented to the GMEC and at an open seminar for faculty and staff. Recommendations for improvements will be addressed and reported to the faculty and incorporated into the Surgical Education Committee resolution items.

CHAPTER 4

DEFINITION AND SCOPE OF SPECIALTY TRAINING:

*T*he goal of a surgical residency program is to prepare the resident to function as a qualified

practitioner of surgery at a high level of performance typical of a board-certified specialist. The education of surgeons for the practice of general surgery encompasses education in basic sciences, training in cognitive and technical skills, development of clinical knowledge, and maturity in the acquisition of surgical judgment. The educational program includes the fundamentals of basic science as applied to clinical surgery, including: wound healing, physiological homeostasis, hematological disorders, oncology, genitourinary physiology, surgical endocrinology, nutrition, fluid and electrolyte balance, shock, metabolic response to injury including burns, musculoskeletal biomechanics and physiology, immunobiology and transplantation, applied surgical anatomy, and surgical pathology.

The *General Surgical Resident Curriculum* constructs its professional training toward competency with objective measures of development, which are included in each curriculum unit. The core competencies were structured with summary curriculum goals descriptive of the desired outcomes of surgical education. When competencies are viewed in conjunction with the objective criteria in each unit, one has a combination of indicators of what is essential for resident learning. The general educational areas in this surgical resident curriculum from which competencies and specific criteria exist, including:

- Integration of theory and practice

- Application of surgical skills

- Use of critical thinking

- Exercise of ethical judgment

- Use of appropriate communication

- Recognition of teaching responsibilities

- Development of system management abilities

This curriculum has been updated and modified directly from the Curriculum developed for the Association of Program Directors in Surgery blended with the Intercollegiate Surgical Curriculum Project from the United Kingdom and the prior Surgical Curriculum. Additions have included the integration of the ACGME competencies project to allow for complete teaching and assessment. The assessment program incorporates the ACGME competencies.

Overview

The proposed curriculum model is:

➤ service-led - providing surgeons fit-for-purpose to work within the clinical practice at Health Systems

➤ modular – permitting trainees to be accredited to provide specific services/skills at particular levels, and not merely at the end of training

> flexible - allowing resident's to alter their career paths and to take time out for personal commitments and interests.

> modern – representing a significant shift from established surgical thinking to incorporate new proposals from the ACGME, ABS and APDS.

Overview of the scope of General Surgery

General Surgery is a large core specialty dealing with high volumes of emergency admissions and a wide range of elective procedures. The majority of consultant general surgeons practice electively in one or more subspecialist areas while managing emergencies in general surgery.

The subspecialties of general surgery taught within the system include:

- Breast Surgery
- Colorectal Surgery
- Trauma and Critical Care
- Surgical Oncology
- Transplant
- Vascular Surgery
- General and Acute Care Surgery
- Pediatric Surgery
- Plastic Surgery
- Cardiothoracic Surgery

1. **Transplantation.** Transplant surgery experience is provided by a one-month rotation in the PGY-3 year on the Transplantation Service at the Hospital. This service is a busy renal and hepatic transplant service. Our residents perform many vascular access procedures and have including the suture renal transplant anastomoses. The resident will learn the principles of immunology, immunosuppression and the technical aspects of organ transplantation.

2.   **Burns.** Each PGY-1 resident spends one month on the burn service at the Burn Center. During this time, the resident actively participates in the resuscitation and long-term treatment of severely burned patients. Residents learn the fundamentals of burn care and become proficient with skin grafting techniques.

Program Components

Clinical Resources

Clinical problems are of sufficient variety and volume to afford the residents adequate experience in the diagnosis and management of adult and pediatric disorders.

Continuity of Care

All residents have the opportunity to develop competence in the preadmission care, hospital care, operative care, and follow-up care (including rehabilitation) of patients. Opportunities for resident involvement in all aspects of care of the same patient are maximized. Each patient in the general surgery clinic is assigned to a junior and senior resident. All aspects of patient care are scheduled and coordinated by their assigned residents for procedures and follow up.

Non-operative Outpatient Experience

Residents have adequate experience in non-operative outpatient diagnosis and care, including multiple areas of medical care and patients of all age groups. Each week residents have at least one or two half days of outpatient clinical experience in physician offices or hospital clinics with a minimum of 10 patients per session on all clinical rotations. Residents are directly supervised by faculty and instructed in pre- and post-operative assessment as well as the operative and non-operative care of general and subspecialty patients. Opportunities for resident involvement in all aspects of outpatient care of the same patient maximized. Surgical Critical Care is taught as a formal course of study in ICU management with a syllabus and educational objectives.

Progressive Responsibility

Residents must have the opportunity to assume increasing responsibility for patient care, under direct faculty supervision (as appropriate for each resident's ability and experience), as they progress through a program.

Basic Surgical Skills

Instruction in basic motor skills including experience in the proper use of surgical instruments and operative techniques is a basic part of the training program. Evaluation of new or experimental techniques and/or materials is emphasized. The application of basic motor skills is integrated into daily clinical activities in the operating room. The process of skills education starts in the surgical simulation laboratory with basic techniques and procedures. Competencies are assigned, reviewed and approved each year and increased with sequential completion.

Residents Scholarly Activities

The program provides an opportunity for residents to participate in research or other scholarly activities, and residents must participate actively in such scholarly activities.

Resources for scholarly activity by residents includes computer and data analysis services, statistical consultation services, research conferences, faculty expertise and supervision, support personnel, time, and funding.

To develop the abilities to critically evaluate medical literature, research, and other scholarly activity, resident education includes instruction in experimental design, hypothesis testing, and other current research methods, as well as participation in clinical research.

Resident Duty Hours and the Working Environment

Providing residents with a sound didactic and clinical education is carefully planned and balanced with concerns for patient safety and resident well-being. The program ensures that the learning objectives of the program are not compromised by excessive reliance on residents to fulfill service obligations. Didactic and clinical education has priority in the allotment of resident's time and energy. Duty hour assignments recognize that faculty and residents collectively have responsibility for the safety and welfare of patients.

Supervision of Residents

1.   All patient care must be supervised by qualified faculty. The program director must ensure, direct, and document adequate supervision of residents at all times. Residents must be provided with rapid, reliable systems for communicating with supervising faculty.

2.   Faculty schedules must be structured to provide residents with continuous supervision and consultation.

3.   Faculty and residents are educated to recognize the signs of fatigue, and adopt and apply policies to prevent and counteract its potential negative effects. An instructional program is provided to assist in resident and staff education.

4.   Resident supervision is conducted in accordance with Health System Policy.

BASIC SCIENCES CURRICULUM

Basic science education includes substantial instruction in anatomy, biomechanics, pathology, and physiology. The basic science program must also include resident education in embryology, immunology, pharmacology, biochemistry, and microbiology.

(1)   Instruction in anatomy includes study and dissection of animal and simulation specimens by the residents and lectures or other formal sessions.

(2)   Instruction in pathology must include organized instruction in correlative pathology in which gross and microscopic pathology are related to clinical and roentgenographic findings.

(3)   Instruction in biomechanics is presented in seminars or conferences emphasizing principles, terminology, and application particularly to orthopedics.

(4)   Organized instruction in the basic medical sciences is integrated into the daily clinical activities by clearly linking the pathophysiologic process and findings to the diagnosis, treatment, and management of clinical disorders.

(5)   Organized instruction in the appropriate use and interpretation of radiographic and other imaging techniques must be provided for all residents.

Basic Science is held every Friday from 7 to 8 am. It is moderated by the Program Director or Assistant Program Director or faculty. Based on resident recommendations the Basic Science course is a resident mentored lecture with subject review by questions based on a basic science test. Curriculum sources include O'Leary "Physiologic Basis of Surgery", Norton "Essential Practice of Surgery", Sabiston "Textbook of Surgery"

Training Services Chart
Service Structure

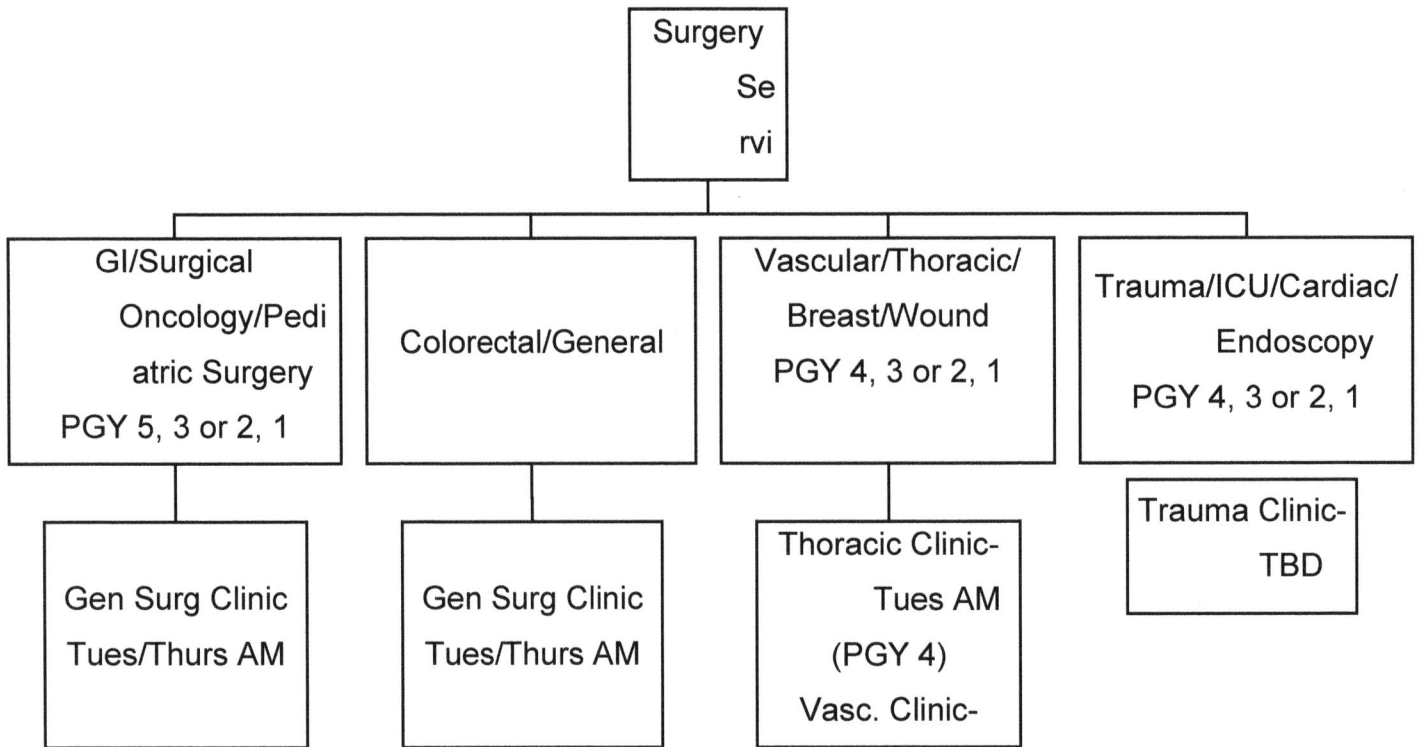

Figure 1. Service Structure

- During PGY4 away months (Trauma)
    - GI/Surg Onc Pediatric will combine w/ Colorectal/General to be comprised of PGY 5, 3a or 2a, 3b or 2b, 1, 1
    - PGY 5 from Surg. Onc replaces PGY4 Trauma/ICU/Cardiac
- During PGY 3 + 2 away months (Transplant/Burn)
    - Colorectal/General service will be comprised of PGY 5, 1
- During intern Ortho/anesthesia rotation months
    - Trauma/ICU/Cardiac/Endoscopy comprised of PGY4, 3 or 2

FIGURE 2. ROTATIONAL DESIGN

	JUL	AUG	SEP	OCT	NOV	DEC	JAN	FEB	MAR	APR	MAY	JUN
PGY 5	red	grey	green	blue	trauma	red	blue	blue	green	blue	red	green
PGY 5	grey	grey	green	trauma	green	green	green	trauma	trauma	trauma	trauma	green
PGY 5	green	green	blue	red	green	green	path	path	path	elective	elective	elective
PGY 4	vegas	red	elective	blue	trauma	red	green	green	blue	trauma	red	blue
PGY 4	trauma	vegas	red	elective	blue	trauma	red	red	green	blue	green	trauma
PGY 4	blue	trauma	vegas	green	elective	blue	blue	trauma	transplant	green	blue	blue
PGY 3	trauma	red	grey	grey	grey	trauma	trauma	transplant	grey	grey	trauma	trauma
PGY 3	grey	grey	trauma	grey	red	grey	trauma	transplant	trauma	trauma	trauma	trauma
PGY 3	grey	grey	trauma	trauma	trauma	grey	grey	grey	transplant	red	blue	grey
PGY 2	surg ed	surg ed	surg ed	burn	burn	burn	blue	blue	green	green	red	grey
PGY 2	green	green	green	green	red	red	blue	green	green	grey	blue	blue
PGY 2	red	green	green	blue	blue	green	green	trauma	trauma	green	trauma	grey
PGY 1	blue	blue	green	green	green	trauma	trauma	grey	grey	grey	red	red
PGY 1	green	green	trauma	trauma	trauma	grey	grey	red	blue	green	trauma	blue
PGY 1	trauma	trauma	grey	red	red	blue	blue	blue	blue	blue	green	green
PGY 1	grey	grey	red	blue	blue	green	red	green	green	trauma	trauma	trauma
PGY 1	red	red	blue	blue	grey	green	green	trauma	trauma	grey	grey	grey

Months on each rotation

	PGY 1	PGY 2	PGY 3	PGY 4	PGY 5
trauma	2	2	4	2	2
blue	2	2		2	2
green	2	3	2	2	2
gold	2				
red	2	1	1	2	2
grey	2	2	4	2	2
path					1
surg ed		1			
elective			1	1	1
away				1	1

elective should be endoscopy for PGY 4's and elective for PGY 5's

CHAPTER 5

ACGME COMPETENCIES

*O*VERVIEW

The underlying structure of the curriculum is the ACGME competencies format. What follows is the outline of the competencies, which are then further specified by PGY levels with accompanying behavioral goals and practices demonstrating implementation. To support this approach, the resident study guide is provided as a suggestion to the pace for the acquisition of the required knowledge. The final section is an outline of the expectations for the finished product of resident training.

Patient Care that is compassionate, appropriate, and effective for the treatment of health problems and the promotion of health. Accessible areas include:
History and physicals, medical decisions, management plans, procedures, preventative medicine, empathy, priorities, patient safety, quality assurance

Patient care that is compassionate, appropriate, and effective for the treatment of health programs and the promotion of health. Residents are expected to:

communicate effectively and demonstrate caring and respectful behaviors when interacting with patients and their families;

a. gather essential and accurate information about their patients;

b. make informed decisions about diagnostic and therapeutic interventions based on patient information and preferences, up-to-date scientific evidence, and clinical judgment;

c. develops and carries out patient management plans;

d. counsel and educate patients and their families;

e. demonstrates the ability to practice culturally competent medicine;

f. use information technology to support patient care decisions and patient education;

g. performs competently all medical and invasive procedures considered essential for the area of practice;

h. provide health care services aimed at preventing health problems or maintaining health;

i. work with health care professionals, including those from other disciplines, to provide patient-focused care.

Medical Knowledge about established and evolving biomedical, clinical, and cognate (e.g. epidemiological and social-behavioral) sciences and the application of this knowledge to patient care. Accessible areas include:

Conditions, treatments, outcomes, new advances

Medical Knowledge about established and evolving biomedical, clinical, and cognate sciences, as well as the application of this knowledge to patient care. Residents are expected to:

a. demonstrate an investigatory and analytic thinking approach to clinical situations

b. know and applies the basic and clinically supportive sciences, which are appropriate to surgery.

Practice-Based Learning and Improvement that involves investigation and evaluation of their own patient care, appraisal and assimilation of scientific evidence, and improvements in patient care. Accessible areas include:

Assess local and regional practices verses national, ethnic differences, using current literature, assess applicability, literature review, IT resources, teaching, assessment patterns of care, teaching.

Practice-based learning and improvement that involves the investigation and evaluation of care for their patients, the appraisal and assimilation of scientific evidence, and improvements in patient care. Residents are expected to:

    a.   analyzes practice experience and performs practice-based improvement activities using a systematic methodology;

    b.   locate, appraise, and assimilate evidence from scientific studies related to their patients' health problems;

    c.   obtains and uses information about their own population of patients and the larger population from which their patients are drawn;

    d.   applies knowledge of study designs and statistical methods to the appraisal of clinical e. use information studies and other information on diagnostic and therapeutic effectiveness; technology to manage information, access on-line medical information, and support their own education;

    f.   facilitates the learning of students and other health care professionals.

Interpersonal and Communication Skills that result in effective information exchange and teaming with patients, their families, and other health professionals. Accessible areas include: Patient and family communications, communication with associates, teamwork, counseling.

Interpersonal and communication skills that result in the effective exchange of information and collaboration with patients, their families, and other health professionals. Residents are expected to:

    a.   creates and sustains a therapeutic and ethically sound relationship with patients;

b.   use effective listening skills and elicit and provide information using effective nonverbal, explanatory, questioning, and writing skills; and

c.   work effectively with others as a member or leader of a healthcare team or other professional group.

Professionalism, as manifested through a commitment to carrying out professional responsibilities, adherence to ethical principles, and sensitivity to a diverse patient population. Accessible areas include:

Focus on respect, integrity, accountability, reliability, confidentiality, informed consent Professionalism, as manifested through a commitment to carrying out professional responsibilities, adherence to ethical principles, and sensitivity to patients of diverse backgrounds. Residents are expected to:

a.   demonstrate respect, compassion, and integrity; a responsiveness to the needs of patients and society that supersedes self-interest, accountability to patients, society and the profession and a commitment to excellence and ongoing professional development;

b.   demonstrate a commitment to ethical principles pertaining to provision or withholding of clinical care, confidentiality of patient information, informed consent, and business practices;

c.   demonstrate sensitivity and responsiveness to patient's culture, age, gender, and disabilities;

d.   demonstrate sensitivity and responsiveness to fellow health care professional's culture, age, gender, and disabilities.

Systems-Based Practice, as manifested by actions that demonstrate an awareness of and responsiveness to the larger context and system of health care and the ability to effectively call on system resources to provide care that is of optimal value. Accessible areas include:

Focus on standards of practice, delivery differences, access to care differences, cost issues, assess system problems, cooperation with hospital services, advocacy, and technology.

Provide a Systems-based practice, as manifested by actions that demonstrate an awareness of and responsiveness to the larger context and system of health care, as well as the ability to call effectively on other resources in the system to provide optimal health care. Residents are expected to:

a. understands how their patient care and other professional practices affect other healthcare professionals, the healthcare organization, and the larger society and how these elements of the system affect their own practice;

b. knows how types of medical practice and delivery systems differ from one another, including methods of controlling healthcare costs and allocating resources;

c. practice cost-effective health care and resources allocation that does not compromise quality of care;

d. advocate for quality patient care and assist patients in dealing with system complexities;

e. know how to partner with health care managers and healthcare procedures to assess, coordinate, and improve health care and know how these activities can affect system performance.

ACGME Competency Junior Levels I-II

Patient Care

In the junior levels, the resident will learn to effectively communicate in a respectful manner with the patient and their family. They learn to provide information regarding the procedure, risks, and benefits involved for the typical type of case.

The junior levels; the resident will learn to focus on the different features in medical history particular to surgical disease including, <u>urgency of the chief complaint,</u> prior acuity of the history of present illness, past medical history and critical features from the review of systems. The resident will <u>learn critical risk factors</u> related to specific disease states.

The junior level resident will learn and <u>understand the protocols</u> for treating patients, managing them both preoperatively and postoperatively.

To perform and document a relevant history and examination on culturally diverse patients.

The junior level resident will learn to explain <u>the effect of the procedure on the patient</u> postoperatively and the course for the typical type of postoperative patient.

The junior level resident will understand basic text book related information regarding decision making, concerns for common complications.

In the junior level, the surgical skills expected of the resident obtained are: understand the different types of techniques and procedures, the use of surgical equipment and products know the appropriate <u>incisions</u> required for appropriate exposure.

The junior level resident will learn baseline measures related to preventing further accentuation of health problems, such as proper follow-up, proper palliation of disease, and proper anticipation of complications related to disease.

The junior level resident will learn how patient progress through with their procedures and protocols, the critical evaluation and decision points regards to patient's undergoing surgery.

Medical Knowledge

The junior level resident will be assessed for the ability to evaluate, determine appropriate testing, and analytically evaluate patients The junior level resident will begin to understand the basic epidemiology of surgical related disease.

The junior level resident will be expected to learn baseline textbook information and have web access for the Surgery online curriculum.

Practice-based Learning and Improvement

Junior level resident will learn to appreciate patient care practices and perform practice-based care by learning from current practices, the variability that is typical in patients. They will learn the standards of patient care from best-practiced guidelines promoted by the American College of Surgeons, American Heart Association, and American College of Chest Physicians.

The junior level resident will learn to access the ACS, APDS and Surgery websites, and other surgery and evidence based medicine information systems such as Cochrane, Center for Evidenced Based Medicine or AHRQ. They will use the provided textbooks, video and online materials to review the latest scientific data for surgical disease.

The junior level resident will be educated as to the patient dynamics and demographics that are particular to their area of practice and how they compare with national guidelines regarding health indicators, such as activity and obesity, and learn basic differentiation from these patient populations as it affects risks and patient outcomes and recovery.

The junior level resident will be schooled in basic study design, in statistical methods as they discuss clinical studies for therapeutic effectiveness in surgical disease.

The junior level resident will demonstrate that they have access on-line information utilizing the Surgery website, ACS Surgery, and Information Services resources to further support information technology in regards to surgical disease.

The junior level resident will teach and present to medical students and health care professionals, provide insight and support and educational conferencing through rounds and didactics brought to conferences.

Interpersonal Communication Skills

The junior level resident will be assessed and be required to have an appropriate and communicative educational relationship with their patients, to provide advice and support of information regarding disease. With on-service rounds and direct patient interviews, the resident will be evaluated and instructed on how to provide affective listening skills, explanatory information, interpret non-verbal communication, and demonstrate good documentation skills in regards to specific surgical disease, uncommon surgical disease, thoracic disease, and end-stage disease.

The junior level resident will demonstrate that she/he is a team member, interacting with faculty, other fellows, nurse practitioners, physician assistants, nurses, and auxiliary staff and form a baseline for standard surgical problems.

Professionalism

The junior level resident will be expected to demonstrate through interaction and rounds that they have the utmost integrity and their considerate compassion for their patients with surgical disease.

The junior level resident will present and participate in didactic conferences on ethical principles regarding withholding of care, patient confidentiality, informed consent and business practices for surgical disease. Through conferences and didactic sessions and patient rounds the fellows will be instructed as to the diversity of patients and the need for appropriate sensitivity and responsiveness as it relates to age, culture, gender, and disabilities for patients with surgical disease.

System-based Practices

The junior level resident will be introduced to protocols and team organization, the importance of providing patient care in the setting with other health care professionals and consultants, the organization as a whole, and also the local society within which they practice for surgical disease.

In interacting with patients both on the floor and during the discharge process, the junior level resident will learn the basic differences between medical practice in urban and rural areas and different delivery systems related to payer problems that would affect postoperative support for patients with surgical disease.

The junior level resident will be introduced to cost effectiveness and research allocation from basic problems and surgical disease.

The junior level resident will be a primary patient advocate as a service supervisor for patients with surgical disease and end-stage problems.

The junior level resident will be introduced to the basic system-related guidelines to provide additional administrative and institutional support for patients with basic problems in surgical disease.

ACGME Competency Resident – Senior Levels III to V

Patient Care

The senior resident will present and provide detailed information and specific data regarding specific procedures in surgical disease to patients in a professional and scientifically based manner. They'll learn how to describe intricacies in regards to complex surgical disease, staging techniques following cancers, and end-stage options for patients for organ failure.

The senior level resident will suggest and implement patient management plans based on previously noted protocols, and adjust these plans in consultation with their attending staff for complex surgical repairs, uncommon surgical disease, resections and explorations, and chronic disease treatments.

The senior level resident will understand the importance of counseling and education in patients for each specific procedure for which they have undergone, and identify the critical times to emphasize communication and education as it relates to the individual procedures for specific surgical disease, procedures and explorations, and surgery for chronic disease.

The senior level resident will have in-depth knowledge beyond textbook information but including current reviews and recent studies to provide additional information regarding patient decisions and education for surgical repairs, uncommon surgical surgery, thoracic resections and explorations, and end-stage procedures for chronic disease.

The senior level resident will perform the appropriate procedures for clinical competency, including access and endoscopies for specific surgical disease.

The senior resident will have in-depth knowledge based on recent articles and studies to provide patients with education regarding appropriate follow-up and management of specific surgical disease, appropriate palliative approaches toward preventing progression of surgical disease, appropriate advise on the effects of surgery, appropriate follow-up and management of adjunctive therapies for malignancies, and appropriate management follow-up for immunosuppression disease, immunosuppression related to transplant.

The senior resident will appreciate the needs and additional benefits of associated health care professionals and consultants to provide additional information and expertise to a patient who has undergone specific surgical repairs, resections, and transplantation.

Medical Knowledge

The senior level resident will demonstrate by his experience in assessing and managing clinically situations, knowledge of recent updates and studies to apply to current clinically situations that are pertinent to common and uncommon surgical disease, and end-stage disease. She/he will also learn how to modify and change protocols based of the same types of information to improve overall patient care in each one of these practices.

Practice-based Learning and Improvement

The senior level resident will apply previously learned information and synthesize best-practiced guidelines for current therapy for specific medical abnormalities with specific case presentation for different organ disease, malignancies, and end-stage disease in a situation specific manner. The senior level resident is expected to have developed a significant sum of knowledge and a maturity in regards to understanding scientific studies above the text book learning that are applicable to current practice for common and uncommon surgical disease, thoracic disease, and chronic problems.

The senior resident will have, through experience and exposure to patients from their area of practice, learn to apply practice information that will improve the overall response patients in the region for all types of surgical problems.

The senior resident, based on presentations and didactic studies and conferences, will have a fine understanding of specifics regarding statistical techniques and methods, flaws, and problems with the current studies in the field of surgical surgery as they apply to diagnosis and therapeutic effectiveness.

The senior resident will apply and use the web based materials available through the ACS, APDS and Surgery websites for prerequisite and requisite curriculum to not only improve his information but to organize his/her activities as a surgeon.

The senior resident will actively guide and instruct students in topics related to surgery with specific in-depth information regarding how these processes relate to patients, and at the same time communicating this information to other health care professionals.

Interpersonal Communication Skills

The senior resident will develop a more mature and appropriate interaction with the patients and their families reflecting both his additional knowledge and understanding the disease process, the hardship and difficulties related to procedures in surgery.

The senior resident by his/her active interaction with families and activities will further exploit his/her understanding of the knowledge and interaction with patients be expected to interact and explain disease processes related to surgery at a high level and provide documentation; specific pointed and well organized, regarding common and uncommon surgical disease and end stage chronic problems.

The senior resident will take more of a leadership role in working with the entire team of care providers ranging from consultants and associated residents on other services, to physician assistants, nurse practitioners, and nurses interacting with them directing care with advice and supervision from his/her attending staff.

Professionalism

The senior resident will demonstrate a high degree of maturity and reflect the appropriate respect, compassion, and integrity as it is appropriate for handling patients as if he/she was a faculty member, and to provide the same type of professionalism and accountability to the patients and their families that would be expected from an established attending surgeon.

The senior resident will understand the ethics and principals regarding patient confidentiality of information, informed consent, business practices, and the withdrawing of care in appropriate circumstances and explain those processes in an organized and precise manner typical of someone experienced in the area of surgery.

The senior resident will adjust his/her behavior and responsiveness to patients demonstrating the appreciation of their culture, age, gender, and disabilities after having an experienced exposure to patients with multiple problems in surgery.

System-based Practice

The senior resident will not only work as a local team leader providing care and support, but in addition he/she will be looked upon as a representative and active component of the health care organization locally and become active in larger activities, such as the American College of

Surgeons Residents Association and will be encouraged to gain experiences with global and regional activities in the field of surgery. As part of his/her education, the senior resident will become trained to understand the differences between different types of health care delivery systems, the effects of controlling health care costs and how that affects resource allocation through discussing different health care systems as it applies to each different activities in surgery. As the senior resident becomes more experienced with providing care and seeing cases, he'll become apprised of the importance of providing cost effect health care and resource allocation in a fashion that avoid compromise in the quality of care. The senior resident by his/her experience and additional exposure to patients with surgical problems will become able to further enhance the patient's ability to deal with hospital systems and their complexities in the different environments she'll be working in, to provide quality patient care.

The senior resident will work with health care managers and providers on new protocols and procedures to initiate and change health care that will improve overall system performance based on his/her prior knowledge.

OVERVIEW OF CLINICAL GOALS AND EXAMPLES
JUNIOR LEVEL - YEARS I AND II

Overview of the Initial Stages:

For most General Surgical trainees, the initial stage of training will follow medical school. At this stage the trainee will focus on evaluation of surgical patients and will therefore gain skills in the assessment of the patient with an acute abdomen and the traumatized patient. Having gained skills in caring for the acutely unwell patient in medical school, these will be built upon to achieve competency in the preoperative assessment, perioperative care and postoperative management of the general surgical patient. Basic surgical skills will be honed mainly in outpatient procedures and Local Anesthetic cases as part of every general surgeon's armamentarium.

The aims, content and levels of competence to be attained for the specialty specific topics are defined in detail in the syllabus.

- Treat patient with acute appendicitis from start to finish

- Assessment, resuscitation and management of patients with acute abdomen
- Recognition and management of severe and necrotizing superficial infections
- Recognize and treat strangulated hernia
- Safely assess the multiply injured patient (includes ATLS certification)
- Identify and manage the majority of abdominal injuries
- Provision of specialist surgical support in the management of conditions affecting the reticulo-endothelial and haemopoetic systems
- Recognize benign lesions of skin and subcutaneous tissues and treat these where appropriate.
- Recognize and appropriately treat malignant skin lesions
- Diagnosis and management, including operative management of primary and recurrent abdominal wall hernia
- Diagnosis and management of perforated peptic ulcer
- Endoscopic diagnosis of upper GI hemorrhage, endoscopic management of some cases, operative management of cases where endostasis has failed
- Basic management of patients with esophagogastric disorders, including motility disorders, diagnosis and assessment of malignancy of the esophagus and stomach
- Diagnosis and management of acute gallstone disease, including operation
- Management of patients with straightforward hepatopancreatobiliary disorders e.g. gallstones. Diagnosis and investigation of malignancy of the biliary tract, pancreas and liver.
- Diagnosis and the medical and surgical treatment of common benign anorectal diseases; Hemorrhoids, fissure, low fistula, pilonidal sinus
- Appropriate diagnosis and emergency treatment of benign colon diseases – diverticular disease, volvulus, lower GI bleeding
- Diagnosis and the medical and surgical treatment of colonic neoplasia.
- Diagnosis of rectal cancer
- Diagnosis and the emergency medical and surgical treatment of inflammatory bowel disease
- Assess and manage acute breast infection
- Assessment and primary management of varicose veins

- Ability to assess published evidence in relational to clinical practice and ability to teach others

OVERVIEW OF THE INTERMEDIATE STAGE - YEARS III AND IV

The intermediate phase includes further training in emergency surgery and minor surgery but also some more subspecialist surgery, with the opportunity to be exposed to all of the major subspecialties. There should also be the opportunity for a limited exposure to one of the smaller subspecialties such as pediatrics, transplant or remote and rural surgery.

These areas could be covered either by specific attachments to emergency/day case/subspecialist cases or by working in an outside rotation, where practice is more general and emergency exposure gained throughout the entire period. This would depend on the local situation. Cases in which treatment competence it expected with limited additional support include:

Blunt and penetrating injuries

Abdominal injuries especially splenic, hepatic and pancreatic injuries

Acute Appendicitis

Peritonitis

Assessment of the acute abdomen

Acute presentation of gynecological disease

Acute intestinal obstruction

Strangulated hernia

Gastrointestinal bleeding

Superficial sepsis, including necrotizing infections

Skin lesions

Abdominal wall

Conditions affecting the reticulo-endothelial and haemopoetic systems

Elective hernia

Venous thrombosis and embolism

Genetic aspects of surgical disease

Perforated peptic ulcer

Upper GI hemorrhage

Acute gallstone disease

Liver trauma

Injuries to the biliary tract

Acute pancreatitis

Liver metastases

Stomas

Inflammatory Bowel disease

Functional disorders

Benign colon

Colorectal neoplasia

Benign anorectal

Chronic lower limb ischemia

Ruptured Abdominal Aortic Aneurysm

Venous disease

Acute limb ischemia

Neck swellings

Acute breast infection

Renal transplantation

SENIOR YEAR - V

In order to be competent in the general surgery, special focus must be spent in both upper and lower GI surgery. However it must be emphasized that sufficient competency and experience to be competent covering general surgical emergencies will not be gained overall until the final chief year has been completed. Even at this stage it is anticipated that certain complex cases will require additional consultation with more experienced or subspecialist consultants.

At the completion of training, the resident can:

- Treat patient with acute appendicitis from start to finish

- Assessment, resuscitation and management of patients with acute abdomen
- Recognition and management of severe and necrotizing superficial infections
- Recognize and treat strangulated hernia
- Safely assess the multiply injured patient (includes ATLS certification)
- Identify and manage the majority of abdominal injuries
- Provision of specialist surgical support in the management of conditions affecting the reticulo-endothelial and haemopoetic systems
- Recognize benign lesions of skin and subcutaneous tissues and treat these where appropriate.
- Recognize and appropriately treat malignant skin lesions
- Diagnosis and management, including operative management of primary and recurrent abdominal wall hernia
- Diagnosis and management of perforated peptic ulcer
- Endoscopic diagnosis of upper GI hemorrhage, endoscopic management of some cases, operative management of cases where endostasis has failed
- Basic management of patients with esophagogastric disorders, including motility disorders, diagnosis and assessment of malignancy of the esophagus and stomach
- Diagnosis and management of acute gallstone disease, including operation
- Management of patients with straightforward hepatopancreatobiliary disorders e.g. gallstones. Diagnosis and investigation of malignancy of the biliary tract, pancreas and liver.
- Diagnosis and the medical and surgical treatment of common benign anorectal diseases – Hemorrhoids, fissure, low fistula, pilonidal sinus
- Appropriate diagnosis and emergency treatment of benign colon diseases, diverticular disease, volvulus, lower GI bleeding
- Diagnosis and the medical and surgical treatment of colonic neoplasia.
- Diagnosis of rectal cancer
- Diagnosis and the emergency medical and surgical treatment of inflammatory bowel disease
- Assess and manage acute breast infection

- Assessment and primary management of varicose veins
- Ability to assess published evidence in relational to clinical practice and ability to teach others make sound ethical and legal judgments appropriate for a qualified surgeon.
- Respect the cultural and religious needs of patients and their families and provide surgical care in accordance with those needs.
- Manage surgical disorders based on a thorough knowledge of basic and clinical science.
- Utilize appropriate skill in those surgical techniques required of a qualified surgeon.
- Use critical thinking when making decisions affecting the life of a patient and the patient's family.
- Collaborate effectively with colleagues and other health professionals.
- Teach and share knowledge with colleagues, residents, students, and other health care providers.
- Teach patients and their families about the patient's health needs.
- Be committed to scholarly pursuits through the conduct and evaluation of research.
- Be prepared to manage complex programs and organizations.
- Provide cost-effective care to surgical patients and families within the community.
- Value lifelong learning as a necessary prerequisite to maintaining surgical knowledge and skill.

Goals by level:

PGY-1

Medical Knowledge	Patient Care	Operative skills, Practice Based	Communication, Professionalism, System Based
The PGY-1 residents completing the General Surgery rotation are expected to demonstrate knowledge in the following areas:	Each PGY-1 completing a General Surgery rotation should be able to:	The PGY-1 General Surgery resident completing a General Surgery rotation is expected to:	The PGY-1 resident is expected to:
Pathology as it is related to General Surgery	Perform a comprehensive history and physical exam, and document this appropriately	Understand the functions of surgical instruments	Discuss physical examination and diagnosis with senior residents and attending physician
Treatment continuum of patients with surgical disease.	Provide adequate pre- and post-operative care with adequate documentation.	Demonstrate the proper use of sterile technique when performing or assisting with operative procedures	Be prepared to present each patient in an organized manner during rounds.
Anatomy of the abdomen, chest, neck, vascular tree	Appropriately diagnose medical and surgical conditions, recognizing urgent and emergent situations and responding appropriately	Perform bedside procedures such as IV insertion, ABG collection, NGT insertion.	Tactfully discuss the nature of medical condition and prognosis with patient and family.
Physiology, fluid and electrolytes			Discuss diagnosis of terminal illness or trauma with patients/family with an attending physician present.
Pharmacology of antibiotics, antihypertensives, diuretics, analgesics, etc.	Understand indications for obtaining laboratory and radiologic tests.	Operative skills expected of the PGY-1 resident include the ability to:	Demonstrate the leadership principles that relate to successful management of patient care.
Demonstrate continued progress in attaining competency in basic	Accurately interpret and manage laboratory tests, ABGs, X-rays etc.	Tie knots effectively. Suture a complex	Develop and implement plans for study,

and clinical sciences.

Understand and explain basic ethical principles inherent in surgical practice

Diagnose and treat routine surgical situations in preparation for operative intervention.

Share data obtained from a comprehensive physical exam with colleagues.

Understand when help is needed.

wound. Use scalpel, forceps, and scissors effectively. Understand the use of electrocautery

The PG 1 resident is expected to perform the following surgical procedures will minimal assistance:

- Breast biopsy
- Appendectomy
- Hernia repair
- Abscess drainage
- Endotracheal Intubation
- Central venous access
- Insertion of peripheral IV

reading, and research that promote personal and professional growth, and that are consistent with program requirements.

Identify and use available resources to survey current surgical research.

Demonstrate an understanding of the socioeconomic, cultural, and managerial factors inherent in providing cost-effective health care.

Goals by level:

PGY-2

Medical Knowledge	Patient Care	Operative skills, Practice Based	Communication, Professionalism, System Based
In addition to all objectives in the PGY1 level,	In addition to all objectives in the PGY1 level,	In addition to all objectives in the PGY1 level,	In addition to all objectives in the PGY1 level,
The PGY-2 resident should be knowledgeable in:	The PGY-2 resident is expected to:	The PGY-2 resident is expected to:	The PGY-2 resident should demonstrate the ability to:
Physiology of the GI tract	Understand the appropriate diagnostic tests for patients presenting with surgical complications	Independently perform routine surgical procedures with minimal supervision, including:	Provide appropriate health teaching to patients scheduled for surgical intervention.
Pathology of gastric and colon disease			
Principles of wound healing and wound management	Use available data from basic and social sciences when planning pre-operative, intra-operative, and postoperative care for new patients.	Appendectomy	Function in an effective collaborative role with faculty and other residents.
		Hernia repair	
The PGY-2 resident should show an improving knowledge base of general surgical principles.		Cholecystectomy	
		Understand principles of adequate surgical exposure.	Function in a leadership role by using the problem-solving approach in planning care for patients and families.
The PGY-2 resident should demonstrate the ability to relate scientific knowledge and research findings to care of patients.	Discuss with team members the ethical aspects of surgical intervention.		
		Demonstrate the ability to use laparoscopic instruments effectively	
	Diagnose an acute abdomen and prepare for the OR		Act as consultant to the emergency department and inpatient services
		Demonstrate the ability to perform the following procedures	

accurately:

Chest tubes

Arterial lines

Pulmonary artery
catheterization

Goals by level:

PGY-3

Medical Knowledge	Patient Care	Operative skills, Practice Based	Communication, Professionalism, System Based
In addition to the expectations of the PGY-1 and 2 levels,	In addition to the expectations of the PGY-1 and 2 levels,	In addition to the expectations of the PGY-1 and 2 levels,	In addition to the expectations of the PGY-1 and 2 levels,
The PGY-3 resident should be knowledgeable in:	The PGY-3 resident is expected to:	The PGY-3 resident is expected to:	The PGY-3 resident
Pathology of malignant disease	Independently make decisions concerning pre- and post-op care for complicated patients.	Be generally facile with laparoscopic instruments	Should effectively provide pre and post-operative teaching to patients requiring surgical intervention and their families.
Pharmacology including cancer chemotherapy		Understand the principles of gastrointestinal anastomosis and fascial closure	
Wound healing and wound management	Use critical thinking in making decisions about management of care	Understand principles of adequate surgical exposure	Should demonstrate an ability to tactfully discuss challenging clinical situations, patient status changes, and terminal illness with patients and families.
The PGY-3 resident should understand and be able to incorporate ethical concepts in the planning and discussion of pre-operative, intra-operative, and post-operative care of patients and families.	Provide critical care with minimal supervision Understand the appropriate diagnostic and treatment approaches for inflammatory and malignant disease.	Understand and manage intraoperative emergencies (i.e. Bleeding, enterotomy) Understands infections and use of drains. Display competency and function as surgeon	Must demonstrate appropriate skill in teaching other residents and other health care professionals.
The PGY3 resident should			

understand and be able to explain risk status classification, and answer questions regarding potential risks of operative procedures.

in a majority of the following surgeries:

Laparoscopic cholecystectomy for acute cholecystitis

Right colectomy with primary anastomosis

Laparotomy for small bowel obstruction

Breast lumpectomy with node sampling

Goals by level:

PGY-4

Medical Knowledge	Patient Care	Operative skills, Practice Based	Communication, Professionalism, System Based
In addition to the expectations of the PGY-1, 2, and 3 residents,	In addition to the expectations of the PGY-1, 2, and 3 residents	In addition to the expectations of the PGY-1, 2, and 3 residents	In addition to the expectations of the PGY-1, 2, and 3 residents
The PGY-4 resident should be knowledgeable in:	The PGY-4 resident is expected to:	The PGY-4 resident is expected to:	The PGY-4 resident is expected to:
Pathology of inflammatory and malignant disease	Direct the care of multiple pre- and post-op patients.	Be generally facile with laparoscopic approaches for advanced laparoscopic procedures	Interact appropriately with multiple consultants, ED physicians, referring physicians, and nursing staff.
Infectious disease diagnosis and management	Understand and is able to apply the principles of surgical critical care.	Understand principles and use of stapling devices.	Collaborate with residents, faculty, and other health professionals to provide comprehensive health care for patients.
Pharmacology and nutrition	Understand all operative approaches to a surgical or vascular problem and is able to pick the most appropriate.	Understand the principles of gastrointestinal and/or vascular anastomosis.	
The PGY-4 resident should demonstrate the knowledge to evaluate standards for surgical practice.	Understand the indications for non-operative management of potential surgical problems.	Understand and manage intraoperative emergencies (i.e. laparotomy, enterotomy)	Understand the need for and promote multidisciplinary care for the patient.
	Understand indications for surgical	With minimal assistance, plan the	Tactfully discuss complex surgical problems and prognosis with

intervention for blunt and penetrating trauma, and selects the appropriate procedure.

The PG 4 resident is expected to provide independent management throughout the spectrum of care for each patient that he/she is following.

progression of advanced surgical cases (i.e. Whipple) from start to completion.

Display competency and function as surgeon in a majority of the following surgeries with minimal assistance:

Total gastrectomy

Thyroidectomy

Fem-pop bypass.

Pancreatic resection

patient and family.

Should be participating at an increased level in the teaching program, including both the formal conference program and the teaching of junior level residents and in serving as teaching assistant to the PGY-1, 2 and 3 residents.

Goals by level:

PGY-5

Medical Knowledge	Patient Care	Operative skills, Practice Based	Communication, Professionalism, System Based
In addition to the expectations of the PGY-1-4 levels	In addition to the expectations of the PGY-1-4 levels	In addition to the expectations of the PGY-1-4 levels	In addition to the expectations of the PGY-1-4 levels
The PGY-5 resident should be knowledgeable in:	The PGY-5 resident is expected to:	The PGY-5 resident is expected to:	The PGY-5 chief resident is expected to:
Pathology of inflammatory and malignant disease	Completely coordinate the care of the surgical or trauma patient in the inpatient setting.	Be facile with laparoscopic approaches for advanced laparoscopic procedures	Manage a population of surgical patients in the clinic with minimal supervision.
Infectious disease diagnosis and management	Coordinate services for follow-up rehabilitation and care.	Understand principles and use of stapling devices.	Provide leadership to residents and medical students in the management of patients with complex surgical conditions.
Pharmacology and nutrition	Provide coordination of care for patients in the outpatient setting.	Understand indications for and independently perform gastrointestinal and/or vascular anastomosis.	
The PGY-5 resident will demonstrate a high level of scientific, clinical, and technical knowledge and skill during evaluation and operative procedures.	Able to direct the care of multiple pre- and post-op patients.		Conduct independent research and assist junior residents in planning clinical research proposals.
Effective decision-making in the management of care for all types of surgical patients and their families.	Understand and is able to apply the principles of surgical critical care.	Understand and independently manage intraoperative emergencies (i.e. laparotomy, enterotomy)	Program responsibilities for each chief resident include ongoing involvement in:
	Understand all operative approaches to a	Independently plan and	

Evaluating knowledge gained from original literature in preparation for life-long.

surgical or vascular problem and is able to pick the most appropriate.

Understand the indications for non-operative management of potential surgical problems.

Understand indications for intervention for blunt/ penetrating trauma, selects the appropriate procedure.

execute the progression of advanced surgical cases (i.e. Whipple) from start to completion.

Display competency and function independently as surgeon in the following cases:

Parathyroidectomy
Pancreato-duodenectomy AP resection

Colon resection for diverticulitis

Schedules/vacations

Evaluations of faculty, residents, and rotation structure

Solving of problems including personnel and attending-resident interaction issues.

RESIDENT STUDY PROGRAM AND OBJECTIVES

Basic Science

All Residents will read a basic Science Text Per year

O'Leary

For the junior residents PGY1- 2 this will be chapter presentation with preparation of a study guide (Chapters submitted to surgery server).

For the senior residents this will include an ABSITE Review of wrong answers to address in the Conference (Summary submitted to surgery server).

The examination questions will be from Access Surgery or the Score portal

All lectures will be filmed.

A Basic Science Exam will be given at the end of the year. The results will be scored and included in the resident's annual assessment

Clinical Science

All residents will follow the Access Surgery reading schedule corresponding to their lecture in addition to the level specific reading program.

Curriculum. PGY 1-2

These residents will read our introductory materials (House staff Manual, Residency Curriculum, Copes) and

The Surgical Review-Atluri.

Surgical Recall

PGY 3-4

These residents will read:

One standard Text:

    Sabiston

    Greenfield

    Schwartz

One clinical Guide:

    Cameron

Rush University Review

Each resident will prepare a study guide for each chapter.

PGY 5

The Chiefs will read:

Surgical Decision Making

Selected Readings in Surgery

They will additionally be reviewing for Mock Oral Exams, the ABSITE Review Course and review the Surgical Curriculum. Each chief will prepare a study guide for the selected reading sections.

Final Resident Goals

At the completion of training, the resident can:

Make sound ethical and legal judgments appropriate for a qualified surgeon.

Respect the cultural and religious needs of patients and their families, and provide surgical care in accordance with those needs.

Manage surgical disorders based on a thorough knowledge of basic and clinical science.

Utilize appropriate skill in those surgical techniques required of a qualified surgeon.

Use critical thinking when making decisions affecting the life of a patient and the patient's family.

Collaborate effectively with colleagues and other health professionals.

Teach and share knowledge with colleagues, residents, students, and other health care providers.

Teach patients and their families about the patient's health needs.

Be committed to scholarly pursuits through the conduct and   evaluation of research.

Be prepared to manage complex programs and organizations.

Provide cost-effective care to surgical patients and families within the community.

Value lifelong learning as a necessary prerequisite to maintaining surgical knowledge and skill.

CHAPTER 6

ROTATIONAL GOALS AND OBJECTIVES

*P*art of the complexity of residency training and assessment is that specialty specific medical

knowledge and service obligations are not always completely aligned. To provide for proper

resident assessment, goals and objectives must be modified based on the specialty service and

activities. To assess the faculty with this approach, the goals and objectives will be grouped by

rotation referring back to the core or specialty chapters in the curriculum to allow for cross

reference.

Gastrointestinal/Surgical Oncology

The rotational specific objectives and goals by junior and senior levels are outlined in the

Curriculum in Chapters Minimally Invasive Surgery, Surgical Oncology, Endocrine Surgery,

Abdominal Surgery, Alimentary Tract Surgery, Liver, Biliary Tract and Pancreas Surgery, Head

and Neck Surgery

Colorectal/General Surgery

The rotational specific objectives and goals by junior and senior levels are outlined in the Curriculum in Chapters Minimally Invasive Surgery, Endocrine Surgery, Abdominal Surgery, Alimentary Tract Surgery, Liver, Biliary Tract and Pancreas Surgery, Surgical Endoscopy, Surgical Genetics

Vascular/Thoracic/Breast/Wound

The rotational specific objectives and goals by junior and senior levels are outlined in the Curriculum in Chapters Wound Healing, Breast Surgery, Vascular Surgery, Cardiothoracic Surgery, and Surgical Genetics

Trauma/Critical Care/Cardiac Surgery

The rotational specific objectives and goals by junior and senior levels are outlined in the Curriculum in Chapters Surgical Critical Care, Trauma, Burn injury, Cardiothoracic Surgery

Pediatric Surgery

The rotational specific objectives and goals by junior and senior levels are outlined in the Curriculum in the Chapter on Pediatric Surgery

Transplant

The rotational specific objectives and goals by junior and senior levels are outlined in the Curriculum in Chapters Surgical Immunology and Organ Transplantation

Burns/Reconstructive Surgery

The rotational specific objectives and goals by junior and senior levels are outlined in the Curriculum in Chapters Surgical Critical Care, Trauma, and Burn injury, Surgical Infections, Metabolism, Plastics and Reconstruction.

Trauma Senior Service

The rotational specific objectives and goals by junior and senior levels are outlined in the Curriculum in Chapters Surgical Critical Care, Trauma, Chapter, Burn injury, Epidemiology

Chapters not specifically addressed in rotational assignments will be covered in the overall conduct of surgery on each rotation and/or during the specific experience on the subspecialty services and anesthesia

CHAPTER 7

EDUCATIONAL POLICIES

*T*he follow section provides some standard policies that would be applicable to any surgical

program. These policies form part of the structure of the working residency program; they should be reviewed annually for compliance with the ACGME and to assure complicity for the medical institution clinical care manual and practice bylaws.

SUPERVISION OF SURGICAL RESIDENTS AT THE HOSPITAL: POLICY STATEMENT

PURPOSE:

To establish policies and procedures for providing proper supervision of all residents working at The Hospital. These include delineation of the minimum requirements for supervision, documentation of supervision, and requirements for monitoring the level or degree of supervision.

GENERAL POLICY:

Attending physicians, as members of the Medical Staff are responsible for the care provided to all patients regardless of the location that such care is provided. In such a role, they must be familiar with each patient for whom they are responsible. Fulfillment of such responsibility requires personal involvement with each patient and each resident who is providing care as part of the training experience.

Each staff patient will be assigned an attending physician whose name will be clearly identified in the patient's record. It is recognized that other staff practitioners may, at times, share responsibility for the care of the patient and provide supervision instead of, or in addition to, the assigned practitioner.

Within the scope of the training program, all residents, without exception, will function under the supervision of an attending physician at all times unless they have made application to and have been granted privileges through the medical staff credentialing process.

Every residency program will assure adequate supervision for each resident at all times. A responsible attending physician is available to the resident in person or by telephone and is able to be present within a reasonable period of time, if needed. Each service or division posts a "call schedule" indicating the resident(s) and responsible practitioner(s) to be contacted for all patient care eventualities.

Each residency training program is so structured as to encourage and permit residents to assume increasing levels of responsibility commensurate with their individual progress in experience, skill, knowledge, and judgment.

Each training program adheres to current accreditation requirements as set forth by the ACGME (Accreditation Council for Graduate Medical Education). For all matters pertaining to the training programs including the level of supervision provided, it is expected that the requirements of the ACGME will be incorporated into the assessments of the resident's capacity to assume increasing levels of appropriate responsibility.

RESPONSIBILITIES

The Departmental Chiefs have responsibility for ensuring individual program implementation and compliance. They are responsible to the medical center administration and board of directors for the quality of the residency training programs and the quality of care provided by staff practitioners and residents in their respective departments. They will assure a high quality program and attain the following standards:

1. Review each resident's compliance with documentation requirements for the assignment of graduated levels of responsibility.

2. Review each resident with respect to compliance with hospital and departmental rules and regulations, especially as it pertains to the performance of procedures, documentation of patient attendance and medical record completion. The departmental chief will conduct this review with the appropriate division directors and the departmental executive committee. Staff practitioners are responsible for providing appropriate supervision to assigned residents and will evaluate those residents assigned to their service.

3. Ensure that staff practitioners are appropriately fulfilling their responsibilities to provide supervision to residents and that ongoing evaluations are conducted. The chief must assess the staff practitioner's discharge of supervisory responsibilities from personal observations and from evaluations and interviews with residents.

GENERAL SUPERVISION

Medical staff members direct the care of the patient and provide the appropriate level of supervision based on the nature of the patient's condition, the likelihood of major changes in the management plan, the complexity of care, and the experience and judgment of the resident under supervision. It is a cardinal principal that responsibility for the care of each patient lies with the staff practitioner to whom the patient is assigned and who supervises all care rendered by residents. Every patient, whether inpatient or outpatient, will have a staff practitioner designated as the staff physician in charge of the patient's care, and the physician's name will be appropriately recorded in each patient's medical record. For outpatients followed in more than one clinic, a staff practitioner from each clinic will be responsible for the care rendered in that clinic.

Generally, direct personal contact between the staff practitioner and residents should take place daily and staff practitioners must enter daily notes in the patient's chart, verifying concurrence of diagnosis and treatment. Such notes will be written as prescribed in the Medical Staff Rules and Regulations. In all cases where the provision of supervision is reflected within the resident's progress note, the note shall include the name of the staff practitioner with whom the case was discussed and the nature of that discussion. Legible countersignatures of the staff physician are required on admission histories and physicals and verification of discharge diagnoses.

Medical staff supervising residents must review all proposed major diagnostic, therapeutic, surgical and all other invasive procedures, significant revisions in treatment plans, and/or changes in the patient's level of care, and note their concurrence with these proposed actions in writing within the patient's medical record. Except in the instance of emergency situations, such approval must be obtained prior to initiating any surgical procedure or significant revision in a patient's treatment plan.

At the time of admission of a teaching patient, either staff or private, or if there is a significant change in the status of a teaching patient, a resident may evaluate the patient and discuss the patient's circumstances via telephone with an appropriate staff practitioner. The attending staff practitioner will then enter a confirming progress note the next workday.

At a minimum, prior to discharge, the staff practitioner will evaluate the patient's response to the treatment or procedure and discuss with the patient the consequence or outcome of the procedure. Evidence of such evaluation will be documented via a progress note.

During all working hours of an outpatient clinic, there must be coverage by a staff practitioner credentialed in the discipline represented by the clinic. Chiefs must prepare a monthly schedule to reflect staff coverage for each clinic within his/her service. Chiefs must ensure that residents perform and/or interpret only those diagnostic tests and procedures for which they have demonstrated competence and have been privileged.

It must be assured by the resident's supervising physician that the appropriate information is present within the patient's medical record at the time of transfer to another service, or upon receipt of a patient from another service. Evidence of this assurance will be documented in the patient's record.

It must be assured by the supervising practitioner that discharge or transfer of the patient from the hospital or clinic, and its attendant documentation, is appropriate based on the specific circumstances of the patient's diagnosis and treatment.

PROCEDURAL SUPERVISION:

The degrees of supervision vary with the relative risk of any patient care activity. Almost all diagnostic and treatment procedures and treatments carry some risk. Some have greater risks than others. The degrees of risk to achieve benefit may be directly proportional to the seriousness of the condition threatening the patient's well-being; hence, those procedures and/or treatments with the highest risk usually require the highest level of supervision. Those procedures, which are high risk usually, require a written informed consent. Those procedures and activities with minimal risk usually do not require specific informed consent and require lesser degrees of supervision.

1.   Procedures with <u>MINIMAL RISK</u>. No written informed consent is required. Prior training   is expected but continued specific close supervision may not be required. This includes:

a.   The performance of a history and physical exam and daily follow-up with appropriate documentation in the medical record;

b.   The prescribing and administration of medications, either oral or parenteral, etc. except for procedural sedation or cancer chemotherapy;

c.   The application of simple splints or bandages, etc.

d.   The performance of certain x-ray procedures such as simple views of the abdomen, chest, and limbs, etc.

2.   Procedures with <u>LOW RISK</u>, which are moderately complex and require prior training and supervision to a satisfactory level of skill and proficiency. Some of these require informed consent. They include procedures such as:

    a.   insertion of NG tube or rectal tube

    b.   venipuncture

    c.   lumbar puncture

    d.   bone marrow aspirations

    e.   skin excisions

    f.   aspirations of joints

    g.   paracentesis

    h.   I&D of abscesses and wound debridement

    i.   suturing of minor lacerations

    j.   prescribing of antiarrythmia medication

    k.   prescribing procedural sedation

3.   Procedures with <u>MODERATE RISK</u> but performed outside of the operating room, but frequently performed in specially prepared areas, some technically complex. All require informed consent. They include procedures such as

    a.   needle biopsy of organs

    b.   placement of central lines and Swan Ganz catheters

    c.   thoracentesis

    d.   placement of chest tube

    e.   simple surgical procedures (e.g., I&D) performed in the operating room

4.   <u>HIGH RISK</u> procedures. A high-risk treatment or procedure is one that has significant risk of possible adverse outcome based on the patient's condition or the risks of the procedure/ treatment.

    a.   most procedures in the operating room

b.   cardiac catheterization lab procedures

c.   administration of cancer chemotherapy

d.   electroconvulsive therapy

e.   the withholding or withdrawal of life sustaining treatment.

In cases involving invasive procedures and/or surgical operations, the staff practitioner will be responsible for authorizing the performance of such invasive procedures or performing and/or directing the performance of a procedure, and for having obtained appropriately informed consent.

Medical staff members supervising residents are responsible for assuring that all diagnostic (particularly invasive procedures), therapeutic and surgical procedures which are high risk or technically complex and performed by residents on patients assigned to them are the appropriate therapy, properly prescribed/ordered, properly initiated or executed, medically monitored, fully explained to the patient, documented, properly supervised, executed and evaluated.

(1)   For all surgical procedures considered <u>HIGH RISK</u>, except in case of life threatening emergency, a staff practitioner will be scrubbed and present in the procedure/operating room.

(2)   For all <u>MODERATE RISK</u> procedures, the staff practitioner is present in the procedural suite or in the hospital and is available for immediate consultation unless the resident has been credentialed to independently perform the procedure, has previously discussed the procedure with the responsible attending physician, and been approved to perform the procedure on the patient in question.

(3)   For all <u>LOW RISK</u> and <u>MINIMAL RISK</u> procedures, the staff practitioner is not usually present, but is available to residents for consultation and support via telephone or in person.

SUPERVISION DURING AN EMERGENCY

An "emergency" is defined as a situation where immediate care is necessary to preserve the life of or prevent serious impairment of the health of a patient. In such situations, any resident, assisted by medical center personnel shall, consistent with the informed consent, be permitted to do everything possible to save the life of the patient or to save a patient from serious harm. The appropriate staff practitioner will be contacted and apprised of the situation as soon as possible. The resident will document the nature of this discussion in the patient's record.

In emergency cases, the resident must consult with and obtain approval from a staff practitioner who will be available to assist or advise as appropriate. In such cases, the staff practitioner will determine, based on the circumstance of the case and the resident's level of experience, whether to be physically present in the procedural/operating room or to be available by telephone. If circumstances do not permit the staff practitioner to write a pre-procedural note, the resident's note will include the name of the responsible staff practitioner, and will indicate that the details of the case, including the proposed procedure, were discussed with and approved by the staff practitioner. In such cases, a staff practitioner must see the patient and countersign the resident's pre-procedural note within 24 hours.

RESIDENT EVALUATIONS AND ADVANCEMENT: GENERAL POLICY STATEMENT

Each resident will be evaluated on the basis of clinical judgment, knowledge, technical skills, humanistic qualities, professional attitudes, behavior and overall ability to manage the care of a patient. Evaluations of residents within a specific program will occur at intervals determined by the program director. Each staff practitioner will also evaluate each resident on the basis of his or her clinical interactions. Such evaluations will be ongoing and will occur more formally at intervals determined by the program director. If at any time a resident's performance is judged to be detrimental to the care of a patient(s), the program director will take immediate action such as is appropriate to assure the safety of the patient(s), up to and including dismissal from the program.

Residents, as part of their training program, will be given progressive responsibility for the care of the patient. A resident may act as a teaching assistant to less experienced residents. Assignment of the level of responsibility must be commensurate with their acquisition of knowledge and development of judgment and skill, and consistent with the requirements of the accrediting body.

Residents may be assigned graduated levels of responsibility to perform procedures or conduct activities without a supervisor present and/or act as a teaching assistant to less experienced residents based on a process of assessing a resident's knowledge, skill, experience and judgment. The determination of a resident's assigned level of responsibility for performing procedures or activities without a supervising attending present and/or act as a teaching assistant will be based on documented evidence of the resident's clinical experience, judgment, etc., and on evaluations by staff practitioners and the departmental chief.

Documentation of a resident's graduated level of responsibility is based upon evidence of the resident's clinical experiences, judgment, knowledge, and technical skill and will be filed in the resident's file and entered in the electronic database as required. Resident files will be maintained in the office of the relevant service chief and will include:

(1)   A specific statement identifying the evidence on which such a determination is made;

(2)   The types of diagnostic or therapeutic procedures the resident may perform and those for which the resident may act as a teaching assistant; and,

(3)   The concurrence of any necessary specialty director or other appropriately credentialed physician.

During the performance of such procedures or operations, a staff practitioner will provide an appropriate level of supervision. Determination of this level of supervision dependent on level of credentialing, the discretion of the individual staff practitioner and is a function of the experience and competence of the resident, and of the complexity of the specific case.

As a general rule, residents at the PGY (Post Graduate Year) 1 will be closely supervised at all levels of complexity higher than "minimum risk". The assigned level of PGY-2 and higher residents will depend on their achieved skill, knowledge and competence. The supervision provided by the staff practitioner may be less if a resident assigned to act as a teaching assistant is present. Such determination shall be made by the staff practitioner on a case-by-case basis considering the resident's level of skill, knowledge and judgment, and the complexity of the specific case. If during the course of the procedure/operation, the resident requests the presence of the responsible staff practitioner, the practitioner will proceed expeditiously to the bedside.

The terms resident, house staff, medical staff, and practitioner are used as defined in the Medical Staff Bylaws. The Medical Staff Bylaws and Rules and Regulations, as well as individual departmental rules and regulations may contain duplicative or more focused language regarding the supervision of house staff and should be interpreted in the context of this document which represents overall institutional policy.

POLICY ON SLEEP DEPRIVATION AND STRESS

Enclosed is the department policy statement regarding sleep deprivation and stress. The policy is meant to define the problem, outline the approach to addressing these issues and propose a monitoring mechanism. Supplemental material that review sleep deprivation studies and how it affects medical practice is included.

Materials provided

1.   DVD-Sleep and Sleep Disorders.. Jack Parker, MD WVU

2.   Parshuram CS et al. CMAJ 2004; 170:965-70

3.   Stress management

4.   Stress reduction techniques

Please review the enclosed material and return this attestation

I have reviewed the enclosed material and policy regarding Sleep Deprivation and Stress.

Signed

_____   Date _____

POLICY: SLEEP DEPRIVATION AND FATIGUE

Part of the General Surgical Residency program in addition to the educational mission is to monitor fatigue and sleep deprivation in our trainees. The following policy reflects the Department of surgery's approach to address this concern.

Signs and Symptoms

Individuals affected by extreme fatigue or sleep deprivation may exhibit decreased short-term memory, irritability, depression, headaches, and sensitivity to noise or light.

Residents exhibiting these symptoms will be:

Relieved of active service

Assessed for systemic diseases such as fibromyalgia and sleep disorders

Formally reviewed by the department chairman

Returned to active service after medical clearance and demonstration of additional education regarding severe fatigue and sleep deprivation.

Those residents that feel that they are exhibiting symptoms or significant fatigue or suffering from sleep deprivation will be required to notify their attending staff and remove themselves from clinical service.

The surgical faculty should review the status of their residents and if in their judgment the resident's behavior or symptoms demonstrate signs of significant fatigue or sleep deprivation, they should relieve the resident of their service obligations and notify the service director.

Additionally, surgery residents must leave after 30 straight hours of service unless it endangers patient care. A call room will be provided for sleep or rest during the day
at all clinical sites for surgery

Education

The residents and surgery surgical staff are required to read the policy statement, and review the enclosed material regarding fatigue and sleep deprivation.

Monitoring Procedures

The following monitoring procedures have been instituted

    a.   Monthly audit of Residents hours by the program director

    b.   Faculty review of fatigue and sleep deprivation indicators

    c.   OR monitoring- Assessment by program director of residents related operative performance including:

        1)   Preoperative patient preparation

        2)   Opening incisions

        3)   Wound closure

    d.   with a special consideration of: evening or night cases, increased activity periods, and weekends.

    e.   Mortality and Morbidity conference citation of sleep deprivation related impact on patient care.

REVIEW

Sleep deprivation and Fatigue

Background: Scientific Studies

Sleep deprivation and Fatigue has been shown to affect brain function. In studies on volunteers after 35 hours of sleep deprivation fMRI assessment demonstrates changes in cerebral pathways used for normal function[1], with impairment of short-term memory. The prefrontal cortex is most affected by fatigue and sleep deprivation. The cognitive functions, which most clearly exhibit these changes, are memory, planning, organizing, timing, adjustment, and verbal fluency. Fortunately, other studies have demonstrated that the brain is able to overcome these affects briefly[2] and that complex and lengthy critical reasoning and rule-based tasks are more resilient to sleep deprivation[3]

Signs and Symptoms

Individuals affected by extreme fatigue or sleep deprivation may exhibit decreased short-term memory, irritability, depression, headaches, and sensitivity to noise or light.

Residents exhibiting these symptoms should be:

Relieved of active service

Assessed for systemic diseases such as fibromyalgia and sleep disorders

Formally reviewed by the department director

Returned to active service after medical clearance and demonstration of additional education regarding severe fatigue and sleep deprivation.

Treatment and Recovery

Surgery residents that experience symptoms of severe fatigue or sleep deprivation must be evaluated for systemic illnesses such as fibromyalgia or sleep disorders, which manifest in the same symptom complexes. To recover from extended periods of sleep deprivation requires sleep, not rest or reduced actives. Sleep deprived residents must sleep for a minimum of 4 to 6 hours before being allow to return to the service.

Support Material

All those involved with individuals exposed to significant fatigue or sleep deprivation should review the following additional material.

REFERENCES

1.   Drummond et al Nature 2000; 403:655-657.

2.   Horne et al, Acta Psychologica 1985; 58:133-139.

3.   Harrison, Y et al Organis. Behav. Hum. Decision Process 1999; 78:128-145.

4.   Parshuram CS et al. CMAJ 2004; 170:965-70

ACGME Policy Addendum

FOR INSERTION INTO THE COMMON PROGRAM REQUIREMENTS FOR ALL CORE AND SUBSPECIALTY PROGRAMS BY JULY 1, 2003

Resident Duty Hours and the Working Environment

Providing residents with a sound academic and clinical education must be carefully planned and balanced with concerns for patient safety and resident well-being. Each program must ensure that the learning objectives of the program are not compromised by excessive reliance on residents to fulfill service obligations. Didactic and clinical education must have priority in the allotment of residents' time and energies. Duty hour assignments must recognize that faculty and residents collectively have responsibility for the safety and welfare of patients.

1. Supervision of Residents

    a. Qualified faculty must supervise all patient care. The program director must ensure, direct, and document adequate supervision of residents at all times. Residents must be provided with rapid, reliable systems for communicating with supervising faculty.

    b. Faculty schedules must be structured to provide residents with continuous supervision and consultation.

    c. Faculty and residents must be educated to recognize the signs of fatigue and adopt and apply policies to prevent and counteract the potential negative effects.

2. Duty Hours

    a. Duty hours are defined as all clinical and academic activities related to the residency program, i.e., patient care (both inpatient and outpatient), administrative duties related to patient care, the provision for transfer of patient care, time spent in-house during call activities, and scheduled academic activities such as conferences. Duty hours do not include reading and preparation time spent away from the duty site.

b.   Duty hours must be limited to 80 hours per week, averaged over a four-week period, inclusive of all in-house call activities.

c.   Residents must be provided with 1 day in 7 free from all educational and clinical responsibilities, averaged over a 4-week period, inclusive of call. One day is defined as one continuous 24-hour period free from all clinical, educational, and administrative activities.

d.   Adequate time for rest and personal activities must be provided. This should consist of a 10-hour time period provided between all daily duty periods and after in-house call.

3.   On-Call Activities

The objective of on-call activities is to provide residents with continuity of patient care experiences throughout a 24-hour period. In-house call is defined as those duty hours beyond the normal workday when residents are required to be immediately available in the assigned institution.

a.   In-house call must occur no more frequently than every third night, averaged over a four-week period.

b.   Continuous on-site duty, including in-house call, must not exceed 24 consecutive hours. Residents may remain on duty for up to six additional hours to participate in didactic activities, transfer care of patients, conduct outpatient clinics, and maintain continuity of medical and surgical care as defined in Specialty and Subspecialty Program Requirements.

c.   No new patients, as defined in Specialty and Subspecialty Program Requirements, may be accepted after 24 hours of continuous duty

d.   At-home call (pager call) is defined as call taken from outside the assigned institution.

e.   The frequency of at-home call is not subject to the every third night limitation. However,   at-home call must not be so frequent as to preclude rest and reasonable personal time for each resident. Residents taking at-home call must be provided with 1 day in 7 completely free from all educational and clinical responsibilities, averaged over a 4-week period.

f.   When residents are called into the hospital from home, the hours residents spend in-house are counted toward the 80-hour limit.

g.   The program director and the faculty must monitor the demands of at-home call in their programs and make scheduling adjustments as necessary to mitigate excessive service demands and/or fatigue.

4.   Moonlighting

a.   Because residency education is a full-time endeavor, the program director must ensure that moonlighting does not interfere with the ability of the resident to achieve the goals and objectives of the educational program.

b.   The program director must comply with the sponsoring institution's written policies and procedures regarding moonlighting, in compliance with the Institutional Requirements III. D.1.k.

c.   Moonlighting that occurs within the residency program and/or the sponsoring institution or the non-hospital sponsor's primary clinical site(s), i.e., internal moonlighting, must be counted toward the 80-hour weekly limit on duty hours.

5.   Oversight

a.   Each program must have written policies and procedures consistent with the Institutional and Program Requirements for resident duty hours and the working environment. These policies must be distributed to the residents and the faculty. Monitoring of duty hours is required with frequency sufficient to ensure an appropriate balance between education and service.

b.   Back-up support systems must be provided when patient care responsibilities are unusually difficult or prolonged, or if unexpected circumstances create resident fatigue sufficient to jeopardize patient care.

6.   Duty Hours Exception

The RRC may grant exceptions for up to 10 % of the 80-hour limit, to individual programs based on a sound educational rationale. However, prior permission of the institution's GMEC is required.

DEPARTMENT OF SURGERY POLICY

RESIDENT PROMOTION

Promotion to the next year of training will entail accomplishing several tasks and meeting employment standards.

Employment Standards

1. No violation of employee code of conduct necessitating disciplinary action
2. No incidents compromising patient safety
3. Observance of annual health required screenings
4. Observance of Departmental guidelines for behavior and resident supervision
5. Maintenance of on an ABSITE score over the 20th percentile
6. Completion of Health line required programs

Annual Residency Accomplishments

1. 90% Attendance of all required conferences (when not on excused leave)
2. Completion of All medical Records required
3. Successful submission of all cases for the PGY year (chiefs-board submission)
4. Successful management of ACGME duty hours requirements
5. Successful completion of all academic examinations
6. 90% attendance of required committee obligations
7. Passing overall score on annual Resident assessment scoring summary
8. Completion of step 3 by end to PGY 3 year
9. Completion of FLS certification

Residents with employment violations or failing to meet annual residency accomplishments may, depending on the violation, be: counseled, be required to have educational/counseling sessions to address the problem with subsequent review, be placed on probation with subsequent review or dismissed from the program.

The standard grievance procedures will be available to residents that disagree with their sited violations.

CHAPTER 8

REFERENCES

Graduate Medical Education Committee, American College of Surgeons. Prerequisite objectives for graduate surgical education: a study of the Graduate Medical Education Committee, American College of Surgeons. J Am Coll Surg 1998;186:50-62.

DaRosa DA, Derossis A. Applying instructional principles to the design of curriculum. In: Distlehorst LH, Dunnington GL, Folse JR (eds). Teaching and Learning in Medical and Surgical Education: Lessons Learned for the 21st Century. Mahwah NJ: Lawrence Erlbaum Associates, Inc., Publishers, 2000;57-68.

Leibrandt TJ, Kukora JS, Dent TL. Integrating educational objectives and the evaluation process in a general surgery residency program. Acad Med 2001;76(7):748-752.

ACS. Prerequisites for graduate surgical education: a guide for medical students and PGY-1 residents. Chicago: American College of Surgeons, 1998.

Blue AV, Griffith CH, III, Wilson J, et al. Surgical teaching quality makes a difference. Amer J Surg 1999;177(1):86-89.

Copeland HL, Hewson MG. Developing and testing an instrument to measure the effectiveness of clinical teaching in an academic medical center. Acad Med 2000;75(2):161-166.

Elliott DL, Skeff KM, Stratos GA. How do you get to the improvement of teaching? A longitudinal faculty development program for medical educators. Teach Learn Med 1999;11:52-57.

Veldenz HC, Dovgan PS, Schinco MS, Tepas JJ, III. M and M conference: enhancing delivery of surgical residency curricula. Current Surgery 2001;58(6):580-582.

Batalden PB, Nelson EC, Roberts JS. Linking outcomes measurement to continual improvement: the serial "V" way of thinking about improving clinical care. Jt Comm J Qual Improv 1994;20:167-180.

Faulkner H, Regehr G, Martin J, et al. Validation of an objective structured assessment of technical skill for surgical residents. Acad Med 1996;71(12):1363-1365.

Leibrandt TJ, Kukora JS, Dent TL. Integrating educational objectives and the evaluation process in a general surgery residency program. Acad Med 2001;76(7):748-752.

Tekian A, McGuire CH, McGaghie WC and Associates. Innovative Simulations for Assessing Professional Competence—from Paper and Pencil to Virtual Reality. Chicago: University of Illinois at Chicago, 1999;254pp.

Wade TP, Kaminski DL. Comparative evaluation of educational methods in surgical resident education. Arch Surg 1995;130:83-87.

CHAPTER 9

REQUISITE CURRICULUM

*O*verview

CONCEPTUAL APPROACH

This approach to the curriculum encompasses two concepts. First it is to complement the extensive and varied subject texts and materials in a manner that prioritizes the learning for implementation to practice. Second, the question or discussion format allows the learner to test competency and retention; this testing is meant to support preparation for clinical rotations and related certification examinations.

ORGANIZATION

The curriculum is organized in sections that start with unit objectives, which are organized according to the ACGME competencies;

Patient Care that is compassionate, appropriate, and effective for the treatment of health problems and the promotion of health.

Medical Knowledge about established and evolving biomedical, clinical, and cognate (e.g. epidemiological and social-behavioral) sciences and the application of this knowledge to patient care.

Practice-Based Learning and Improvement that involves investigation and evaluation of their own patient care, appraisal and assimilation of scientific evidence, and improvements in patient care.

The section is further stratified by junior and senior levels (where appropriate). Each section is an outline of questions or directives such as "discuss" or "identify" related to the specialty section topics that in turn are specific with an outline of detail areas that the resident should understand to be competent in the area of practice. Some sections include specific skills that should be obtained related to the area of study.

References that support a successful response to the questions and directives in the curriculum are provided where appropriate. Additionally, the references provide for additional practice based learning and population related comparisons. To enhance the importance of population specificity and the needs of our aging population, additional sections are provided in the subject area specific to elderly patients and a geriatric population.

SUBJECT AREAS

The concept of the core curriculum stems from the idea that all specialties share the related areas of medical knowledge or patient care to some degree. While some of this content is covered again in the specialty sections and is redundant, in general the core material allows for each specialty related material to be prioritized in the specific section. On a fairly arbitrary basis, subjects were grouped under Interpersonal and Communication Skills, Professionalism and System Based Practice because their base elements most coincided with that particular competency.

CHAPTER 10

CORE CURRICULUM

SECTION 10.1 WOUND HEALING

UNIT OBJECTIVES

Demonstrate an understanding of the physiology of wound healing.

Demonstrate the ability to manage complex wound care in a variety of settings.

Medical Knowledge about established and evolving biomedical, clinical, and cognate (e.g. epidemiological and social-behavioral) sciences and the application of this knowledge to patient care.

Junior Level:

1. Describe the physiological process of normal wound healing, including the healing relationship to:

a.	Anatomy	e.	Microbiology
b.	Physiology	f.	Immunology
c.	Biology	g.	Molecular Biology
d.	Biochemistry		

2. Explain the effect of the following factors on wound healing:

    a. Nutrition

    b. Pathologic metabolic states (including diabetes mellitus)

    c. Hematologic status

    d. Radiation

    e. Immune response

    f. Growth factors

    g. Super oxide radical formation

    h. Pharmacologic manipulation

    i. Infection/sepsis

    j. Chemotherapeutics

    k. Trauma

3. Describe the steps of normal of wound healing, including:

    a. Inflammation   d. Epithelialization

    b. Proliferation   e. Contracture/contraction

    c. Remodeling

4. Discuss the pathophysiology of delayed wound healing due to microbial physiology, virulence, and host defenses.

5. Differentiate between the pathophysiology of thermal, chemical, and electrical burns.

6. Discuss the principles of aseptic technique in uncomplicated cases related to the following procedures:

    a. Incision making   c. Wound closures

    b. Debridement   d. Dressings, splints, and casts

7. Describe the common chemical agents which are classically discussed in relation to burns and their antidotes.

8. Explain the principles of wound care as they relate to:

    a. Debridement   d. Chronic wounds

    b. Traumatic wounds   e. High-pressure injection injury

    c. Burn wounds   f. Medication infiltration

9. Summarize the principles of wound protection and subsequent healing using:

    a. Dressings

        (1) Occlusive   (3) Alginates

        (2) Non-occlusive   (4) Casting

    b. Other wound dressing materials

        (1) Collodium   (5) Dakin's solution

        (2) Petroleum gauze   (6) Acetic acid solution

        (3) Xeroform   (7) Silvadene, sulfamylon

        (4) Scarlet Red   (8) Iodine, Bacitracin

c. The concept of "moist wound healing"

d. Adjunctive therapies: hyperbaric oxygen, electrical stimulation, vacuum assisted wound management, pulse irrigation

10. Discuss potential problems in complicated wound healing, including such challenges as snake, animal, insect, and human bites; electric burns; deep space infections of the hand; penetrating wounds; and radiation.

11. Define and describe the causes of postoperative wound complications such as:

a. Dehiscence

b. Evisceration

c. Fasciitis and abscess formation

12. Discuss the concept of the reconstructive ladder.

13. Describe the microbiology of gangrene and necrotizing fasciitis.

14. Explain the principles associated with the selection of appropriate incisions applying surgical anatomy to include:

a. Blood supply   d. Strength

b. Lines of tension   e. Cosmesis/aesthetics

c. Access

15. Describe the rationale for selection of appropriate wound closure and reconstruction as it relates to wound healing in:

a. Primary and delayed primary closure

b. Secondary healing

c. Skin graft, split and full thickness

d. Local flaps

e. Regional flaps

f. Microvascular flaps

g. Composite grafts

16. Assess the properties and uses of different types of suture material, including those that are absorbable and non-absorbable.

17. Analyze the therapeutic options for treatment of abnormal or delayed wound healing because of:

    a. Host resistance d. Radiation

    b. Infection e. Ischemia

    c. Diabetes mellitus

18. Discuss treatment choices for the following wound healing problems:

    a. Dehiscence c. Hernia

    b. Infection

19. Identify the resources needed to assist with wound healing outside the hospital and outline methods for resource acquisition to include home health care and equipment rental.

20. Describe the use of pressure relief devices and beds to prevent pressure ulcerations.

21. Differentiate between fetal wound healing and adult wound healing. Discuss the possible applications of fetal wound healing.

Patient Care that is compassionate, appropriate, and effective for the treatment of health problems and the promotion of health.

Junior Level:

1. Provide basic care to wounds from abrasions and small lacerations, including acute debridement, closure, and dressing placement.

2. Provide care for complex traumatic injuries considering:

    a. Management of hemorrhage

    b. Acute pain control

    c. When to explore operatively

d. Debridement

e. Acute closure or coverage

f. Secondary reconstruction

3. Evaluate the progress of wound healing.

4. Apply all types of dressings and casts.

5. Make and close common incisions in the outpatient clinic, outpatient emergency department, and in the operating room.

6. Remove casts and complex dressings.

7. Assess thermal and non-thermal burns and initiate treatment.

8. Debride and care for wounds of low to intermediate complexity, including traumatic injuries.

9. Apply all types of complex dressings, including body casts.

10. Make and close incisions of low to intermediate complexity.

11. Debride complex wounds and provide post debridement care of such wounds.

12. Manage wounds of low to intermediate complexity, and alter therapy as indicated.

13. Perform complex procedures for the closure of difficult wounds, including various local and regional skin flaps and grafts.

14. Manage the care of various complex wound complications such as dehiscence, wound infections, and incisional hernias.

15. Analyze the use and need for complex reconstructive flaps and grafts; (e.g., application of the "reconstructive ladder").

Practice-Based Learning and Improvement that involves investigation and evaluation of their own patient care, appraisal and assimilation of scientific evidence, and improvements in patient care.

INFORMATION TECHNOLOGY AND POPULATION COMPARISONS
REFERENCES

Bentz ML. Pediatric Plastic Surgery.   CT: Appleton and Lange, 1998;1-1099.

Cohen IK, Diegelmann RF, Lindblad WJ. Wound Healing: Biochemical and Clinical Aspects. Philadelphia: WB Saunders Co., 1992.

Ellis H. Incisions, closures, and management of the wound. In: Zinner MJ, Schwartz SI, Ellis H (eds), Maingot's Abdominal Operations (10th ed).   CT: Appleton & Lange 1997; 395-426.

Fine NA, Mustoe TA. Wound healing. In: Greenfield LJ (ed), Surgery: Scientific Principles and Practice (2nd ed). Philadelphia: Lippincott-Raven, 1997;78-83.

Lawrence WT. Wound healing biology and its application to wound management. In: O'Leary JP (ed), The Physiologic Basis of Surgery (2nd ed). Baltimore: Williams and Wilkins, 1996;118-140.

Townsend CM, Jr., Beauchamp RD, Evers BM, Mattox KL (eds). Sabiston Textbook of Surgery (16th ed). Philadelphia: WB Saunders Company, 2001.

Young DM, Mathes SJ. Wound healing. In: Miller TA (ed), Modern Surgical Care: Physiologic Foundations and Clinical Applications (2nd ed). St. Louis: Quality Medical Publishing, Inc., 1998;1237-1247.

10.1A WOUND HEALING IN ELDERLY PATIENTS

UNIT OBJECTIVES:

Demonstrate an understanding of the pathophysiological impact that aging imposes on wound healing.

Demonstrate the ability to manage complex and chronic wounds in older patients.

Medical Knowledge about established and evolving biomedical, clinical, and cognate (e.g. epidemiological and social-behavioral) sciences and the application of this knowledge to patient care.

1.   Describe the process of normal wound healing in older patients, highlighting the differences from the adult and child with respect to:

    a.   Physiology

    b.   Microbiology

    c.   Immunology

2.   Explain the effect of the following factors on wound healing in older patients:

    a.   Nutrition

    b.   Metabolic state (including diabetes mellitus)

    c.   Collagen deposition

    d.   Pharmacologic manipulation

    e.   Physical activity/mobility

3.   Explain the principles of wound care as they relate to chronic wounds.

4.   Define and describe the causes of postoperative wound complications such as:

    a.   Dehiscence

    b.   Evisceration

    c.   Fasciitis

5.   Describe the rationale for selection of appropriate wound closure and reconstruction as it relates to geriatric wound healing in:

a. Primary and delayed primary closure

b. Secondary healing

c. Skin graft, split and full thickness

d. Local flaps

e. Regional flaps

f. Microvascular flaps and transfers

g. Tissue substitutes and adjuncts

6. Analyze the therapeutic options for treatment of abnormal or delayed wound healing in elderly patients because of:

a. Host resistance

b. Infection

c. Diabetes mellitus

d. Ischemia

7. Identify the resources needed to assist with chronic wound healing outside the hospital and outline methods for resource acquisition to include home health care and equipment rental.

8. Describe the use of pressure relief devices and beds to prevent pressure ulcerations.

Patient Care that is compassionate, appropriate, and effective for the treatment of health problems and the promotion of health.

1. Provide basic care to chronic wounds and pressure ulcers, including acute debridement and dressing placement.

a. Identify the clinical stages of pressure ulceration.

b. Evaluate the progress of wound healing.

c. Apply all types of dressings and casts.

d. Remove casts and complex dressings.

2. Perform wound debridement, and be able to provide post debridement care to debrided wounds.

3. Perform procedures for the closure of difficult wounds in older patients, including frequently used local and regional skin flaps and grafts.

4. Manage the care of various complex wound complications such as dehiscence, wound infections, and incisional hernias.

5. Analyze the pros and cons of complex reconstructive options in older patients' chronic wounds.

6. Be able to instruct other health care professionals in basic evaluation, prevention, and dressing care of chronic wounds or pressure ulcers.

Practice-Based Learning and Improvement that involves investigation and evaluation of their own patient care, appraisal and assimilation of scientific evidence, and improvements in patient care.

INFORMATION TECHNOLOGY AND POPULATION COMPARISONS
REFERENCES

Chicarilli ZN: Pressure sores in the elderly. In: Katlic MR (ed). Geriatric Surgery: Comprehensive Care of the Elderly Patient. Baltimore: Urban and Schwarzenberg, 1990; 549-586.

Evans JM, Andrews KL, Chutka DS, Fleming KC, Garness SL. Pressure Ulcers: Prevention and management. Mayo Clin Proc 1995;70:789-799.

Fine NA, Mustoe TA. Wound healing. In: Greenfield LJ (ed), Surgery: Scientific Principles and Practice. Philadelphia: Lippincott-Raven, 1997;78-83.

Gerstein AD, Phillips TJ, Rogers GS, Gilchrest BA: Wound healing and aging. Derm Clin 1993;11(4):749-757.

Kerrigan CL, Daniel RK: Pressure sores in the elderly. In: Meakins JL, McClaran JC. (eds), Surgical Care of the Elderly. Chicago: Year Book Medical Publishers, Inc., 1988;485-498.

Thomas DR, Allman RM (eds). Pressure ulcers. Clinics in Geriatr Med 1997; August.

Van der Kerkhof PCM, Van Bergen B, Spruijt K, Kuiper JP: Age-related changes in wound healing. Clinical and Experimenta

SECTION 10.2   FLUID AND ELECTROLYTE HOMEOSTASIS

UNIT OBJECTIVES:

Demonstrate an understanding of normal fluid and electrolyte homeostasis.

Demonstrate the ability to maintain homeostasis by recognizing and correcting fluid and electrolyte derangements.

Medical Knowledge about established and evolving biomedical, clinical, and cognate (e.g. epidemiological and social-behavioral) sciences and the application of this knowledge to patient care.

1.   Describe body water volumes and distribution.

2.   Indicate the normal electrolyte distribution of cell water and extracellular fluid to include the following:

    a.   Sodium   e.   Calcium

    b.   Potassium   f.   Magnesium

    c.   Chloride   g.   Phosphate

    d.   Bicarbonate

3.   Outline the normal electrolyte content of body fluids such as blood, extracellular fluid (ECF), urine, saliva, gastric juice, bile, and pancreatic fluid.

4.   Identify water and electrolyte changes in response to various stress situations such as:

    a.   Diseases, including trauma and burns

    b.   Operative therapy

    c.   Non-operative therapy

5.   Analyze water and electrolyte disorders affecting the hospitalized elderly by discussing the etiology and treatment of such conditions as:

    a.   Water overload

    b.   Plasma volume depletion

    c.   Changes in serum sodium levels

d.   Changes in serum potassium levels

6.   Describe the role of the following hormones in fluid and electrolyte homeostasis:

    a.   Vasopressin (ADH)   e.   Steroids

    b.   Renin   f.   Adrenocorticotrophic hormone

    c.   Angiotensin   (ACTH)

    d.   Aldosterone

7.   Apply the physiology of water and sodium imbalance to the following:

    a.   Salt and water depletion (depletion of extracellular fluid volume [ECFV]

    b.   Salt and water excess (expansion of ECFV)

    c.   Hyponatremia (hypo-osmolarity)

    d.   Hypernatremia (hyperosmolarity)

8.   Explain the treatment for water and sodium imbalance, including the use of and complications from diuretics and fluid restrictions.

9.   Summarize normal potassium physiology, the causes and consequences of depletion and excess, and the treatment for potassium imbalance.

10.   Discuss the complexities of calcium, phosphorus, and magnesium excesses and deficiencies in such situations as:

    a.   Metastatic breast cancer

    b.   Hepatic failure

    c.   Hyperparathyroidism

    d.   Milk-alkali syndrome

    e.   Eclampsia

11.   Illustrate treatments for high or low calcium, phosphorus, and magnesium in the instances listed directly above.

12.   Discuss the changes that affect water and sodium regulation, related to patient age and renal maturity, to include:

    a.   Concentrating ability

b.   ADH secretion

c.   Ability to conserve sodium

d.   Secretion of atrial natriuretic peptide

13.   Outline the pathophysiology of fluid and electrolyte problems in cardiac, aortic, and peripheral revascularization, including reperfusion injury.

Patient Care that is compassionate, appropriate, and effective for the treatment of health problems and the promotion of health.

1.   Use patient fluid balance data as general measures of fluid homeostasis.

2.   Estimate the patient's state of sodium and water balance by history and physical examination in the following locations/situations:

a.   Emergency department

b.   Pre- and post- operative patients

c.   In conjunction with nutritional considerations in patients on long-term total parenteral nutrition (TPN).

3.   Provide fluid and electrolyte orders to nursing staff for such situations as:

a.   Sepsis

b.   Burns

c.   Major surgery requiring transfusion

d.   Ascites

e.   Cardiac failure

f.   Malnutrition

g.   Fistulas (high output intestinal)

h.   Hypertrophic pyloric stenosis

4.   Coordinate orders involving nutrition, acid-base, and electrolyte problems.

5.   Apply fluid and electrolyte principles to the following special applications:

a.   Neonates   c.   Geriatric patients

  b. Infants   d. Cardiac bypass patients

6. Manage outpatients and inpatients with hypo- and hyper- kalemia.

7. Manage patients with hypo- and hyper- calcemia.

Practice-Based Learning and Improvement that involves investigation and evaluation of their own patient care, appraisal and assimilation of scientific evidence, and improvements in patient care.

INFORMATION TECHNOLOGY AND POPULATION COMPARISONS

REFERENCES

Abrams WB, Beers MH, Berkow R (eds). Water and electrolyte disorders. The Merck Manual of Geriatrics (2nd ed). Whitehouse Station, NJ: Merck Research Laboratories, Merck & Co., Inc., 1995;16-34.

Brandt MM, Bessey PQ. Electrolyte disorders. In: Cameron JL (ed), Current Surgical Therapy (6th ed). St. Louis: Mosby, 1998;1115-1121.

Cobbs EL, Duthie EH, Jr, Murphy JB (eds), Homeostasis. Geriatrics Review Syllabus: A Core Curriculum in Geriatric Medicine (4th ed). Dubuque IA: Kendall/Hunt Publishing Company, 1999.

Fabri PJ. Fluid and electrolyte physiology and pathophysiology. In: Miller TA (ed), Modern Surgical Care: Physiologic Foundations and Clinical Applications (2nd ed). St. Louis: Quality Medical Publishing, Inc., 1998;38-53.

Fenves AZ, Emmett M. Fluids and electrolytes. In: O'Leary JP (ed), The Physiologic Basis of Surgery (2nd ed). Baltimore: Williams and Wilkins, 1996;75-83.

Glynn L, Meyer A. Fluid and electrolyte therapy. In: Cameron JL (ed), Current Surg Therap (6th ed). St. Louis:Mosby, 1998;1057-1062.

Wait R, Kahng KU, Dresner LS. Fluids and electrolytes and acid-base balance. In: Greenfield LJ, Mulholland M, Oldham KT, Zelenock GB, Lillemoe KD (eds), Surgery: Scientific Principles and Practice (2nd ed). Philadelphia: Lippincott-Raven, 1997; 242-59

SECTION 10.3 ACID-BASE HOMEOSTASIS

UNIT OBJECTIVES:

Demonstrate an understanding of the biochemistry and physiology of acid-base homeostasis. Demonstrate the ability to diagnose and effectively treat complex disorders of acid-base balance.

Medical Knowledge about established and evolving biomedical, clinical, and cognate (e.g. epidemiological and social-behavioral) sciences and the application of this knowledge to patient care.

1. Explain hydrogen ion biochemistry and physiology to include:
   a. The Henderson-Hasselbalch equation
      (1) Ventilatory component (pCO_2)
      (2) Renal component (HCO_3^-)
   b. Hydrogen ion production and disposal
   c. Buffering systems
      (1) Acute (bicarbonate)
      (2) Chronic (bone, renal, and pulmonary

2. Relate the biochemistry of membrane gas exchange using the example of gases exchanging over the alveolar/capillary interface.

3. Explain the physiology of hydrogen ion production and renal excretion of hydrogen ions.

4. Describe renal bicarbonate reabsorption and regeneration.

5. Summarize the contributions of the skeleton, kidneys, and lungs in maintaining a normal pH.

6. Classify metabolic acidosis, including "anion gap" and hyperchloremic acidosis.

7. Identify specific causes of metabolic acidosis.

8. Given values for pH, pCO_2, and HCO_3^-, distinguish between compensated and uncompensated metabolic acidosis, respiratory acidosis, metabolic alkalosis, respiratory alkalosis, and mixed abnormalities; derive a differential diagnosis for each.

9. Explain age-associated changes that may occur in certain respiratory and renal regulatory processes that are known to maintain normal pH. How does aging affect:

    a. Ability to hyperventilate in response to acute metabolic acidosis

    b. The kidney's response to an acid load (Describe recovery of the blood pH.)

10. List disorders, common in elderly patients that contribute to acid-base disturbances. Explain the mechanisms that can lead to acid-base disturbances associated with:

    a. Heart failure   d. Renal disease

    b. Anemia   e. Pulmonary disease

    c. Sepsis   f. Diabetes mellitus

11. Identify specific acid-base disturbances in elderly patients caused by such frequently used drugs as:

    a. Salicylates

    b. Diuretics

    c. Laxatives

12. Relate metabolic alkalosis to the following:

    a. Chloride-responsive alkalosis

    b. Chloride-resistant alkalosis

    c. Paradoxic aciduria

13. Predict the importance of primary diseases and their complications to the evaluation of patient risk for:

    a. Shock

    b. Bowel obstruction

    c. Sepsis

14. Analyze the acid-base problem and its cause in specific clinical situations, and determine an appropriate course of therapy for the following conditions:

    a. "Medical" problems such as:

	(1)	Diabetic ketoacidosis	(4)	Renal insufficiency
	(2)	Lactic acidosis	(5)	Respiratory failure
	(3)	Renal tubular acidosis		

b.   "Surgical" problems such as:

    (1)   Pyloric stenosis

    (2)   Gastric outlet obstruction

    (3)   Fistulas

    (4)   Ureteroileal conduit

    (5)   Shock

15.   Why are disturbances of acid-base balance common in elderly patients? Explain by discussing the implications of:

a.   Impaired homeostatic mechanisms

b.   High prevalence of drug use and disease

16.   Summarize the adverse effects of acid-base disturbances on the following body systems:

a.   Central nervous system / intracranial pressure

b.   Renal physiology

c.   Pulmonary physiology

Patient Care that is compassionate, appropriate, and effective for the treatment of health problems and the promotion of health.

1.   Diagnose and treat acid-base disturbances of all types.

2.   Diagnose and treat complex and combined problems in acid-base disturbances as a component of overall care.

3.   Manage complex situations in the intensive care unit where acid-base abnormalities coexist with other metabolic derangements, including:

a.   Fluid and electrolytes   c.   Renal disease

b.   Total parenteral nutrition   d.   Pulmonary disease

Practice-Based Learning and Improvement that involves investigation and evaluation of their own patient care, appraisal and assimilation of scientific evidence, and improvements in patient care.

INFORMATION TECHNOLOGY AND POPULATION COMPARISONS: SEPSIS

REFERENCES

Abrams WB, Beers MH, Berkow R (eds). Acid-base regulation. The Merck Manual of Geriatrics (2nd ed). Whitehouse Station, NJ: Merck Research Laboratories, Merck & Co., Inc., 1995:32-34.

Buechter KJ, Byers PM. Nutrition and metabolism. In: O'Leary JP (ed), The Physiologic Basis of Surgery (2nd ed). Baltimore: Williams and Wilkins, 1996;100-117.

Cobbs EL, Duthie EH, Jr, Murphy JB (eds), Age related physiologic changes. Homeostasis. Geriatrics Review Syllabus: A Core Curriculum in Geriatric Medicine (4th ed). Dubuque IA: Kendall/Hunt Publishing Company, 1999.

Lindeman RD. Renal and electrolytic disorders. In: Duthie E, Katz P (eds). Practice of Geriatrics (3rd ed). Philadelphia: WB Saunders, 1998;546-562.

Wait R, Kahng KU, Dresner LS. Fluids and electrolytes and acid-base balance. In: Greenfield LJ, Mulholland M, Oldham KT, Zelenock GB, Lillemoe KD (eds), Surgery: Scientific Principles and Practice (2nd ed). Philadelphia: Lippincott-Raven, 1997;242-266.

Web reference http://www.tmc.tulane.edu/anes/acid

SECTION 10.4. METABOLISM

UNIT OBJECTIVES:

Demonstrate an understanding of the metabolic basis of substrate utilization and the disease states caused by specific alterations in intermediary metabolism.

Demonstrate the ability to apply this understanding of metabolism by integrating it with direct application to the management of patients.

Medical Knowledge about established and evolving biomedical, clinical, and cognate (e.g. epidemiological and social-behavioral) sciences and the application of this knowledge to patient care.

Section 1: Energy

1. Describe the principles of energy conversion to mechanical work and the efficiency of energy conversion and thermal balance.
2. Define basic energy units such as the calorie and the kilocalorie.
3. Discuss the routes of heat loss and their relationship to energy balance.
4. Relate oxygen consumption and carbon dioxide production to thermogenesis, energy production, and measurement of energy balance by indirect calorimetry.
5. Explain the respiratory quotient, its usefulness in determining substrate utilization patterns, and its relationship to respiratory function.
6. Define basal and resting metabolic rates and their relationship to body weight, size, age, and sex.
7. Predict daily energy requirements using metabolic rate equations.
8. Discuss the effects of ambient temperature, injury, burn, infection, pain, fear, anxiety, and starvation on energy requirements.
9. Integrate the above knowledge with prediction equations to estimate metabolic demands of critically-ill patients (e.g., the Harris-Benedict Equation).
10. Discuss how different substrates (carbohydrates, fats, and proteins) contribute to specific disease processes.

Section 2: Temperature and Fuel Homeostasis

117

1. Describe how the brain controls body temperature and alters temperature set point in response to stress and other factors.

2. Describe the mediators that influence temperature set point and the febrile response; explain their relation to changes in oxygen consumption.

3. Explain the differences between endogenous, exogenous, and bacterial pyrogens. Summarize their relation to post-traumatic fever and other disease processes resulting in fever.

Section 3: Hormonal Control of Body Fuels

1. Identify the hormones responsible for storage and mobilization of energy. Describe their effects.

2. Explain the metabolic effects of glucagon and insulin on protein, fat, and carbohydrate metabolism.

3. Explain the effects of catecholamine release during stress and the results of these effects on metabolism of glucose, fat, and protein as well as heat production.

4. Summarize the causes of negative nitrogen balance following injury, and explain the role of glucocorticoids on protein metabolism.

5. Discuss the systemic effects of corticosteroids on the body's response to injury and infection.

6. Describe the function of growth hormone and thyroid hormone as anabolic or catabolic mediators.

Section 4: Intermediary Metabolism

1. Explain the processes involved in carbohydrate metabolism, including glycogen synthesis and degradation, glycolysis, and gluconeogenesis.

2. Summarize the following metabolic processes:

    a.   Protein synthesis and degradation

b. Role of alanine and glutamate in deamination

c. Urea cycle

3. Explain the metabolism of lipids, including:

a. Synthesis
b. Catabolism
c. Formation of ketone bodies
d. Role of the tricarboxylic acid cycle

4. Describe the role of macrophages and cytokines in response to stress and metabolism.

5. Summarize the metabolic responses to short-term starvation that maintain euglycemia.

6. Identify the changes in fuel oxidation and substrate utilization that occur during fasting.

7. Describe the alanine and Cori cycles, and relate them to alterations in renal, hepatic, and cardiopulmonary function during adaptation to long-term starvation.

8. Explain the routes of nitrogen loss during starvation, injury and infection. Describe the effects of glucose, fat, and protein on nitrogen metabolism in these situations.

9. Describe the changes in body composition that occur with:

a. Bed rest
b. Complicated and uncomplicated operations
c. Trauma
d. Sepsis

10. Explain how protein metabolism is affected by hormonal regulators. Summarize its relationship to oxygen consumption, temperature regulation, and energy balance.

11. Summarize the hormonal regulation of gluconeogenesis after trauma and during critical illness.

12. Describe the caloric contribution of endogenous substrates, and analyze the association between tissue loss and weight loss.

13. Compare the differences between the alterations in intermediary metabolism occurring with hypothermia and intense exercise with those in trauma, infection, and prolonged critical illness.

Section 5: Implications for the Elderly Patient

1. Describe the changes in calorie requirements, basal metabolic rate, and fat stores in elderly patients.

2. Discuss impaired glucose tolerance and renal excretion in the elderly patient.

3. Name specific vitamin and mineral deficiencies in older people and their causes and effects.

4. Describe the problem with decreased total body water and its impact in the elderly patient.

5. What is the prevalence and cause of protein-calorie malnutrition in the geriatric population; what is the impact on abdominal surgery?

6. How does the temperature set point differ in elderly patients, and how does the presentation of peritonitis differ?

Patient Care that is compassionate, appropriate, and effective for the treatment of health problems and the promotion of health.

1. Determine daily energy requirements of critically-ill patients using established formulas accounting for varied metabolic demands.

2. Utilize metabolic cart and indirect calorimetry to calculate metabolic needs in similar patients. Discuss the efficacy and limitations of this method.

3. Calculate nitrogen balance status in critically-ill patients, and alter metabolic supply and demand to establish positive balance.

Practice-Based Learning and Improvement that involves investigation and evaluation of their own patient care, appraisal and assimilation of scientific evidence, and improvements in patient care.

INFORMATION TECHNOLOGY AND POPULATION COMPARISONS: SEPSIS
REFERENCES

Amaral JF, Caldwell MD. Metabolic response to starvation, stress, and sepsis. In: Miller TA (ed), Modern Surgical Care: Physiologic Foundations and Clinical Applications (2nd ed). St. Louis: Quality Medical Publishing, Inc., 1998;1-37.

Buechter KJ, Byers PM. Nutrition and metabolism. In: O'Leary JP (ed), The Physiologic Basis of Surgery (2nd ed). Baltimore: Williams and Wilkins, 1996;100-117.

Civetta JM, Taylor RW, Kirby RR. Critical Care (3rd ed). Philadelphia: Lippincott-Raven Co., 1997.

Powers JS, Billings FT, Jr. Management of perioperative problems in the aged. In: Adkins RB, Jr., Scott HW, Jr. (eds), Surgical Care for the Elderly (2nd ed). Philadelphia: Lippincott-Raven Publishers, 1998;33-50.

Reuben DB, Greendale GA, Harrison GG. Nutrition screening in older persons. J Am Geriatr Soc 1995;43:415-425.

Rosenthal RA, Andersen DK. Physiologic considerations in the elderly surgical patient. In: Miller TA (ed), Modern Surgical Care: Physiologic Foundations and Clinical Applications (2nd ed). St. Louis: Quality Medical Publishing, Inc., 1998;1362-1384.

Smith BE. Anesthetic considerations in elderly patients. In: Adkins RB, Jr., Scott HW, Jr. (eds), Surgical Care for the Elderly (2nd ed). Philadelphia: Lippincott-Raven Publishers, 1998;51-76.

Souba WW, Austen WG, Jr., Nutrition and metabolism. In: Greenfield LJ, Mulholland M, Oldham KT, Zelenock GB, Lillemoe KD (eds), Surgery: Scientific Principles and Practice (2nd ed). Philadelphia: Lippincott-Raven, 1997;42-66.

SECTION 10.5. NUTRITION

UNIT OBJECTIVES:

Demonstrate a working knowledge of the methods of nutritional assessment and routes of nutritional support.

Demonstrate an understanding of the metabolic consequences of surgical disease and the need for nutritional support.

Demonstrate an understanding of the unique nutritional concerns for specific clinical conditions.

Recognize the need for artificial nutritional support and arrange enteral nutrition.

Medical Knowledge about established and evolving biomedical, clinical, and cognate (e.g. epidemiological and social-behavioral) sciences and the application of this knowledge to patient care.

1.   Discuss risk factors contributing to malnutrition in the hospitalized patient, including:

    a.   Low nutritional reserve

    b.   Extensive preoperative studies

    c.   Lack of oral (PO) intake secondary to underlying disease

    d.   High stress conditions

2.   Summarize the characteristics of the indicators for nutritional assessment, including:

    a.   Weight loss greater than 10% of body weight

    b.   Serum albumin less than 3.4 gm/dl

    c.   Impaired immunologic response: anergic response and total lymphocyte count (TLC) less than 1500/cc

    d.   Specific physical signs

3.   Analyze methods of nutritional assessment using:

    a.   Pertinent history

    b.   Anthropomorphic measurements

     c.   Laboratory measurements

     d.   Immunologic measurements

4.   Analyze and be prepared to explain potential problems associated with primary nutritional problems affecting older people, including:

     a.   Protein-energy undernutrition

     b.   Vitamin deficiencies

     c.   Trace mineral deficiencies

     d.   Obesity

5.   Explain methods of calculating energy requirements, including:

     a.   Simple estimate (resting: 20 kcal/kg-d; moderate stress: 30 kcal/kg-d; severe stress: 40 kcal/kg-d)

     b.   Harris-Benedict Equation

     c.   Nitrogen balance

     d.   Basal metabolic cart

6.   Analyze the metabolic responses to starvation and stress/trauma.

7.   Provide general guidelines for determining nutritional composition:

     a.   Non-protein calorie to protein ratio

     b.   Protein requirements

     c.   Carbohydrate/fat balance

     d.   Ventilation issues (effect on respiratory quotient)

8.   Summarize factors that can lead to problems in elderly patients, resulting from effects of mild vitamin deficiencies, especially in those institutionalized elderly patients that are associated with:

     a.   Cognitive impairment

     b.   Poor wound healing

     c.   Anemia

     d.   Bruising

e.   Increased risk of infections

f.   Increased risk of developing certain cancers

9.   Discuss the indications, contraindications, and benefits of enteral feedings: describe sites of delivery and potential complications and their treatment.

10.   Discuss the indications, contraindications, and disadvantages of parenteral feeding; describe the details of initiating total parenteral nutrition (TPN), monitoring delivery, and managing potential complications.

11.   Summarize content and rationale for special formulations used in patients with:

a.	Congestive heart failure	d. Respiratory failure
b.	Liver failure	e. Glucose intolerance
c.	Renal failure	

12.   Explain recent advances in surgical nutrition, including:

a.	Role of glutamine	c. Growth factors
b.	Role of arginine	d. Omega-3 fatty acids

13.   Analyze the potential implications of nutritional deficiencies in certain disease states, and define the role of nutritional components in preventing acquired and malignant disease.

14.   The following examples are conditions that can result from protein-energy undernutrition. Discuss the significance of each to the elderly surgical patient:

a.	Cognitive dysfunction	c. Pressure sores
b.	Decreased muscle strength	d. Altered thyroid function

Patient Care that is compassionate, appropriate, and effective for the treatment of health problems and the promotion of health.

1.   Perform nutritional assessment of hospitalized patients.

2.   Select appropriate methods of nutritional support, and provide necessary monitoring.

3.   Calculate nutritional requirements for patients with:

a.	Malignancy	c. Pancreatitis

b.	Stress/trauma	d.	Enterocutaneous fistula

4. Insert enteral and parenteral tubes and lines.

5. Manage nutritional support in patients with specific clinical conditions listed above.

6. Recognize and correct the subtle caloric and vitamin imbalances in patients receiving TPN.

7. Perform operative gastrostomies, jejunostomies, and percutaneous endoscopic gastrostomies.

8. Recognize and treat complications of enteral and parenteral feeding, including:

a.	Diarrhea	d.	Fatty metamorphosis of liver
b.	Dehydration	e.	Glucose intolerance
c.	Line sepsis		

9. Become familiar with the use of the "SCALES" protocol for evaluating risk of malnutrition in elderly patients, using these variables:

a. Sadness

b. Cholesterol level

c. Albumin level

d. Loss of weight

e. Eating problems

f. Shopping and food preparation problems

g. Effects of malnutrition, both excess and depletion

Practice-Based Learning and Improvement that involves investigation and evaluation of their own patient care, appraisal and assimilation of scientific evidence, and improvements in patient care.

INFORMATION TECHNOLOGY AND POPULATION COMPARISONS: SEPSIS

REFERENCES

Alpers DH, Clouse RE, Stenson WF. Manual of Nutritional Therapeutics (2nd ed). Boston: Little, Brown and Co., 1988.

Abrams WB, Beers MH, Berkow R (eds). Nutrition.. The Merck Manual of Geriatrics (2nd ed). Whitehouse Station, NJ: Merck Research Laboratories, Merck & Co., Inc., 1995;7-16.

Bower RH. Nutrition support in the surgical patient. In: Cameron JL (ed), Current Surgical Therapy (6th ed). St. Louis: Mosby, 1998;1062-1067.

Buechter KJ, Byers PM. Nutrition and metabolism. In: O'Leary JP (ed), The Physiologic Basis of Surgery (2nd ed). Baltimore: Williams and Wilkins, 1996;100-117.

Goldstein R. Nutrition and aging. In: Adkins RB, Jr., Scott HW, Jr. (eds), Surgical Care for the Elderly (2nd ed). Philadelphia: Lippincott-Raven Publishers, 1998;117-130.

Herrmann VM, Daly JM. Surgical nutrition. In: Miller TA (ed), Modern Surgical Care: Physiologic Foundations and Clinical Applications (2nd ed). St. Louis: Quality Medical Publishing, Inc., 1998;54-82.

Morley JE, Miller DK. Malnutrition in the elderly. Hospice Practice 1992;27(7):95-116. Rolandelli RH, Ullrich JR. Nutritional support in the frail elderly surgical patient. In: Zenilman ME, Roslyn JJ (eds), Surgery in the elderly patient, Surg Cl of N Amer 1994;74(1):79-91.

Sax HC. Nutrition support in the critically ill. In: Cameron JL (ed), Current Surgical Therapy (6th ed). St. Louis: Mosby, 1998;1143-1045.

Souba WW, Austen WG, Jr., Nutrition and metabolism. In: Greenfield LJ, Mulholland M, Oldham KT, Zelenock GB, Lillemoe KD (eds), Surgery: Scientific Principles and Practice (2nd ed). Philadelphia: Lippincott-Raven, 1997;42-66.
http://www.clinnutr.org

White JV, Ham RJ. Nutrition. In: Ham RJ, Sloan PD (eds), Primary Care Geriatrics: A Case-Based Approach (3rd ed). St. Louis: Mosby, 1997;108-127.

SECTION 10.6 HEMATOLOGY

UNIT OBJECTIVES:

Demonstrate knowledge of the physiology of hematopoiesis and the cellular constituents of blood.

Demonstrate an understanding of how common hematologic disorders affect the surgical patient.

Demonstrate an understanding of the normal and abnormal mechanisms of hemostasis, coagulation, and fibrinolysis.

Demonstrate a familiarity with hypercoagulable states and their implications for care of surgical patients.

Demonstrate an understanding of transfusion therapy, its indications, and potential complications.

Understanding of practice in the prevention and management of venous thrombosis and Embolism

Prophylaxis: Use of common methods of prophylaxis against venous thrombosis and embolism.

Medical Knowledge about established and evolving biomedical, clinical, and cognate (e.g. epidemiological and social-behavioral) sciences and the application of this knowledge to patient care.

Section One: Blood Physiology

1.   Describe the fundamental components of hematopoiesis, including the development of lymphocytes and hematopoietic cells from multipotent cells.
2.   Discuss the structure, function, production, and degradation of hemoglobin.
3.   Discuss the structure, function, lifespan, metabolic activity, and degradation of red blood cells (RBC's).
4.   Outline and compare the common congenital and acquired anemias, such as those associated with:
    a.   Decreased RBC production
    b.   Excessive RBC destruction, including hemoglobinopathies

5.   Briefly discuss polycythemia and implications for surgical patients.

6.   Describe hemoglobin S disease (sickle cell disease), and understand the implications of this and related disorders for surgical management.

7.   Discuss the fundamental roles of the following in inflammation, immune response, and infection:

   a.   Granulocytes (polymorphonuclear leukocytes [PMN's], basophils, eosinophils)

   b.   Lymphocytes

   c.   Monocytes

8.   Discuss platelet production and physiology, and relate these to common problems such as autoimmune thrombocytopenia (ITP).

9.   Discuss the effect of common drugs on hemostasis.

Section Two: Hemostasis, Coagulation, and Fibrinolysis

1.   Discuss the phases of normal hemostasis, including:

   a.   Primary hemostasis (vasoconstriction and platelet aggregation/activation)

   b.   Secondary hemostasis (activation of the coagulation cascade and formation of a fibrin clot).

2.   Categorize the fundamental cellular and molecular events involved in platelet activation.

3.   Identify and describe the endogenous procoagulants and anticoagulants in blood.

4.   Diagram the intrinsic, extrinsic, and common coagulation pathways and their sites of activation.

5.   Describe and explain the delicate interaction of the following forces in the control of coagulation:

   a.   Blood flow   c.   Thrombomodulin

   b.   Endothelium   d.   Fibrinolysis

6.   Discuss indications for and methods of conducting common tests of coagulation and hemostasis, such as:

   a.   Partial-thromboplastin time (APTT)

      b.   Prothrombin time (INR)

      c.   Thrombin time

      d.   Bleeding time

      e.   Platelet aggregation studies

7. Indicate the mode of action and site of action for the following common drugs affecting blood clotting:

      a.   Heparin

      b.   Coumadin

      c.   Aspirin and other non-steroidal anti-inflammatory drugs (NSAID's)

8. Identify congenital coagulopathies and summarize considerations made in the diagnosis and management in patients with these disorders undergoing elective surgery.

9. Identify and discuss pathophysiology and the management of common acquired disorders of coagulation (coagulopathies) associated with stress, trauma, surgery, and co-morbid disease, including:

      a.   Disseminated intravascular coagulation (DIC)

      b.   Dilutional thrombocytopenia

      c.   Mechanical circulation

      d.   Vitamin K deficiency

      e.   Uremia

      f.   Liver failure

      g.   Hypothermia

10. Differentiate between the features, diagnosis, and management of the known hypercoagulable states, including:

      a.   Protein C deficiency

      b.   Protein S deficiency

      c.   Antithrombin III deficiency

      d.   Antiplatelet antibody production

      e.   Factor V Leiden

11. Discuss various aspects of pharmacologic therapy to modify hemostasis, including:

   a. Agents which affect platelet function

   b. Heparin

   c. Coumadin-type drugs

   d. Hirudin

   e. Epsilon aminocaproic acid and other antifibrinolytic agents

12. Describe methods to reverse or modify the activities of heparin and Coumadin-type drugs.

13. Discuss management of the anticoagulated patient referred for elective surgery.

14. Discuss fibrinolytic therapy, indications and complications.

Section Three: Transfusion Therapy

1. Discuss the clinical and economic rationale for blood component transfusion therapy.

2. Briefly describe the method of preparing, handling, and use of additives for the following blood components:

   a. RBC's   d. Cryoprecipitate

   b. Platelets (PLT's)   e. Granulocytes

   c. Fresh frozen plasma (FFP) f. Factor concentrates

3. Point out the indications for blood component transfusion at your hospital consistent with National Institutes of Health (NIH) consensus recommendations.

4. Understand the elements of informed consent for blood transfusion.

5. Discuss factors that influence the decision to transfuse.

6. Explain the principles of blood typing and transfusion therapy, including indications and complications to include the following:

   a. Major and minor blood group antigens and their laboratory evaluation

   b. Blood components and indications for transfusion

   c. Risks of transfusion, diagnosis, and therapy of transfusion complications

   d. Indications for and methods of autotransfusion and autologous blood donation

e.   Complications resulting from blood transfusion, including relative risk of viral infections

7.   Explain the significance of the following:
    a.   Major and minor blood group antigens
    b.   Role of autoantibodies
    c.   Difference between blood screening, typing, and compatibility testing

8.   Discuss cardinal features of the following immediate transfusion reactions, including their diagnosis and management:
    a.   Febrile
    b.   Allergic
    c.   Hemolytic

9.   Assess the incidence and risk of transfusion-related infections such as:
    a.   Acquired Immune Deficiency Syndrome (AIDS)
    b.   Cytomegalovirus (CMV)
    c.   Hepatitis

10.   Define the methods, indications, and benefits of autologous blood donation.
11.   Illustrate the application of erythropoietin, granulocyte-colony stimulating factor, and similar agents to the surgical patient with co-morbid disease.
12.   Explain the mechanics, application, and limitations of intraoperative autotransfusion.
13.   Describe indications for DDAVP in patients with coagulation disorders.

Section Four: Hematologic Considerations in Elderly Patients
    1.   Describe changes in the hematopoietic and coagulation systems associated with aging.
    2.   List chronic diseases that influence the hematopoietic or coagulation systems that are prevalent in elderly patients.
    3.   List common drugs prescribed to elderly patients who are prone to alter hematopoietic reserve or coagulation.

Patient Care that is compassionate, appropriate, and effective for the treatment of health problems and the promotion of health.

1. Outline a cost-effective strategy to identify preoperative patients at risk for abnormal bleeding based on:

    a. History of bleeding diathesis

    b. Magnitude of surgery

    c. Potential for vascular involvement

2. Evaluate patients with known hematologic disorders.

3. Recommend and perform preoperative, intraoperative, and postoperative interventions to minimize morbidity in patients with hematologic disorders.

4. Diagnose and definitively treat unexpected intra- and post- operative hemorrhage.

5. Assess risks and perform vascular access procedures in patients with anemic, neutropenic, and coagulopathic disorders.

6. Recognize and treat immediate transfusion reactions.

7. Discuss with patient and family the risks, benefits, and alternatives to blood component transfusion.

8. Participate in the surgical care of patients undergoing splenectomy, liver biopsy, and nodal staging for hematologic disease

9. Identify patients at risk for developing deep venous thrombosis (DVT) and prophylax against DVT, using pharmacologic and mechanical methods.

10. Manage patients on chronic anticoagulation therapy who require elective surgery.

11. Discuss pathophysiology of hemoglobin S disease (sickle cell disease) and its surgical implications.

12. Manage patients with hemoglobin S disease requiring surgery.

13. Manage patients on fibrinolytic therapy.

14. Methods of investigation for suspected thromboembolic disease

15. Anticoagulation, heparin and warfarin

16. Role of V/Q scanning, CT angiography and thrombolysis

17. Place of pulmonary embolectomy

18. Knowledge of methods of prevention, mechanical and pharmacological

Practice-Based Learning and Improvement that involves investigation and evaluation of their own patient care, appraisal and assimilation of scientific evidence, and improvements in patient care.

Recognition of patients at risk for DVT

1. Diagnosis:
2. Awareness of symptoms and signs associated with pulmonary embolism and DVT
3. Role of duplex scanning, venography and d-dimer measurement
4. Treatment: Initiate and monitor treatment

INFORMATION TECHNOLOGY AND POPULATION COMPARISONS: TRAUMA

REFERENCES

Bell WR, Braverman PE. Abnormal operative and postoperative bleeding. In: Cameron JL (ed), Current Surgical Therapy (6th ed). St. Louis: Mosby, 1998;1086-1091.

Clagett GP, Anderson FA, Helt J, Levine MN, Wheeler HB. Prevention of venous thromboembolism. Fourth ACCP Consensus Conference of Antithrombotic Therapy. Chest 1995;108(4):312S-334S.

Colman RW, Hirsh J, Marder VJ, et al. (eds). Hemostasis and Thrombosis: Basic Principles and Clinical Practice (4th ed). Philadelphia: Lippincott Williams & Wilkins, 2001.

Jackson MR, Clagett GP. Hemostasis and thrombosis in the surgical patient. In: Miller TA (ed), Modern Surgical Care: Physiologic Foundations and Clinical Applications (2nd ed). St. Louis: Quality Medical Publishing, Inc., 1998;173-196.

Mannucci PM. Hemostatic drugs. New England Journal of Medicine 1998;339:245-253.

Peterson P, Hayes TE, Arkin CF, Bovill EG, et al. The preoperative bleeding time test lacks clinical benefit. College of American Pathologists' and American Society of Clinical Pathologists' Position Article. Arch Surg 1998;133:134-139.

Scott-Conner CEH, Brunson CD. The pathophysiology of the sickle hemoglobinopathies and implications for perioperative management. Am J Surg 1994;168:268-274.

Scott-Conner CEH, Rock WA, Jr, Spence R, et al. Hemostasis, thrombosis, hematopoiesis, and blood transfusion. In: O'Leary JP, Capote LR (eds). The Physiologic Basis of Surgery (3rd ed). Philadelphia: Lippincott Williams and Wilkins, 2002.

SECTION 10.7 CLINICAL LABORATORY

UNIT OBJECTIVES:

Demonstrate an understanding of the pathogenesis of benign and malignant surgical disease.

Develop competency in the diagnosis and management of human organ pathology.

Demonstrate a working understanding of the principles of surgical pathology.

Demonstrate competence in the acquisition and interpretation of surgical specimens.

Apply clinical and laboratory data to diagnose disease processes and to institute appropriate
disease management.

Medical Knowledge about established and evolving biomedical, clinical, and cognate (e.g.
epidemiological and social-behavioral) sciences and the application of this knowledge to patient
care.

1.   Describe appropriate containers for storing blood and other body fluids during laboratory
        transport to sites where common serum chemistry studies are to be performed.

2.   Discuss the relative sensitivity, specificity, and accuracy of common laboratory studies.

3.   Demonstrate competency in interpreting:

        a.   Abnormal urinalysis

        b.   Abnormal thyroid function studies

        c.   Steroid suppression tests

4.   Outline the standard components of a coagulation profile, including the common clinical
        conditions associated with their abnormalities.

5.   Identify significant components for each of the following:

        a.   A complete blood count

        b.   The meaning of "left shift"

        c.   Common clinical conditions causing elevations in each component

6.   Analyze causes for artificially abnormal laboratory values, including:

        a.   Specimen hemolysis

        b.   Impact of hyperglycemia

        c.   Impact of hypoalbuminemia

7. Identify potential adverse effects of repeated phlebotomies, and discuss potential remedies for the following concerns:
    a. Patient pain
    b. Anemia
    c. Thrombophlebitis
    d. Arterial thrombosis
    e. Patient and hospital costs

8. Discuss the typical presentation of microbiologic data, and the importance of the following:
    a. Specimen identification and timing of sample
    b. Organism identification
    c. Drug sensitivity profile
    d. Minimum inhibitory concentration
    e. Beta-lactam resistance
    f. Resistance
    g. Colonization
    h. Contaminated specimen

7. Explain the importance of laboratory quality control in the hospital and outpatient setting. Clarify the meaning of role reference laboratory.

Patient Care that is compassionate, appropriate, and effective for the treatment of health problems and the promotion of health.

1. Identify the indications for routine preoperative laboratory studies, recognize clinically significant abnormalities, and provide appropriate management.
2. Manage the postoperative course of patients, using relevant laboratory studies (including their indication, relevance to clinical condition, and continued need).

3. Manage the anticoagulation status of patients using heparin and Coumadin, while considering the patient's Prothrombin time (PT) and partial thromboplastic time (PTT).

4. With the assistance of medical consultation, investigate and diagnose a new coagulation defect in a surgical patient.

5. Modify patient's infectious disease treatment plan using data from a microbiology report.

SECTION 10.8 SURGICAL PATHOLOGY

Medical Knowledge about established and evolving biomedical, clinical, and cognate (e.g. epidemiological and social-behavioral) sciences and the application of this knowledge to patient care.

1.   Discuss the indications, contraindications, and limitations of the following biopsy techniques:

    a.   Fine-needle aspiration (FNA)

    b.   Stereotactic biopsy

    c.   Core biopsy

    d.   Incisional biopsy

    e.   Excisional biopsy

2.   Explain the methods of handling and transporting tissue obtained by the methods listed above.

3.   Describe the role of needle aspiration in the diagnosis and management of:

    a.   Breast pathology

    b.   Thoracic pathology

    c.   Abdominal pathology

    d.   Thyroid pathology

    e.   Head and neck malignancy

4.   Discuss principles and indications for the following methods of tissue preparation:

    a.   Hematoxylin and eosin stains

    b.   Immunohistochemistry

    c.   Specific stains (enolase, argentaffin)

    d.   Polymerase chain reaction

5.   Discuss the use and interpretation of genetic analysis of neoplastic tissue, including:

    a.   Ploidy status

    b.   Mitotic activity

c. Cell-cycle phase

d. Describe the basic principles of:

e. Pathogenesis of reversible and irreversible cell injury

f. Acute and chronic inflammatory responses

2. Discuss the pathogenesis, clinical significance, signs and symptoms, and therapy for:

a. Derangements of normal wound healing

b. Fluid and hemodynamic derangements including shock, edema, congestive heart failure

c. Disorders of coagulation and hemostasis, including complications of: hemorrhage, disseminated intravascular coagulation (DIC), deep venous thrombosis (DVT), pulmonary embolism (PE)

d. Disorders of the immune system, especially hypersensitivity reactions and autoimmune disease

e. Infectious diseases involving bacteria, viruses, fungi, or parasites

f. Neoplastic disease

Patient Care that is compassionate, appropriate, and effective for the treatment of health problems and the promotion of health.

1. Recognize the early signs and symptoms and initiate therapy for the following:

a. Alterations of normal wound healing including infection and disruption

b. Fluid and hemodynamic derangements

c. Disorders of coagulation and hemostasis

d. Disorders of the immune system

e. Infectious diseases involving bacteria, viruses, fungi, or parasites

f. Neoplastic disease

2. Participate in deciding the appropriate surgical procedure for benign and malignant disease.

3. Monitor patients for possible postoperative complications and institute appropriate diagnostic studies and therapy for such conditions as:

    a. Wound infections

    b. Atelectasis/respiratory compromise

    c. Cardiac dysrhythmias/myocardial infarction

    d. Ileus

    e. Urinary retention

    f. Deep venous thrombosis/pulmonary embolus

    g. Systemic infection

4. Teach medical students and more junior residents about basic pathologic principles while on rounds and in the operating room.

Patient Care that is compassionate, appropriate, and effective for the treatment of health problems and the promotion of health.

1. Perform FNA, core, incisional, and excisional biopsies; and discuss the results and implications of each with the attending surgeon, the pathologist, and then the patient.

2. Review and discuss the details of a surgical pathology report with the attending surgeon.

3. Discuss intraoperative gross findings, and guide differential diagnosis formulation with the surgical pathologist and surgical team.

4. Review intraoperative frozen section and postoperative permanent section histology with the surgical pathologist and surgical team.

5. Participate in autopsies performed for deaths following acquired disease and trauma.

6. Participate in a multidisciplinary conference including surgeon, pathologist, radiologist, and oncologist by discussing pertinent patient history, operative findings, pathophysiology, and proposed treatment.

Practice-Based Learning and Improvement that involves investigation and evaluation of their own patient care, appraisal and assimilation of scientific evidence, and improvements in patient care.

INFORMATION TECHNOLOGY AND POPULATION COMPARISONS

REFERENCES

Cotran RS, Kumar V, Collins T, Robbins SL. Robbins SL. Robbins Pathologic Basis of Disease (6th ed). Philadelphia: WB Saunders Co., 1999;1-1425.

Abrams WB, Beers MH, Berkow R (eds). Organ systems. The Merck Manual of Geriatrics (2nd ed). Whitehouse Station, NJ: Merck Research Laboratories, Merck & Co., Inc., 1995;419-1350.

Rosenthal RA, Andersen DK. Physiologic considerations in the elderly surgical patient. In: Miller TA (ed), Modern Surgical Care: Physiologic Foundations and Clinical Applications (2nd ed). St. Louis: Quality Medical Publishing, Inc., 1998;1362-1384

SECTION 10.9 SURGICAL INFECTIONS

UNIT OBJECTIVES:

Demonstrate an understanding of the principles of infection, acquisition, diagnosis, and treatment.

Demonstrate an understanding of the typical presentation and treatment of common surgical infections.

Demonstrate an understanding of methods used to minimize infectious complications in surgical patients.

Demonstrate an understanding of techniques to minimize risk of viral infection spread, including hepatitis and HIV/AIDS.

Recognition of peritonitis and initiation of treatment.

Medical Knowledge about established and evolving biomedical, clinical, and cognate (e.g. epidemiological and social-behavioral) sciences and the application of this knowledge to patient care.

Section One: Mechanisms of Infection, Surgical Hazards, and Epidemiology

1.   Discuss the mechanisms of infection acquisition in surgical patients, to include: 1) mode of transmission, 2) patient risk factors, and 3) methods of prevention:

      a.   Community--acquired

      b.   Procedure--related

      c.   Nosocomial

2.   Explain the role of bacterial inoculum and virulence as well as local and systemic adjuvant factors that contribute to infection and abscess formation.

3.   Discuss how the host defenses of dissemination, inflammation, and loculation participate in the coordinated inflammatory response to infection and subsequent abscess formation.

4.   Demonstrate an understanding of and correct technique for hand washing as the single most important method for preventing infectious disease transmission.

5. Analyze the infectious disease risks to which patients and surgeons are exposed, considering the most common infections and the use of universal precautions to minimize disease transmission.

6. Understand the operating room wound classification system as it applies to infection rate surveillance.

7. Understand the role and purpose of hospital surveillance and/or infection control management groups.

8. Understand the impact of "surgeon-related" factors to surgical infections such as: length of operation, handling of tissues, electrocautery, choice of suture, hair clippings.

9. When elderly persons mount a "significant fever" of 38.5°C (101°F) or greater, severe life-threatening bacterial infection is oftentimes present. Summarize the factors involved in and frequency of occurrence of the following factors in the febrile elderly patient:

    a. Altered mental status   e. Respiratory rate

    b. Leukocytosis   f. Serum glucose

    c. Rapid change in functional status   g. Serum sodium

    d. Appetite

10. More than half of the occurrences of bacteremia in persons 65 and older are hospital acquired. Discuss the significance of the following organisms to elderly patients who, as a group, experience increased infection associated with morbidity and mortality:

    a. Gram-positive cocci (coagulase-negative staphylococci, Staphylococcus aureus, enterococci)

    b. Gram-negative bacilli (E. coli, Klebsiella species)

11. Explain the older adult's susceptibility to pneumonia, summarizing effects of the following factors:

    a. Age-related changes in pulmonary reserve (e.g., alterations in lung volumes, elasticity, and compliance ventilation)

    b. Diminished cough

    c. Airway collapse

    d. Comorbid conditions (interfering with gag reflexes and ciliary transport)

e.   Aspiration of oropharyngeal flora

f.   Hematogenous spread of microbes

Section Two: Surgical Infections

1.   Describe the mode of transmission, diagnosis, and treatment of typical infections seen in surgical patients, including:

     a.   Those common to all patients (pneumonia, urinary tract infections [UTI], skin infections)

     b.   Those uniquely cared for by surgeons (complex soft tissue, diabetic foot ulcers, postoperative abdominal abscesses, dehiscences)

2.   Suggest common sources of postoperative fever; outline a diagnostic approach and proposed plan of intervention.

3.   Differentiate between the following types of postoperative pneumonia, discussing patient risk factors, unique diagnostic clues, and treatment strategies:

     a.   Non-ventilatory-associated

     b.   Ventilatory-associated

     c.   Aspiration-acquired

4.   Demonstrate an understanding of intra-abdominal abscesses, paying particular attention to:

     a.   Etiology   c.   Surgical management

     b.   Bacterial participation   d.   Therapy failure

5.   Differentiate cellulitis, lymphangitis, lymphadenitis, and fasciitis from cutaneous abscess; describe the management of each.

6.   Discuss the pathophysiology, diagnosis, and treatment of necrotizing fasciitis with special attention to risk factors and physical examination findings.

7.   Outline the Advanced Trauma Life Support (ATLS) guidelines for tetanus prophylaxis; describe treatment principles for Clostridium tetani infection.

8.	Summarize characteristics of those fungal infections of surgical significance, differentiating between community-acquired, nosocomial, and opportunistic infections.

9.	Describe the RNA and DNA viruses of surgical significance, indicating their prevalence and modes of transmission.

10.	Outline the management strategies for the diagnosis and treatment of infected catheters, implantable devices, and surgical hardware.

Section Three: Use of Antibiotics in Surgery

1.	Summarize indications for prescribing prophylactic antibiotics associated with:

	a.	Clean procedures (hernia, vascular, thyroid)

	b.	Clean-contaminated procedures (GI, GU, Oropharyngeal)

	c.	Contaminated procedures

	d.	Implantable devices

		(1)	Vascular grafts

		(2)	Orthopedic hardware

		(3)	Soft tissue implants and synthetic reinforcements (breast, hernia)

2.	Analyze situations where prophylactic antibiotics are discouraged:

	a.	Burns

	b.	Post-splenectomized patient

	c.	Early aspiration

3.	Discuss the importance of timing and dosing for prophylactic antibiotic use; analyze antibiotic use in older patients, and analyze potentially adverse consequences of their use.

4.	Justify the empirical first-line approach to antibiotic use in the treatment of surgical infections and early intra-abdominal infection.

5.	Summarize the method by which microbiologic data are gathered, interpreted, and applied to altering antibiotic choice, dose, and duration.

6.	Discuss the mechanism of action, mechanism of resistance, applications, side effect profile, and costs of the following antimicrobials:

	a.	Penicillin and derivatives

b.	Cephalosporin	g.	Aztreonam
c.	Vancomycin	h.	Sulfonamides
d.	Erythromycin and derivatives	i.	Anti-fungal agents
e.	Metronidazole	j.	Aminoglycosides
f.	Quinolones	k.	Anti-virals

7. Demonstrate an understanding of the general pharmacology of antibiotics, pharmacologic changes that occur in the septic patient, and describe the effect of local environment on volume of distribution and protein binding.

8. Differential diagnosis of peritonitis, Anatomy of abdomen and pelvis
   Pathophysiology and treatment of intraperitoneal sepsis, generalized sepsis and septicemia shock
   Conditions which do not require surgery

Patient Care that is compassionate, appropriate, and effective for the treatment of health problems and the promotion of health.

1. Appropriately diagnose and treat common infections seen in surgical patients.
2. Make an appropriate and timely diagnosis for simple and complex infections in the postoperative patient; alter therapy as dictated by clinical, radiologic, and microbiologic response.
3. Competently diagnose and treat necrotizing fasciitis, and Clostridium perfringens infections.
4. Prepare patients for elective surgery by providing effective parenteral and enteral prophylactic antibiotics when indicated.
5. Coordinate the treatment of aggressive soft tissue infections to include:
   a. Early operative debridement and re-debridement as necessary
   b. Urinary and fecal diversion when necessary
   c. Antibiotic management
   d. Postoperative critical care, including fluid and nutrition management

6. Identify sources of implantable device infection; confirm diagnosis; and appropriately treat such infections.

7. Practice the effective use of universal precautions, including meticulous hand washing to minimize infection transmission risk from health care professional (HCP) to patient, and vice versa.

8. Contact the office of epidemiology, infection control, or the resident supervisor when breaches in techniques of universal precautions have been committed.

9. Work with members of the infectious disease specialty team in the management of complex surgical wounds.

10. Peritonitis

    a.   History and exam

    b.   Recognition of severity of illness

    c.   Investigation

    d.   Resuscitation including antibiotics, invasive monitoring

    e.   Treat symptoms

    f.   Timing of intervention

    g.   Recognition of success/failure of nonoperative treatment

11. Ability to perform emergency laparotomy

12. Recognition of management of complications

13. Laparotomy

14. Gastro/duodenum-perforated PU closure

Practice-Based Learning and Improvement that involves investigation and evaluation of their own patient care, appraisal and assimilation of scientific evidence, and improvements in patient care.

INFORMATION TECHNOLOGY AND POPULATION COMPARISONS REFERENCES

Berk SL. Infectious diseases. In: Cobbs EL, Duthie EH, Jr, Murphy JB (eds), Geriatrics Review Syllabus: A Core Curriculum in Geriatric Medicine (4th ed). Dubuque IA: Kendall/Hunt Publishing Company, 1999; 233-241.

Drebin JA, Mundy LM. Surgical wound infection. In: Cameron JL (ed), Current Surgical Therapy (6th ed). St. Louis: Mosby, 1998;1078-1082.

Dunn D. Infection. In: Greenfield LJ, Mulholland M, Oldham KT, Zelenock GB, Lillemoe KD (eds), Surgery: Scientific Principles and Practice (2nd ed). Philadelphia: Lippincott-Raven, 1997;159-182.

Durham RM, Mazuski JE. Surgical infection: principles of management and antibiotic usage. In: Miller TA (ed), Modern Surgical Care: Physiologic Foundations and Clinical Applications (2nd ed). St. Louis: Quality Medical Publishing, Inc., 1998;149-172.

Fry DE. Surgical infection. In: O'Leary JP (ed), The Physiologic Basis of Surgery (2nd ed). Baltimore: Williams and Wilkins, 1996;184-227.

Howard RJ. Surgical infections. In: Schwartz SI (ed), Principles of Surgery (6th ed). New York: McGraw-Hill, Inc., 1994:145-174.

Mandell GL, Douglas RG, Bennett JE. Mandell, Douglas and Bennett's Principles and Practices of Infectious Diseases (4th ed). New York: Churchill Livingstone, Inc., 1995.

Meakins JL (ed). Surgical Infections: Diagnosis and Treatment. New York: Scientific American, Inc., 1994.

Omann GM, Hinshaw DB. Inflammation. In: Greenfield LJ, Mulholland M, Oldham KT, Zelenock GB, Lillemoe KD (eds), Surgery: Scientific Principles and Practice (2nd ed). Philadelphia: Lippincott-Raven, 1997;130-158.

SECTION 10.10 SHOCK AND RESUSITATION

UNIT OBJECTIVES:

Demonstrate an understanding of the pathophysiology of shock, common surgical etiologies, and its categorizations.

Demonstrate an understanding of the mechanisms and pathophysiology of cardiopulmonary arrest.

Demonstrate the ability to manage the treatment of shock and cardiopulmonary arrest.

Medical Knowledge about established and evolving biomedical, clinical, and cognate (e.g. epidemiological and social-behavioral) sciences and the application of this knowledge to patient care.

1. Define shock, categorize it based upon type, explain the etiology and pathophysiology of each type of shock:
    a. Cardiogenic
    b. Hypovolemic
    c. Distributive (septic, anaphylactic, neurogenic, and adrenal insufficiency mediated)
    d. Obstructive (cardiac tamponade, tension pneumothorax, pulmonary embolus)

2. Summarize the clinical presentation and hemodynamic parameters associated with each type of shock using clinical terms, such as heart rate, respiratory rate, and blood pressure and filling pressures.

3. Propose an algorithm for diagnosing and initiating treatment for each shock type.
    a. Cardiogenic
    b. Hypovolemic
    c. Distributive (septic, anaphylactic, neurogenic, and adrenal insufficiency mediated)
    d. Obstructive (cardiac tamponade, tension pneumothorax, pulmonary embolus)

4.   Discuss the pathophysiology, including the mechanism of arrest, for each of the following situations:

   a.   Acute myocardial infarction

   b.   Acute dysrhythmia

   c.   Congestive heart failure

   d.   Hypovolemic shock (blood loss, dehydration)

   e.   Burns

   f.   Hemorrhagic shock (non-traumatic)

   g.   Septic shock

   h.   Anaphylactic shock (envenomation, drug related)

   i.   Acute adrenal insufficiency

   j.   Penetrating or blunt trauma

      (1) Tension pneumothorax

      (2) Pericardial tamponade

      (3) Hemorrhagic shock

   k.   Hypothermia

   l.   Substance abuse

   m.   Electrical injury

   n.   Suffocation

   o.   Acute stroke

5.   Explain the indications for and the pharmacokinetics of each of the following drugs:

   a.   Lidocaine   j.   Vasopressin

   b.   Digoxin   k.   Nitroglycerin

   c.   Metoprolol   l.   Amrinone

   d.   Diltiazem   m.   Milrinone

   e.   Pronestyl   n.   Levophed

   f.   Amiodarone   o.   Phenylephrine

   g.   Dopamine   p.   Epinephrine

   h.   Dobutamine

   i.   Adenosine (Adenocard®)

6.   Summarize the indication and appropriate technique for cardiac support, pressors, and Circulatory Assist Devices (IABP, LVAD, RVAD).

7.   Outline the signs and symptoms of acute airway obstruction and define the appropriate intervention in adult and pediatric patients.

8.   Outline the surgical house staff role on the "code team."

9.   Explain the physiological impact of mechanically assisted ventilation on the cardiovascular/respiratory system.

10.   Analyze methods for initiating and maintaining ventilator/ weaning support.

11.   Describe the indications and potential complications for the following surgical interventions:

    a.   Bag mask ventilation, endotracheal intubation (oral and nasal)

    b.   Cricothyrotomy

    c.   Thoracostomy tube

    d.   Central venous catheter

    e.   Peripheral vein cutdown

    f.   Arterial line

    g.   Pulmonary artery catheter

    h.   Diagnostic peritoneal lavage (DPL)

    i.   Resuscitative thoracotomy

    j.   Pericardiocentesis

    k.   Thoracentesis

    l.   Ultrasound

    m.   Wound exploration

12.   Review the importance of serial physical examinations, hemodynamic monitoring, and serial laboratory evaluations, including urine output and lactic acidosis, in assessing patient response to specific resuscitation treatment.

13.   Outline the clinical and laboratory indications for transfusion of the following blood products:

    a.   Packed red cells

b.   Fresh frozen plasma

c.   Platelets

d.   Cryoprecipitate

e.   Whole blood

f.   Specific clotting factor concentrates (VIII, IX, XII)

g.   Recombinant erythropoietin

14.   Analyze the potential complications from use of the above products.

15.   Older patients represent a special population, presenting key differences in emergency situations. Analyze and use examples to describe the significance of the following characteristics that are more frequent in the older patient:

a.   Vague, imprecise symptoms

b.   Atypical disease presentation

c.   Co-morbidity

d.   Polypharmacy (multiple organ specific physician's input)

e.   Possibility of cognitive impairment

f.   Diagnostic tests with different normal values (age adjustments for normal values)

g.   Likelihood of decreased functional reserve

h.   Inadequate social support systems

16.   Describe the role and indications (if any) for the following products in acute resuscitation:

a.   Recombinant activated Protein C

b.   Hespan and similar products

c.   Albumin

17.   Assess the indications, guidelines, and potential complications of the following cardiovascular drugs:

a.   Dopamine

a.   Dobutamine

b.   Phenylephrine

c.   Vasopressin

   d.   Epinephrine

   e.   Norepinephrine

   f.   Amrinone

   g.   Nitroglycerine

   h.   Esmolol

   i.   Nipride

   j.   Diltiazem

18.   Analyze and explain factors involved in blood pressure overestimation in the older patient (pseudohypertension, arteriosclerosis, arm size cuff discrepancies).

Patient Care that is compassionate, appropriate, and effective for the treatment of health problems and the promotion of health.

1.   Complete and pass Advanced Cardiac Life Support (ACLS), Advanced Trauma Life Support (ATLS), and Fundamentals of Critical Care Support (FCCS) training.

2.   Manage the unconscious patient (seizure).

3.   Serve on the code team and the trauma team.

4.   Recognize and manage airway obstruction.

5.   Perform endotracheal and nasotracheal intubation.

6.   Use disposable airway equipment, (e.g., bags, gloves) as transmissible infection precautions.

7.   Perform Cricothyrotomy and tracheostomy.

8.   Manage mechanical ventilator equipment.

9.   Manage flail chest (pneumothorax, hemothorax, obstructive shock states).

10.   Manage carbon monoxide poisoning.

11.   Diagnose cardiac arrest and rhythm disturbances

12.   Apply closed chest cardiac massage (CPR).

13.   Perform closed chest defibrillation.

14. Perform venous access procedures, including subclavian and jugular and femoral vein catheterizations and saphenous vein cutdown.

15. Determine the indication, dosage, contraindications, and method of administration of the following medications:

    a.   Morphine

    b.   Lidocaine and Procainamide

    c.   Propranolol

    d.   Atropine

    e.   Diltiazem

    f.   Epinephrine and norepinephrine

    g.   Dopamine and Dobutamine

    h.   Amrinone

    i.   Adenosine (Adenocard ®)

    j.   Cardiac glycosides

    k.   Nitroglycerin and nitroprusside

    l.   Furosemide, Mannitol, Bumex, Diamox

    m.   Sodium bicarbonate

    n.   Calcium

    o.   Amiodarone

    p.   Labetalol

16. Estimate volume requirements in acute trauma, burns, and hemorrhage; and institute replacement therapy.

17. Control external blood loss.

18. Perform pulmonary artery catheterization, including determining catheter position by pressure wave recording and electrocardiogram (EKG).

19. Manage cardiogenic and septic shock.

20. Use pneumatic antishock garments.

SECTION 10.11 SURGICAL IMMUNOLOGY

UNIT OBJECTIVES:

Demonstrate an understanding of general immunological principles and their application to surgical practice.

Demonstrate an understanding of the principles of care for patients with abnormal immune function who are undergoing general surgery procedures.

Demonstrate an understanding of the emerging field of molecular biology and the novel immune therapies having potential application to clinical surgery.

Medical Knowledge about established and evolving biomedical, clinical, and cognate (e.g. epidemiological and social-behavioral) sciences and the application of this knowledge to patient care.

Section One: General Immunologic Principles

1.   Describe the basic concepts of the human immune system, including:

   a.   Cells involved in host defense

   b.   Central roles of lymphocytes and macrophages

   c.   Their derivation from pluripotent stem cells

2.   Summarize the major activities of the macrophage, its products of secretion, and its role as the antigen-presenting cell (APC).

3.   Describe the ontogeny, function, and role in cellular immunity and graft rejection of the T-lymphocyte; demonstrate understanding of the T-cell receptor and its interaction with the human leukocyte antigen (HLA) complex.

4.   Summarize the events in T-cell activation, including the roles of CD4+ and CD8+ cells and the release of involved interleukins.

5.   Explain the development, differentiation, and function of B-lymphocytes in the formation of antibodies; outline and describe the functional anatomy of an immunoglobulin molecule.

6. Describe the immune functions of the spleen, liver, thymus, and bone marrow; summarize the impact of their manipulation on the immune system.

7. Describe immunological changes which occur in the elderly patient compared to a younger patient.

Section Two: Defenses against Infection

1. Describe the resident flora, mechanical barriers, local hormones, and chemicals of the epithelium in the following tracts involved in the body's defenses against infection:

    a. Gastrointestinal

    b. Respiratory

    c. Genitourinary

2. Describe the body's response to infection when:

    a. There has been no prior antigenic contact

    b. There has been prior contact

        (1) Passive and active immunization

        (2) T-cell memory activation

3. Explain the therapeutic and prophylactic roles of intravenous immunoglobulin and viral vaccines.

4. Distinguish between several known congenital and acquired immunodeficiency states, including sepsis and severe burns.

5. Describe tests of cellular immune integrity, including skin and laboratory tests of lymphocyte function.

Section Three: Clinical Immunology

1. Describe the mechanism of action and potential side effects of current immunosuppressive agents; state the rationale for their use and timing in transplantation and in other medical applications:

    a. Prednisone

    b. Cyclosporine

    c.   Azathioprine

    d.   Tacrolimus (FK5O6)

    e.   Mycophenolatemofetil (RS6144)

    f.   Monoclonal antibody (Moab) use for induction

2.   Differentiate between agents used to treat acute transplant rejection:

    a.   Steroids

    b.   Radiation therapy

    c.   Poly- and mono- clonal antibodies

3.   Summarize the role and preparation of monoclonal antibodies in the treatment of neoplastic lesions. Describe their application to clinical pathology and diagnostic and therapeutic oncology. Describe side effects and their treatment.

4.   Explain the preparation, quality control, and application of polyclonal antibodies. Describe side effects and their treatment.

5.   Outline an approach to the management of infection in immunocompromised patients resulting from:

    a.   Iatrogenic immunosuppression secondary to drugs

    b.   Natural immune deficiency states

    c.   Impaired immunity secondary to cancer

6.   Formulate a plan for management of immunosuppression in patients with severe surgical morbidity or complications.

Section Four: Trends in Immunology and Molecular Biology

1.   Recognize new and investigational immunosuppressive drugs used for non-transplant medical conditions.

2.   Summarize the current rationale and clinical status of novel oncologic treatments using biologic modifiers and immunomodulation; analyze their potential limitations and side effects.

3.   Explain the manipulation of gene transplantation and describe several clinical applications currently being investigated.

4.   Discuss the growing importance of molecular biology and the basic techniques of recombinant DNA technology to investigate problems in immunology, oncology, and pathology.

5.   Explain the significance of transgenic animals, their creation, and potential application to experimental and clinical transplantation.

Patient Care that is compassionate, appropriate, and effective for the treatment of health problems and the promotion of health.

1.   Participate in the perioperative management of immunosuppressive agents in chronically-medicated patients undergoing general surgery.

2.   Plan and perform elective surgery in immunosuppressed patients with attention to minimizing infectious risks; perform emergent surgical intervention (treatment of perforated viscous) in similar high-risk patients.

3.   Optimize patients' immune state secondary to systemic compromise following major surgery, burns, trauma, and malnutrition.

4.   Recognize and treat wound infections and other complex disorders in chronically immunosuppressed patients undergoing elective and emergent surgery.

5.   Monitor drug levels and side effects in immunosuppressants.

6.   Participate in the care of patients receiving immunostimulatory medications (e.g., IV immunoglobulin [IVIG], granulocyte stimulating factor).

7.   Describe differences in survival rate which occur in elderly patients compared to younger patients. Consider the following factors:

   a.   Differences in work-ups that occur in elderly patients.

   b.   Complications in elderly versus younger patients

SECTION 10.12. GERIATRIC SURGERY

UNIT OBJECTIVES:

Be prepared to manage or co-manage the health care needs of prospective surgical geriatric patients.

Medical Knowledge about established and evolving biomedical, clinical, and cognate (e.g. epidemiological and social-behavioral) sciences and the application of this knowledge to patient care.

I. PRINCIPLES OF NORMAL AGING

The resident will acquire a working knowledge of general principles of aging while recognizing the considerable heterogeneity of patients age 65 and older.

The general principles will include the study of:

1.   Demography of aging

2.   Biology of aging relative to age-related physiologic changes

3.   Preventive geriatrics: health maintenance

The resident will be prepared to recognize, interpret, and manage the principal elements in the Psychology of aging that present as the patient's psychologic status, cultural value system, and personally-preferred lifestyle.

Elements of the Psychology of aging will include applying principles of:

1.   Neuropsychiatric aging: brain-behavior relationships (dementia, acute delirium/changes in mental states)

2.   Hypothalamic function and regulation of body temperature

The resident will be prepared to identify age-related physiologic changes and apply that knowledge during surgical counseling and decision-making.

Age-related physiologic changes will encompass:

1. Aging relative to tissues, organ systems, immune functions, and nutritional needs

2. Endocrine and metabolic alterations (e.g., carbohydrate and insulin metabolism)

3. Changes in laboratory values (e.g., expected changes in normal blood chemistries)

PATHOPHYSIOLOGY IN THE ELDERLY PATIENT

The resident will develop clinical management strategies, considering the unique aspects of geriatric pathophysiology.

Knowledge of disease processes will include the study of:

1. Mortality: leading causes of death for those 65 and older

2. Morbidity: leading causes of disability

3. Factors affecting altered disease presentation

4. Comorbidity: chronic diseases superimposed on acute disease

5. Geriatric syndromes (dementia, failure to thrive, fractures, malnutrition, sleep problems)

The resident will be prepared to analyze and apply information about medication to principles of age-related pharmacokinetics, pharmacodynamics, and adverse drug reactions.

Physiologic and Psychosocial implications will build upon a working knowledge of:

1. Changes in drug metabolism and excretion

2. Adjustment of doses and age-specific side effects

3. Use of psychotropic agents and pain medications

4. Identification of possible adverse drug-drug interactions

5. Significance of financial problems imposed by polypharmacy

III. PREOPERATIVE ASSESSMENT OF THE ELDERLY PATIENT

The resident will modify his/her approach to evaluation and diagnosis in a manner that is effective, efficient, and in accord with the special needs and limitations of the geriatric individual.

Factors to consider will include:

1. Developing attitudes toward and communicating with the elderly; age bias

2. Establishing lines of communication with health care team: personal physician/geriatrician, social worker

The resident will be prepared to obtain and utilize patient data for decision making prior to surgery.

Full geriatric assessment of patient baseline data will include consideration of:

1. Functional capabilities: activities of daily living, mental and physiologic health

2. Psychosocial variables: ethnic factors, cultural mores, social supports, and community relations

3. Differences in health care preferences according to perspectives of patient, referring physician, and surgeon

4. Considering risks to desired surgical outcomes: comorbidity, frailty, and social supports

The resident will be prepared to implement interventions that minimize legal and ethical risks to the patient's individual rights and liberties.

Interventions will require consideration of the following factors:

1. Weighing aggressive approach with patient's right to autonomy: legal right to self-determination and perceptions of quality of life

2. Rights regarding competence and advance directives: informed consent, surrogate decision making, long-term care, extent of care, living wills, and decisions about death

3. Cost: benefit ratio determination

IV. OPERATIVE MANAGEMENT OF THE ELDERLY PATIENT

The resident will monitor and act upon coexisting requirements of care to maintain patient stability.

Monitoring of patient surgical needs will include:

1.   Planning and supporting the selection and management of local, regional, and general anesthetics

2.   Managing conscious sedation

3.   Maintaining body temperature and metabolic homeostasis during surgery

4.   Following Halsted's Principles during surgical intervention

V. PERIOPERATIVE CARE OF THE ELDERLY PATIENT

The resident will determine and act upon the continuing needs of the surgical patient based upon patient communication and interaction, use of patient data, and analysis of surgical outcome. Perioperative decisions will require:

1.   Management of complications such as sepsis, cardiac problems, diabetes, pulmonary and renal failure.

2.   Determining need for prophylaxis for common complications like DVT and PE, aspiration pneumonia

3.   Sustaining patient with homeostasis, fluid management, ventilator support, wound and antibiotic management

4.   Determining management for deconditioning, use of Foley catheters and NG tubes, use of invasive monitoring

5.   Management of directive care issues such as life sustaining mechanisms: supportive care, extent of care issues

VI. LONG-TERM RECOVERY/REHABILITATION OF THE ELDERLY PATIENT

The resident will be prepared to utilize information and resources to maximize positive outcomes.

Data and resource utilization will include application of rehabilitation principles:

1.   Optimizing patient health and maintaining function

2.   Communicating with the patient and family regarding quality of life issues

3.   Directing long-term recovery and rehabilitation for home, community, and/or institutional settings

4.   Applying non-institutional support systems and institutional services for patient and family

VII. FINANCING, UTILIZATION, AND REIMBURSEMENT ISSUES

The resident will be prepared to analyze the continuum of care available to that patient, considering the complex factors inherent to implementation when matching health services to individual needs and resources.

The consideration of factors related to health services will include an analysis of:

1.   Elderly patient rights to benefits: age-based and needs-based services and entitlements

2.   Delivery of health services available to the patient and his/her family

3.   Cost:benefit ratio determination; economic impact of operative procedure

4.   Implications of long-term care: the recovery period, quality of life

Patient Care that is compassionate, appropriate, and effective for the treatment of health problems and the promotion of health.

VIII. PATIENT OUTCOMES

The resident will analyze and utilize his/her surgical data in systematic fashion.

Analysis and utilization of surgical data will include:

1.   Selecting, maintaining, and analyzing a patient outcome database

2.   Comparing patient outcomes with local medical community and national standards

3.   Initiating improvements in patient care based on patient outcome data

SECTION 10.13 MANAGEMENT OF AMBULATORY SURGERY

UNIT OBJECTIVES:

Demonstrate knowledge of the principles and rationale for performing ambulatory surgical procedures where ambulatory surgery is defined as any procedure for which the patient is admitted and discharged on the same day, regardless of type of anesthesia.

Demonstrate the ability to manage surgical conditions in an ambulatory setting.

Medical Knowledge about established and evolving biomedical, clinical, and cognate (e.g. epidemiological and social-behavioral) sciences and the application of this knowledge to patient care.

1.   Discuss the principles and rationale for performing ambulatory surgery on selected patients, including:
   a.   Assessment of patient risk
   b.   Patient selection
   c.   Level of preparation for patients with co-morbid diseases

2.   List those general surgical procedures commonly performed in an ambulatory setting in your community.

3.   Discuss the social and economic issues associated with selecting an ambulatory surgery option.

4.   Describe the anesthesia options available for ambulatory surgery and their possible complications to include:
   a.   Discussion of types of anesthetic
   b.   Delineation of duration of typical local anesthetic action and limitations
   c.   Calculation of dosages, including maximum dosage of typical local anesthetics
   d.   Discussion of techniques of local anesthetics, both field and nerve block
   e.   Consideration of possible adverse reactions
   f.   Outlining of benefits and risks of pharmacologic sedation

5. Analyze the importance of postoperative pain management in the ambulatory setting.

6. Differentiate between intraoperative issues in awake versus anesthetized patients in terms of:

    a. Patient's physical and emotional comfort

        (1) Positioning of patient

        (2) Patient's physical exposure

        (3) Tissue handling

    b. Intraoperative communication with the patient

        (1) Aspects of procedure

        (2) Provide distraction from awareness of procedure via "small talk" or some other means

    c. The need to maintain a sensitive and professional level of communication with other health care workers

7. Discuss postoperative follow-up procedures, including methods for monitoring and managing complications.

8. Outline community resources available to assist ambulatory surgery patients, and describe the methods for accessing these resources.

9. Describe appropriate methods for handling pathology specimens for typical outpatient procedures.

Patient Care that is compassionate, appropriate, and effective for the treatment of health problems and the promotion of health.

1. Complete a preoperative evaluation of a patient as a potential candidate for ambulatory surgery, including consideration of patient risks and treatment options.

2. Counsel patients and their families appropriately about ambulatory surgery and follow-up care, including obtaining informed consent after discussing the risks, benefits, and alternatives to the procedure.

3. Preoperatively prepare a patient with co-morbid diseases for ambulatory surgery.

4. Perform procedures while assuring patient comfort:

    a. Provide adequate local anesthesia and/or adequate sedation

    b. Prevent potentially negative visual and auditory stimuli

    c. Communicate with the patient intraoperatively in a calm and reassuring manner:

        (1) Alert patient to new aspects of the procedure

        (2) Communicate results of the procedure to the patient

        (3) Respond sensitively to patient's concerns regarding level of pain, embarrassment, and procedure's results

5. Maintain a positive, calm, reassuring, and professional atmosphere in the operating room.

6. Perform selected ambulatory surgical procedures such as:

    a. Excision of skin and soft tissue lesions

    b. Breast biopsy

    c. Lymph node biopsy

    d. Vascular access procedures

    e. Incising and draining (I & D) abscesses

    f. Endoscopic procedures

    g. Hernia repairs

    h. Anorectal surgery

    i. Laparoscopic cholecystectomy

7. Arrange for appropriate handling of pathological specimens.

8. Manage unexpected emergencies during the course of ambulatory surgery, such as:

    a. Hemorrhage   d. Chest pain

    b. Anaphylactic shock   e. Pneumothorax

    c. Drug reaction

9. Perform appropriate postoperative examination prior to discharge.

10. Manage postoperative surgery and anesthesia complications.

11. Prescribe necessary follow-up care, including:

a.   Prescribing appropriate postoperative analgesia

b.   Communicating instructions and expectations for follow-up, such as:

    (1)   Pain level and location

    (2)   Possible side effects of medications

    (3)   Level of activity and return to work

    (4)   Wound care and potential problems

    (5)   Timing of follow-up appointment

c.   Arrange for home health and other outpatient services using institutional and community resources

Patient Care that is compassionate, appropriate, and effective for the treatment of health problems and the promotion of health.

Attitudes:

1.   Recognize the concerns of patients and family regarding ambulatory surgery and outpatient follow-up care.

2.   Become attuned to patient's concerns and needs:

a.   Preoperatively

b.   Intraoperatively

c.   Postoperatively

SECTION 10.14. OUTPATIENT SURGERY

UNIT OBJECTIVES:

Maintain continuity in terms of care of the patient with surgical diseases from pre-hospital evaluation through post-surgical management and follow-up.

Develop and hone skills in history taking, physical examination, interpersonal communication, critical appraisal, and self-directed learning.

Medical Knowledge about established and evolving biomedical, clinical, and cognate (e.g. epidemiological and social-behavioral) sciences and the application of this knowledge to patient care.

1.   Delineate the components of and discuss the importance of a focused history and physical examination performed in an outpatient setting on a patient with a surgical disease.

2.   Identify indications for, technical aspects of, and typical results from the following screening tests:

    a.   Stool guaiac   c.   Prostate screening

    b.   Sigmoidoscopy   d.   Mammography

3.   Demonstrate a working knowledge of the natural history of surgical diseases:

    a.   If untreated

    b.   If treated surgically

    c.   If treated non-surgically

4.   Distinguish between different types of biopsy techniques in an outpatient setting.

5.   Specify indications for such common office procedures as:

    a.   Core-needle biopsy/fine-needle aspiration

    b.   Incision and drainage of abscesses (recognize those requiring in-hospital operating room drainage)

    c.   Sigmoidoscopy/anoscopy

    d.   Excision of cutaneous lesions

6. Delineate hospital mechanisms for admitting patients.

7. Estimate costs of hospitalization and various surgeries.

8. Describe the expected appearance of wound sites at various postoperative intervals.

9. Delineate appropriate pain medications and dosages.

10. Specify the need for drains and tubes, stating the types and special requirements for replacement or removal.

Patient Care that is compassionate, appropriate, and effective for the treatment of health problems and the promotion of health.

1. Demonstrate the ability to obtain the essential elements of a focused preoperative history, including assessment of medications.

2. Perform a complete physical examination, paying special attention to assessment of cardiopulmonary risk of surgery.

3. Order appropriate and cost-effective laboratory tests for screening and pre- and post-operative evaluation.

4. Accurately interpret clinical laboratory results, pathology reports, and radiographic studies.

5. Synthesize historical findings, physical examination, and laboratory data for diagnosis.

6. Develop appropriate plans for management.

7. Order appropriate consultations.

8. Appropriately and sensitively counsel the patient and patient's family regarding:

    a. Disease entity (prognosis, treatment options, additional treatment)

    b. Surgical issues

        (1) Operative risks (possible complications, including mortality)

        (2) Operative procedures (preparation, testing, duration of surgery and hospitalization)

        (3) Anesthesia

        (4) Prognosis (curative vs. palliative)

    c. Other treatment options (no treatment [explain natural history of disease] and non-surgical therapy)

      d.   Informed consent

      e.   Community resources

9.   Perform appropriate office procedures.

10.   Arrange patient admission to hospital facility.

11.   Explain the prospective surgical approach to the patient.

12.   Postoperatively, obtain appropriate follow-up history, including:

      a.   General well-being

      b.   Pain control

      c.   Presence of fever

      d.   Nutritional state (ability to eat, nausea)

      e.   Bowel function

      f.   Level of activity

      g.   Compliance with instructions (medications, complications of medication, physical therapy)

13.   Perform appropriate postoperative examination of the surgical site.

14.   Provide appropriate wound care. Identify and manage wound problems, including:

      a.   Superficial wound separation; abdominal dehiscence

      b.   Vascular surgery incisions and wounds (diabetic foot problems and their impact)

      c.   Seromas

      d.   Infections (cellulitis or abscess, determining the need for antibiotics, drainage, office vs. operating room care)

      e.   Lymphoceles

      f.   Incisional hernia

      g.   Foreign body reaction (to sutures, staples)

15.   Ascertain the need for further consultative support, and arrange for patient referral when indicated.

16.   Assess the need for further follow-up, including:

      a.   Arrangement for home nursing evaluation and care

b. Assessment/arrangement for other support (e.g., the homemaker)

c. Prescribing appropriate dietary supplements

d. Hospice care

17. Prescribe appropriate pain medication.

18. Assess patient's ability to maintain level of activity (drive motor vehicle, work, exercise, sexual activity)

19. Appropriately and sensitively communicate with patient and family.

20. Appropriately communicate with referring physicians in a timely fashion regarding patient outcome.

21. Develop the ability to teach in office settings (for nurses, patients, medical students, and junior house officers).

Patient Care that is compassionate, appropriate, and effective for the treatment of health problems and the promotion of health.

ATTITUDINAL OBJECTIVES:

1. Have a working understanding of the role of the surgeon as primary care giver in office and clinical settings.

2. Demonstrate professionalism, empathy, and compassion by showing respect for a patient's privacy and self-esteem during aspects of the physical examination which may be uncomfortable, frightening, or embarrassing for the patient.

3. Demonstrate an awareness of, and respect for, patient autonomy, especially regarding:

a. Decisions about therapy

b. Decisions not to treat

c. Issues of patient compliance

4. Show an awareness of, and respect for, the contributions of other office staff members (nurses, technicians, secretaries).

5. Demonstrate a respect for medical students in office and/or clinic settings.

6. Recognize patient or patient family responsibilities that may affect the timing of surgery.

7. Demonstrate an understanding of, and sensitivity to, patient socioeconomic concerns regarding such issues as:

    a. Insurance and the ability to pay for physician services, hospitalization, and prescribed medications

    b. Possible loss of work time and wages

8. Demonstrate sensitivity and appropriate flexibility regarding patient fears and concerns, including:

    a. Preoperatively

        (1) Anxiety about pain and procedure's findings

        (2) Embarrassment

    b. Intraoperatively

        (1) Pain and individual response to pain

        (2) Modesty

        (3) Comfort

    c. Postoperatively

        (1) Ability to care for self   (3) Level of function

        (2) Drugs   (4) Prognosis

9. Display a working knowledge of the management of the office and the outpatient surgical setting.

Practice-Based Learning and Improvement that involves investigation and evaluation of their own patient care, appraisal and assimilation of scientific evidence, and improvements in patient care.

INFORMATION TECHNOLOGY AND POPULATION COMPARISONS
REFERENCES:

Abrams WB, Beers MH, Berkow R. History and physical examination. Comprehensive geriatric assessment. Establishing therapeutic objectives: quality of life issues. Surgery: preoperative evaluation and intraoperative and postoperative care. In: Abrams WB, Beers MH, Berkow R (eds), The Merck Manual of Geriatrics (2nd ed). Whitehouse Station, NJ: Merck Research Laboratories, Merck & Co., Inc., 1995;205-224; 224-235; 235-238; 321-345.

Annas GJ. Informed consent, cancer, and truth in prognosis. N Engl J Med 1994;330:223-225.

Cobbs EL, Duthie EH, Jr, Murphy JB (eds), Geriatrics Review Syllabus: A Core Curriculum in Geriatric Medicine (4th ed). Dubuque IA: Kendall/Hunt Publishing Company, 1999.

Dunkle RE, Lynch S. Social work: more of the same or something new? In: Seltzer MM (ed), The Impact of Increased Life Expectancy: Beyond the Gray Horizon, New York, NY: Springer Publishing Company; 1995:131-147.

Friedsam HJ. Long-term care in the very long term. In: Seltzer MM (ed), The Impact of Increased Life Expectancy: Beyond the Gray Horizon, New York, NY: Springer Publishing Company; 1995:165-188.

Howard RJ. Finding the cause of postoperative fever. Postgrad Med J 1989;85:223-238.

Laine C, Davidoff F. Patient-centered medicine. A professional evolution. JAMA 1996;275:152-156.

Macpherson DS, Snow R, Lofgren RP. Preoperative screening: value of previous tests. Ann Int Med 1990;113:969-973.

Moore AA, Siu AL. Screening for common problems in ambulatory elderly: clinical confirmation of a screening instrument. Am J Med 1996;100:438.

Narr BJ, Hansen TR, Warner MA. Preoperative laboratory screening in healthy Mayo patients: cost-effective elimination of tests and unchanged outcomes. Mayo Clin Proc 1991;66:155-159.

Powers JS, Billings FT, Jr. Management of perioperative problems in the aged. In: Adkins RB, Jr., Scott HW, Jr. (eds), Surgical Care for the Elderly (2nd ed). Philadelphia: Lippincott-Raven Publishers, 1998;33-50.

Williams GC, Deci EL. The importance of supporting autonomy in medical education. Ann Intern Med 1998;129:303-308.

Woodard LJ, Pamies RJ. The disclosure of the diagnosis of cancer. Primary Care 1992;19:657-663.

SECTION 10.15 BASIC SURGICAL SKILLS

UNIT OBJECTIVES

Acquisition of basic surgical skills in instrument and tissue handling.

Incision of skin and subcutaneous tissue: Ability to incise superficial tissues accurately with suitable instruments.

Closure of skin and subcutaneous tissue: Ability to close superficial tissues accurately.

Knot tying: Ability to tie secure knots.

Hemostasis: Ability to achieve hemostasis of superficial vessels.

Tissue retraction: Use of suitable methods of retraction.

Use of drains: Knowledge of when to use a drain and which to choose.

Tissue handling: Ability to handle tissues gently with appropriate instruments.

Skill as assistant: Ability to assist helpfully, even when the operation is not familiar.

Ability to assess the patient and manage the patient, and propose surgical or non-surgical management through:

Ability to assess the acute abdomen, resuscitate the patient and judge whether immediate operation is necessary.

Ability to manage patient care in the perioperative period.

Medical Knowledge about established and evolving biomedical, clinical, and cognate (e.g. epidemiological and social-behavioral) sciences and the application of this knowledge to patient care.

1.   Incision of skin and subcutaneous tissue:

    a.   Langer's lines

    b.   Healing mechanism

    c.   Choice of instrument

    d.   Safe practice

2.   Closure of skin and subcutaneous tissue: Options for closure

    a.   Suture and needle choice

    b.   Safe practice

      c.   Knot tying:

      d.   Choice of material

      e.   Hemostasis:

      f.   Techniques

      g.   Tissue retraction:

      h.   Choice of instruments

      i.   Use of drains:

           (1)   Indications

           (2)   Types

           (3)   Management/removal

      j.   Tissue handling:

      k.   Choice of instruments

3.   Abdominal anatomy

      a.   Etiology

      b.   Pathophysiology of shock

      c.   Pathophysiology of peritonitis and sepsis

      d.   Differential diagnosis

4.   Preoperative

      a.   Interview

      b.   Investigate

      c.   Assess

      d.   Report

5.   Preoperative assessment and management: Ability to assess the patient adequately prior to operation and manage any preoperative problems appropriately.

6.   Intraoperative care: Ability to conduct safe surgery in the operating theatre environment.

7.   Postoperative care: Ability to care for the patient in the postoperative period.

8.   Blood Products: Appropriate use of blood products.

9.   Antibiotics: Appropriate use of antibiotics.

10. Preoperative assessment and management

    a. Cardiorespiratory physiology

    b. Diabetes mellitus

    c. Renal failure

    d. Pathophysiology of blood loss

11. Pathophysiology of sepsis

    Risk factors for surgery and scoring systems

12. Principles of day surgery

Patient Care that is compassionate, appropriate, and effective for the treatment of health problems and the promotion of health.

1. Incision of skin and subcutaneous tissue:

    a. Ability to use scalpel, diathermy and scissors

    b. Closure of skin and subcutaneous tissue:

    c. Accurate and tension free apposition of wound edges

    d. Knot tying:

        (1) Single handed

        (2) Double handed

        (3) Instrument

            a. Superficial

            b. Deep

2. Hemostasis:

    a. Control of bleeding vessel (superficial)

    b. Diathermy

    c. Suture ligation

    d. Tie ligation

    e. Clip application

3.   Tissue retraction:

    a.   Tissue forceps

    b.   Placement of wound retractors

4.   Use of drains:

    a.   Insertion

    b.   Fixation

    c.   Removal

5.   Tissue handling:

Appropriate application of instruments and respect for tissues

6.   Skill as assistant:

Anticipation of needs of surgeon when assisting

7.   Central line insertion

8.   Recognition of indication for surgery

9.   Ability to perform emergency laparotomy/laparoscopy

10.   Preoperative assessment and management:

    a.   History and examination

    b.   Interpretation of preop investigations

    c.   Management of comorbidity

    d.   Resuscitation

11.   Skill acquisition

    a.   Surgical history and examination (elective and emergency)

    b.   Construct a differential diagnosis

    c.   Plan investigations

    d.   Clinical decision making

12.   Taking consent for intermediate level intervention; emergency and elective

    a.   Written clinical communication skills

    b.   Interactive clinical communication skills: Patient's

      c.   Interactive clinical communication skills: colleagues

13.   Intraoperative care:

      a.   Diathermy, laser use

      b.   Tourniquets

      c.   Principles of local anesthesia

14.   Postoperative care:

      a.   Cardiorespiratory physiology

      b.   Diabetes mellitus

      c.   Renal failure

      d.   Pathophysiology of blood loss

      e.   Pathophysiology of sepsis

      f.   Complications specific to particular operation

15.   Blood Products:

      a.   Components of blood

      b.   Alternatives to use of blood product

16.   Antibiotics:

      a.   Common pathogens in surgical patients

      b.   Antibiotic sensitivities

      c.   Antibiotic side-effects

      d.   Principles of prophylaxis and treatment

17.   Postoperative care:

    Assessment of patient's condition

18.   Postoperative analgesia

      a.   Fluid and electrolyte management

      b.   Monitoring of postoperative patient

      c.   Detection of impending organ failure

d.   Initial management of organ failure

e.   Use of MDT meetings

Practice-Based Learning and Improvement that involves investigation and evaluation of their own patient care, appraisal and assimilation of scientific evidence, and improvements in patient care

1.   Safety in theatre

     a.   Sharps safety

     b.   Radiation use and risks

2.   Infection risks

3.   SIS and Trape Study applications

4.   Clinical Scholar

     a.   Pose a clinical question

     b.   Recognize and identify gaps in knowledge and expertise around a clinical question

     c.   Formulate a plan to fill the gap:

          (1)   Conduct an appropriate literature search based upon a clinical question

          (2)   Assimilate and appraise the literature

          (3)   Develop a system to store and retrieve relevant literature

          (4)   Consult others (physicians and other healthcare professionals) in a collegiate manner

          (5)   Propose a solution to the clinical question

          (6)   Implement the solution in practice. Evaluate the outcome and reassess the solution (re-enter the loop at c-i or c-ii)

          (7)   Identify practice areas for research

SECTION 10.16 SURGICAL GENETICS

UNIT OBJECTIVES

Basic understanding of genetically determined diseases.

Endocrine: Basic understanding of the influence of genetics on endocrine disease.

Colorectal: Basic understanding of the influence of genetics on colorectal cancer development.

Breast: Basic understanding of the influence of genetics of breast cancer development.

Upper GI/HPB: Basic understanding of the influence of genetics in upper GI disease.

Clinical and molecular genetics: Basic understanding of the principles of genetics.

Medical Knowledge about established and evolving biomedical, clinical, and cognate (e.g. epidemiological and social-behavioral) sciences and the application of this knowledge to patient care.

1.   Endocrine:

Principal genetically influenced endocrine diseases and syndromes, MEN I, MEN II, Thyroid, Parathyroid, Pancreas and adrenal

2.   Colorectal:

Outline knowledge of genetic changes which predispose to colorectal cancer including familial adenomatous polyposis, HNPCC and other polyposis syndromes

3.   Breast:

Outline knowledge of genetic changes which predispose to breast cancer; BRCA1, BRCA2, P53

4.   Upper GI/HPB:

Describe the principal of genetically influenced upper gastrointestinal diseases and syndromes, including Duodenal polyposis, familial gastric cancer, Peutz-Jeger syndrome and polycystic disease of the liver

5.   Clinical and molecular genetics:
       a.   Modes of inheritance
       b.   Genetic Testing
       c.   Screening
       d.   Prophylactic intervention
       e.   Therapeutic intervention
       f.   Ethics

Patient Care that is compassionate, appropriate, and effective for the treatment of health problems and the promotion of health.

1.   Patient and family education
2.   Screening testing

Practice-Based Learning and Improvement that involves investigation and evaluation of their own patient care, appraisal and assimilation of scientific evidence, and improvements in patient care

1.   Review of Evidenced Medicine for focused genetic therapy
2.   Understanding of the current state of gene therapy

CHAPTER 11

SPECIALTY BASED

SECTION 11.1 SURGICAL CRITICAL CARE

UNIT OBJECTIVES:

Demonstrate knowledge of the principles associated with the diagnosis and management of critically ill patients, including knowledge of simple and complex multiple organ system normalities and abnormalities.

Demonstrate the ability to appropriately diagnose and treat patients with interrelated system disorders in the intensive care unit.

Diagnosis of gas gangrene and other necrotizing infections

Medical Knowledge about established and evolving biomedical, clinical, and cognate (e.g. epidemiological and social-behavioral) sciences and the application of this knowledge to patient care.

Junior Level:

Complete the coursework and testing to obtain Basic and Advanced Cardiac Life Support (BCLS and ACLS) and Fundamental Critical Care Support (FCCS) and Advanced Trauma Life Support (ATLS) certification.

Section One: Administration

1.   Define and describe the role of the surgeon in the critical care setting to include these aspects:

      a.   Unit administration/management (surgeon as unit director)

           (1)   Triage of patients

           (2)   Economic concerns

           (3)   Data collection and computer usage

           (4)   Infection control and total quality management (TQM) issues

           (5)   Ethical concerns (consent, durable power of attorney, living wills)

           (6)   Local laws for referral to Medical Examiner

           (7)   Management/consultation for specific surgical conditions

> (8)   Coordination of multidisciplinary consultants relating and interpreting information between non-surgical consultants

2. Identify and outline criteria for admitting patients to the intensive care unit (ICU) to include:

    a.   Medical indications (related to specific diseases, e.g., pulmonary, cardiac, renal)

    b.   Surgical indications directly related to specific surgical illness

3. Identify and outline criteria for discharging patients from the ICU, to include:

    a.   Medical indications

    b.   Surgical indications

    c.   Patients unacceptable for ICU (e.g., futile care, do not resuscitate [DNR] orders)

4. Identify and explain the considerations surgeons must make when working with consultants in managing critical care situations.

5. Identify potential Organ, Tissue Donor candidates, as well as the hospital specific procedure for contacting families for potential donation.

Section Two: General Pathophysiology--Body as a Whole

1. Describe the normal physiologic response to a variety of insults such as sepsis, trauma, or surgery by associating the adaptation of the following systems from their pre-stress to post-stress states:

    a.   Respiratory   d.   Metabolic

    b.   Hemodynamic e.   e.   Endocrine

    c.   Renal

2. Describe the concept of the Systemic Inflammatory Response Syndrome (SIRS).

3. Describe prophylactic measures routinely used in critical care such as:

    a.   Gastrointestinal (GI) bleeding prophylaxis, including neutralizing, inhibitory compounds, and surface agents

b. Prophylactic antibiotics (demonstrate differences between true prophylaxis, empiric and therapeutic uses)

c. Pulmonary morbidity prophylaxis (incentive spirometry)

d. Prophylaxis against venous thromboembolic events

e. Aseptic technique

f. Universal precautions

g. Skin care protocols

h. Guide wire catheter changes for work-up of fever or change in clinical status

4. Discuss the pharmacotherapeutics of drugs used for support and treatment of the critically ill patient with emphasis on:

a. Mode of action,

b. Physiologic effects,

c. Spectrum of effects,

d. Duration of action,

e. Appropriate doses,

f. Means of metabolism or excretion,

g. Complications,

h. Cost:

i. The classes of drugs should include:

    (1) Vasopressors

    (2) Vasodilators

    (3) Inotropic agents

    (4) Bronchodilators

    (5) Diuretics

    (6) Antibiotics/antifungal agents

        a. Distinguish between empiric, therapeutic, and prophylactic

        b. Demonstrate knowledge of classes of anti-infectives

j. Antidysrhythmics

k. Antihypertensives :Predict applicability of different classes in a particular situation:

(1)   Use of beta blockers in hypertensive tachycardic patient

(2)   Use of ace inhibitors in hypertensive patient with congestive heart failure

(3)   Use of calcium channel blockers in hypertensive patient with angina

5.   Outline the indications and methods for providing nutritional support by completing the following activities:

     a.   Discuss indications, selection of formulations, cost, route of administration of parenteral versus enteral forms of nutrition

     b.   Explain complications of parenteral and enteral routes of feeding as well as select methods to avoid the complications

     c.   Interpret findings associated with abnormalities in levels of glucose, chloride, sodium, phosphate, magnesium, trace metals/elements, and vitamins in the critically-ill patient receiving enteral or parenteral feedings; prepare recommendations for elderly patients under these same conditions

     d.   Estimate protein calorie requirements for patients of varying degrees of illness, and be able to analyze adequacy of nutritional support using commonly obtainable laboratory values

6.   Outline the principles of postoperative fever with respect to causes, empiric diagnostic modalities, and specific therapy. How useful are these principles when considering the elderly patient?

7.   Describe, apply, and revise appropriate treatment interventions based upon analysis of changes in the patient's clinical and laboratory parameters:

     a.   Adjustment of intravenous fluids with respect to expected stress response, including metabolic, hormonal, cardiovascular, and renal responses to replacement of fluid losses (Describe association between high levels of stress hormones and alterations of glucose metabolism remembering: do not volume resuscitate patients with excessive amounts of glucose.)

     b.   Efficacy of prophylactic measures for PE, stress ulceration and infection

    c.   Adequacy of nutritional support in a patient with multiple sites of protein losses (e.g., fistulas, drain sites, or metabolic stressors [infection, acute lung injury {ALI}, hyperthermia, respiratory failure])

    d.   Analysis and treatment of postoperative fever and methods of treatment

    e.   Events leading to and responsible for initiation of ventilatory support

    f.   Differentiate low cardiac output, hypotensive/hypertensive states in terms of preload, pump, or afterload

    g.   Analysis and treatment of seizures or acute change in mental status, including the role of:

        (1)   ABC's (airway, breathing, circulation); draw electrolytes/blood-urea-nitrogen (BUN)/ creatinine/glucose/calcium, magnesium

        (2)   Glucose/thiamine intravenously

        (3)   Evaluate medication record for new drugs or interactions (Ativan, Versed, phenobarbital, Dilantin [not applicable in the acute event])

    h.   Analysis and treatment of acute respiratory failure from changes in the airway, pump, or lung.

8.   Review the management and diagram a plan for the care of the critically ill surgical patient with multiple medical problems such as:

    a.   Cardiac dysrhythmias

    b.   Pulmonary insufficiency from airway, bellows (pump), or parenchymal problems

    c.   Acute/chronic renal failure with hemodynamic instability or need of specific fluid therapy (TPN), renal replacement therapy, high output GI fistulas

    d.   Diabetes mellitus and its special problems in the realm of nutritional support

    e.   Hemodynamic instability in the face of acute/chronic renal or pulmonary insufficiency

Section Three: Airway-Respiration

1.   Describe the commonly used indications for initiation of ventilation support, including:

    a.   Indications and commonly acceptable values for initiation of mechanical ventilation

b. Evaluation of airway

c. Evaluation of adequacy of thoracic pump (muscle strength)

d. Evaluation of lung parenchymal characteristics (arterial blood gases and chest x-ray)

e. Analysis of commonly used pulmonary values (e.g., tidal volume [Vt], maximum ventilatory volume [MVV], compliance static and dynamic, functional residual capacity [FRC], PEEP, auto PEEP, airway pressures)

f. Indications and commonly acceptable values for weaning from mechanical ventilation

2. Review respiratory physiology, and describe the specific pathology involved in ventilation and perfusion deficits.

3. Discuss the association of airway obstruction with age, giving consideration to each of the following:

a. Repeated disruption of the balance of inflammatory mediators and humeral protection (elastase and antielastase, oxidant and antioxidant)

b. Neutrophil recruitment

c. Tissue repair culminating in inflammatory lung destruction

d. Accumulated environmental oxidant injuries

4. Analyze and compare the principles of ventilator mechanics, including modes of ventilation, triggering mechanisms, and possible uses.

5. Describe the pathophysiology of acute lung injury (ALI, with spectrum from mild to severe ALI, also known as ARDS) and the management of the long-term ventilator-dependent patient to include:

a. Pneumonias (aspiration or nosocomial)

b. Acute renal failure

c. Cardiac failure

d. Prevention of malnutrition or restitution of body stores

e. Systemic Inflammatory Response syndrome (SIRS, MODS- Multiple Organ

Dysfunction Syndrome the most severe form known as MSOF- Multi-System Organ Failure)

    f.   Sepsis

    g.   Skin care problems

    h.   Physical therapy (maintenance of muscle mass and function, prevention of contractions)

    i.   Psychological support for both patient and family

6.   Review management of the following complex respiratory problems: Mechanically ventilated patient with:

    a.   Areas of differing compliance

    b.   Bronchopleural or bronch-esophageal fistula

    c.   Borderline cardiac reserve (non-compliant left ventricle, recent myocardial infarction, valvular dysfunction)

7.   Explain why otherwise healthy elders may be more vulnerable to poor outcomes from diseases affecting diffusion (producing lower oxygen levels, e.g., pneumonia, COPD). Consider these factors in your explanation:

    a.   Heart rate

    b.   Ventilatory response to hypoxia

    c.   Ventilatory response to hypercapnia

8.   Analyze the pros and cons of the use of the following drugs to improve respiratory function:

    a.   Bronchodilators (aerosols vs. parenteral medications)

    b.   Membrane stabilizing agents (cromolyn sodium, steroids)

    c.   Diuretics

    d.   Venodilators

    e.   Analgesics and sedatives

    f.   Mucolytics

Section Four: Circulation

1.   Describe and compare the following cardiac function parameters:

      a.   Preload

      b.   Afterload

      c.   Myocardial contractility

2.   Define the information obtained from the use of the following invasive/non-invasive monitoring devices.

      Specify: which information is directly/indirectly measured or calculated, the accuracy and cost of obtaining the information, and review the hemodynamic principles associated with the use of each device:

      a.   Arterial catheters

      b.   Central venous catheters

      c.   Swan-Ganz catheters

      d.   Intracranial pressure monitors

      e.   End tidal carbon dioxide monitors

      f.   Pulse oximetry

      g.   Peripheral nerve stimulators (for testing adequacy of neuromuscular blockade)

      h.   Foley catheters

      i.   Intestinal pH monitors

      j.   Bioelectric impedance

3.   Outline the protocols for definition of patterns and management of hemodynamically unstable patients, and analyze the selection of appropriate therapy by completing these activities:

      a.   Predict improvements in hemodynamic status with manipulation of definable variables, including fluid and drug therapies.

      b.   Detect and revise therapies based on the use of invasive/non-invasive monitoring devices.

4. Review cardiac function and hemodynamic monitoring from the following standpoints. Interpret changes in accuracy of values obtained from hemodynamic monitoring devices in:

    a. Patients with severe pulmonary insufficiency who have low compliances or high PEEP

    b. Patients with severe valvular insufficiency/stenosis

    c. Various shock states (hypovolemic, septic, spinal, or cardiogenic)

    d. High dose vasopressors

5. Summarize the effects of appropriate volume and drug therapies to manipulate the cardiovascular system in the following patients:

    a. Hypovolemic hypotensive patient

    b. Hypotensive euvolemic patient

    c. Hypotensive hypervolemic patient

    d. Hypotensive oliguric patient

    e. Hypotensive, hypervolemic oliguric patient

    f. Hypovolemic oliguric patient

    g. Hypotensive, oliguric hypoxic patient

6. Discuss the significant patient characteristics in a geriatric population associated with increased risk of thromboembolic disease, including:

    a. Underlying congestive heart failure

    b. Prolonged immobility before surgery

    c. Paralysis

    d. Previous DVT

    e. Hypercoagulable states (due to malignancy or coagulation factor deficiency)

Section Five: Renal

1. Review acid-base and electrolyte abnormalities common in critically-ill patients.

2.   Identify, define, and classify the major categories of acid-base disturbance (metabolic acidosis and/or alkalosis, respiratory acidosis and/or alkalosis) in the context of the patient's altered physiology. Cite common clinical scenarios for their appearance:

   a.   Metabolic acidosis (hypovolemic shock, chloride excess resuscitation, occult ischemia)

   b.   Metabolic alkalosis (contraction alkalosis excessive diuretic use)

   c.   Respiratory acidosis

   d.   Respiratory alkalosis (early sign of sepsis vs. ventilator complication)

3.   Discuss the identification and correction of complex acid-base problems such as choice of intravenous fluids for electrolyte replacement in the:

   a.   Hyperchloremic, metabolically-acidotic patient

   b.   Hypochloremic, metabolically-alkalotic patient

   c.   Stuporous, dehydrated, hyponatremic patient

   d.   Stuporous dehydrated hypernatremic patient

   e.   Patient with central diabetes insipidus

   f.   Hyponatremic, volume overloaded patient with carbon dioxide retention

Section Six: Neurologic

Describe the initial evaluation, ongoing, acute monitoring and long-term management of possible neurologic or behavioral abnormalities occurring in the ICU setting:

   a.   Seizures

   b.   Coma

   c.   Stroke

   d.   Multifactorial effects of "postoperative confusion"

   e.   Delirium

   f.   Brain death

Section Seven: Gastrointestinal/Hepatic

1.   Discuss specific fluid compositions and the effect of the losses of such fluids as gastric, pancreatic, biliary, and succus entericus from intestinal fistulas of various levels. (Fluid

should be described in terms of volume, electrolyte composition, and replacement fluid of choice.)

2. Superficial sepsis, including necrotizing infections

    a. Natural history of condition

    b. Vulnerable individuals

    c. Physiology of associated conditions; diabetes, atherosclerosis, steroid therapy, immunocompromised etc.

    d. Knowledge of bacteriology and toxins involved

    e. Mechanisms of septic shock

    f. Massive blood transfusion complications

    g. Knowledge of appropriate antibiotic therapy

    h. Knowledge of necrotizing fasciitis

Senior Level:

Section Eight: Administration

1. Describe the criteria for predicting preoperatively the patient's need for critical care, including:

    a. Pre-existing disease states (cardiac, pulmonary, or renal)

    b. Operation-specific requirements for postoperative intensive care management

2. Review and interpret the relationships of physicians, nurses, and administrators in managing patients assigned to the ICU.

3. Discuss the value of an interdisciplinary approach to health care for the critically ill, elderly surgical patient. Include consideration of these groups/disciplines, working together:

    a. Surgery   f. Pharmacy

    b. Nursing staff   g. Religion

    c. Family-friends as caregivers   h. Social work

    d. Physical therapy   i. Hospital administration

    e. Medical consultants

4.	Identify new modes of intensive care therapeutics by completing the following activities:

	a.	Predict and analyze the need for a new technology.

	b.	Formulate a plan for the institution of new technologies or therapeutics.

	c.	Critique and revise applicability of new technologies or therapeutics on a cost: benefit ratio.

5.	Summarize the following moral and ethical problems encountered in the ICU:

	a.	The need for organ donation and the identification of potential donors

	b.	Decisions about whom to resuscitate and to what degree

	c.	Care for the mentally incapacitated or incompetent patient

	d.	Dealing with a difficult family and futility of care

	e.	Identifying and interacting with alternate religious/cultural beliefs

Section Nine: General Pathophysiology--Body as a Whole

1.	Discuss the use of sepsis severity scores.

2.	Distinguish between the major characteristics of septic shock and hypovolemic shock:

	a.	Summarize initial evaluation and presentation

	b.	Analyze therapeutic options

	c.	Revise therapeutic options based on clinical parameters obtained from monitoring devices.

3.	Explain the concepts of tissue oxygen supply and demand. Demonstrate the contributions from the following components:

	a.	Calculate oxygen delivery

	b.	Calculate oxygen consumption

	c.	Analyze the effect of cardiac output and varying preload, pump, and afterload to oxygen delivery

	d.	Analyze the contributions of hemoglobin and percent of saturation on oxygen delivery

e. Explain the changes in tissue oxygen delivery and uptake related to pH, temperature, 2, 3-diphosphoglyceride (DPG)

4. Discuss the evaluation and treatment of the following bleeding disorders:
   a. The role of blood vessels, platelets, fibrin cascade, and degeneration in normal hemostasis.
   b. Disseminated intravascular coagulopathy (DIC), defining common causes and therapy.
   c. Thrombocytopenia as a failure of production, accelerated destruction, or dilution
   d. Hemophilia A
   e. Von Willebrand's disease
   f. Idiopathic thrombocytopenia purpura (ITP) and thrombotic thrombocytopenia purpura (TTP) as causes of thrombocytopenia (compare and contrast)
   g. Heparin or Coumadin therapy misapplication
   h. Advanced liver disease
   i. The role of Protein C, S, and lupus circulating anticoagulant and their roles in bleeding disorders

5. Outline the unique problems of the following surgical subspecialties in critical care management:
   a. Neurosurgery   e. Cardiac surgery
   b. Urology   f. Thoracic surgery
   c. Orthopedics   g. Burns
   d. Pediatric surgery   h. Trauma

6. Discuss management of the overall hospital course of the patient with altered physiologic states:
   a. Preoperative considerations specific to their disease
   b. Operative considerations specific to their disease
   c. Postoperative considerations specific to their disease

7.   Outline the nutritional and metabolic components for a patient with specific disease states.

Section Ten: Renal

Discuss the physiologic principles and define specific management aspects associated with the following complex acid-base problems:

a.   Renal tubular acidosis (differentiate between Type I and II)

b.   Management of high output loss states from the gastrointestinal tract in a patient with poor cardiac function

c.   Management of volume excess states associated with eunatremia or hyponatremia

Section Eleven: Gastrointestinal/Hepatic

Review and summarize the management of hepatic and renal failure, including:

a.   Utility/disutility of disease-specific nutritional formulations

b.   Adjustment or elimination of toxic substances (antibiotics, contrast material, narcotics)

c.   Current means for support of renal failure, high dose diuretics, continuous veno-venous hemofiltration (CVVH), continuous veno-venous hemodialysis (CVVHD), dialysis (peritoneal and hemodialysis)

Section Twelve: Endocrine

Describe and specify therapy for the following endocrine-related problems associated with critical care:

a.   Hypothyroidism/hyperthyroidism

b.   Hyperparathyroidism/hypoparathyroidism (changes in calcium and magnesium values)

c.   Adrenal cortical excess (Cushing's disease and syndrome)

d.   Adrenal cortical deficiency states (Addison's disease)

Patient Care that is compassionate, appropriate, and effective for the treatment of health problems and the promotion of health.

<u>Junior Level</u>:

1.   Provide initial evaluation and management of the critically-ill postoperative patient.

2.   Institute the following therapeutic interventions:

    a.   Manage fluid orders

    b.   Determine ventilator settings

    c.   Order pharmacologic support drugs

    d.   Determine the need for and duration of antibiotic therapy

3.   Obtain ACLS, FCCS, and ATLS certification.

4.   Perform the following procedures:

    a.   Orotracheal and nasotracheal intubation, nasogastric and bladder intubation

    b.   Arterial catheter insertion

    c.   Central venous and pulmonary artery catheter insertion

    d.   Placement of tube thoracotomy

    e.   Cricothyrotomy

    f.   Pericardiocentesis

5.   Serve on code and trauma team.

6.   Manage critically ill patients in the intensive care unit:

    a.   Determine need for ventilation and select situation appropriate airway and initial ventilator settings

    b.   Compute initial and ongoing fluid requirements

    c.   Analyze need for operative intervention

    d.   Initiate rehabilitation process after stabilization of injuries, including:

        (1)   Attention to possible altered body habitus

        (2)   Requirements for special devices (physical, occupational, or speech therapy)

        (3)   Maintain nutritional status

        (4)   Provide support, interaction, and information for the family

    e.   Establish intravenous access and maintain with appropriate sterile techniques for evaluation of fever

f.   Determine need for ongoing ICU management

g.   Identify appropriate antibiotic therapy distinguishing between prophylactic, empiric, and therapeutic uses

h.   Monitor hemodynamic data

i.   History and examination for necrotizing infections

j.   Recognition of the early warning signs

k.   Radical excisional surgery

l.   Fournier's gangrene/necrotizing fasciitis/debridement

Senior Level:

1.   Direct all surgical management of patients in the ICU, including taking direct responsibility for admission and discharge.

2.   Manage invasive monitoring catheters, interpret the data obtained, and manipulate the hemodynamic variables toward calculated goals.

3.   Manage the following situations:

     a.   Multiple organ system failure; providing support for failing, failed, or normal organs

     b.   Life threatening surgical infections (e.g., ascending cholangitis, ascending myonecrosis or gangrene)

     c.   Hypovolemic shock

     d.   Renal failure

     e.   Nutritional failure

     f.   Liver failure

4.   Place emergency transvenous/transthoracic access for cardiac pacing.

5.   Perform emergency thoracotomy.

6.   Manage the nutritional and metabolic components of the patient's illness.

7.   Serve on code and trauma teams as a team leader.

8.   Construct a caregiver assessment to include caregiver preparedness, needs, and signs of strain. Consider caregiver emotional support and actual physical care of the patient.

9.   Analyze the special need for caregiver support systems when the patient is elderly.

Practice-Based Learning and Improvement that involves investigation and evaluation of their own patient care, appraisal and assimilation of scientific evidence, and improvements in patient care.

INFORMATION TECHNOLOGY AND POPULATION COMPARISONS
REFERENCES

Abrams JH, Cerra FB. Essentials of Critical Care: Clinical Cases and Practical Solutions. St. Louis : Quality Medical Publishing, Inc., 1993.

Abrams JH, Cerra FB. Essentials of Surgical Critical Care. St. Louis : Quality Medical Publishing, Inc., 1993.

Alia I, Esteban A. Weaning from mechanical ventilation. Crit Care 2000;4(2):72-80.
Bartlett JG, Dowell SF, Mandell LA, et al., Practice guidelines for the management of community-acquired pneumonia in adults. (Infectious Disease Society of America). Clin Infect Dis 2000;31(2):347-382.

Bartlett RH. Critical care. In: Greenfield LJ, Mulholland M, Oldham KT, Zelenock GB, Lillemoe KD (eds), Surgery: Scientific Principles and Practice (2nd ed). Philadelphia : Lippincott-Raven, 1997;215-242.

Bongard FS, Sue DY. Current Critical Care Diagnosis and Treatment. Norwalk CT : Appleton and Lange, 1994.

Cameron JL (ed). Surgical critical care. Current Surgical Therapy (6th ed). St. Louis : Mosby, 1998;1099-1157.

Civetta JM, Taylor RW, Kirby RR. Critical Care (3rd ed). Philadelphia : Lippincott-Raven Co., 1997.

Davella D, Brambilla GL, Delfini R, et al. Guidelines for the treatment of adults with severe head trauma: criteria for surgical treatment (Part III). J Neurosurg Sci 2000;44(1):19-24.

Deitch E. Tools of the Trade and Rules of the Road: A Surgical Guide. Philadelphia: Lippincott Raven, 1997 (Chapt 25 Intubation 233-241, Chapt 26 Vascular Access 242-258, Chapt 27 Troubleshooting Hemodynamic and Monitoring Devices, Chapt 28 Ventilators).

Fundamentals of Critical Care Support Course Textbook (2nd 3d). Anaheim , CA : Society of Critical Care Medicine, 1998.

Gazmuri RJ. Buffer treatment for cardiac resuscitation: putting the cart before the horse? Crit Care Med 1999;27(5):875-876.

Greenburg AG, Simms HH. Pathophysiology of shock. In: Miller TA (ed), Modern Surgical Care: Physiologic Foundations and Clinical Applications (2nd ed). St. Louis : Quality Medical Publishing, Inc., 1998;197-219.

Gueugniaud PY, Carsin H, Bertin-Maghit M. Current advances in the initial management of major thermal burns. Intensive Care Med 2000;26(7):848-856.

Hall JB, Schmidt GA, Wood LDH. Principles of Critical Care (2nd ed). New York : McGraw-Hill, 1998;1-1767.

Hoyt DB, Potenza BM, Cryer HG, et al. Trauma. In: Greenfield LJ, Mulholland M, Oldham KT, Zelenock GB, Lillemoe KD (eds), Surgery: Scientific Principles and Practice (2nd ed). Philadelphia : Lippincott-Raven, 1997;267-422.

Junkerman C, Schiedermaye D. Practical Ethics for Students, Interns, and Residents: A Short Reference Manual (2nd ed). Hagerstown , MD : University Publishing Group, Inc., 1998.

Jurusz DJ, Gilmore JY. Shock and hypoperfusion states. In: O'Leary JP (ed), The Physiologic Basis of Surgery (2nd ed). Baltimore : Williams and Wilkins, 1996;84-99.

Kern KB, Halperin HR, Field J, et al. New guidelines for cardiopulmonary resuscitation and emergency cardiac care: changes in the management of cardiac arrest. JAMA 2001;285(10):1267-1269.

Knudson MM. Definitive care phase: geriatric trauma. In: Greenfield LJ, Mulholland M, Oldham KT, Zelenock GB, Lillemoe KD (eds), Surgery: Scientific Principles and Practice (2nd ed). Philadelphia : Lippincott-Raven, 1997;386-390.

Maier RV. Postoperative respiratory failure. In: Cameron JL (ed), Current Surgical Therapy (6th ed). St. Louis : Mosby, 1998;1103-1108.

Maier RV. Shock. In: Greenfield LJ, Mulholland M, Oldham KT, Zelenock GB, Lillemoe KD (eds), Surgery: Scientific Principles and Practice (2nd ed). Philadelphia : Lippincott-Raven, 1997;182-214.

Ostermann ME, Keenan SP, Seiferling RA, et al. Sedation in the intensive care unit: a systematic review. JAMA 2000;283(11):1451-1459.

Powers JS, Billings FT, Jr. Management of perioperative problems in the aged. In: Adkins RB, Jr., Scott HW, Jr. (eds), Surgical Care for the Elderly (2nd ed). Philadelphia : Lippincott-Raven Publishers, 1998;33-50.

Procaccio F, Stocchetti N, Citerio G, et al. Guidelines for the treatment of adults with severe head trauma: initial assessment; evaluation and pre-hospital treatment; current criteria for hospital admission; systemic and cerebral monitoring (Part I). J Neurosurg Sci 2000;44(1):1-10.

Procaccio F, Stocchetti N, Citerio G, et al. Guidelines for the treatment of adults with severe head trauma: criteria for medical treatment (Part II). J Neurosurg Sci 2000;44(1):11-18.

Richardson CJ, Rodriguez JL. Identification of patients at highest risk for ventilator-associated pneumonia in the surgical intensive care unit. Am J Surg 2000;179(2A Suppl):8S-11S.

Richardson JD. Common pulmonary derangements, respiratory failure, and adult respiratory distress syndrome. In: Miller TA (ed), Modern Surgical Care: Physiologic Foundations and Clinical Applications (2nd ed). St. Louis : Quality Medical Publishing, Inc., 1998;738-764.

Sanders AB, Witzke DB, Jones JS, et al. Principles of care and application of the geriatric emergency care model. In: Sanders AB (ed), Emergency Care of the Elder Person. St. Louis : Beverly Cracom Publications, 1996;59-93.

Sax HC. Nutrition support in the critically ill. In: Cameron JL (ed), Current Surgical Therapy (6th ed). St. Louis : Mosby, 1998;1143-1145.

Shapiro MB , Anderson HL, Bartlett RH, et al. Respiratory failure: conventional and high-tech support. Surg Clin N Am 2000;80(3):871-873.

The Brain Trauma Foundation, The American Association of Neurological Surgeons, The Joint Section on Neurotrauma and Critical Care. Resuscitation of blood pressure and oxygenation. J Neurotrauma 2000;17(6-7):4710478.
http://www.sccm.org

Wertheim WA . Perioperative risk: review of two guidelines for assessing older adults. American College of Cardiology and American Heart Association. Geriatrics 2000;55(7):61-66; quiz 69.

Health Care Financing Administration, 42 CFR, Part 482 [HCFA-3005-F], RIN: 0938-AI95. Medicare and Medicaid Programs; Hospital Conditions of Participation; Identification of Potential Organ, Tissue, and Eye Donors and Transplant Hospitals' Provision of Transplant-Related Data. AGENCY: Health Care Financing Administration (HCFA), HHS.

ACTION: Final Rule

SUMMARY: This final rule addresses only provisions relating to organ donation and transplantation. It imposes several requirements a hospital must meet that are designed to increase organ donation. One of these requirements is that a hospital must have an agreement with the Organ Procurement Organization (OPO) designated by the Secretary, under which the hospital will contact the OPO in a timely manner about individuals who die or whose death is imminent in the hospital. The OPO will then determine the individual's medical suitability for donation. As well, the hospital must have an agreement with at least one tissue bank and at least one eye bank to cooperate in the retrieval, processing, preservation, storage, and distribution of tissues and eyes, as long as the agreement does not interfere with organ donation. The final rule requires a hospital to ensure, in collaboration with the OPO with which it has an agreement that the family of every potential donor is informed of its option to donate organs or tissues or not to donate. Under the final rule, hospitals must work with the OPO and at least one tissue bank and one eye bank in educating staff on donation issues, reviewing death records to improve identification of potential donors, and maintaining potential donors while necessary testing and placement of organs and tissues take place. In addition, transplant hospitals must provide organ-transplant-related data, as requested by the OPTN, the Scientific Registry, and the OPOs. The hospital must also provide, if requested, such data directly to the Department.

DATES: These regulations are effective on August 21, 1998.

SECTION 11.2: TRAUMA

UNIT OBJECTIVES:

Demonstrate an understanding of the pathophysiologic effect of blunt and penetrating trauma.

Demonstrate the ability to effectively manage the surgical care of a patient with complex multisystem injuries.

Demonstrate knowledge of, and the ability to, manage a variety of healthcare services for trauma patients such as pre-hospital transportation, emergency department care, in-hospital care, and rehabilitation.

Closed thoracic injury: Assessment and initial management of blunt injury of the thorax.

Penetrating thoracic injury: Assessment and initial management of penetrating injury of the thorax.

Closed and penetrating abdominal injury: Assessment and initial management of blunt and penetrating injury of the abdomen.

Blunt and penetrating soft tissue and skeletal injury: Assessment and initial management of blunt and penetrating injury of the soft tissues and skeleton.

Medical Knowledge about established and evolving biomedical, clinical, and cognate (e.g. epidemiological and social-behavioral) sciences and the application of this knowledge to patient care.

<u>Junior Level:</u>

1. Describe the anatomy and physiology of all body systems affected by trauma, including the initial functional evaluation of the:

    a. Central nervous system   e. Genitourinary system

    b. Cardiovascular system   f. Extremity function

    c. Pulmonary system   g. Nutritional status

    d. Gastrointestinal system

2. Review the anatomy, physiology, and pathology applicable to the general management of trauma patients, including:

    a. Central nervous system

b.   Musculoskeletal system

c.   Hand/forearm

d.   Ear, nose, and throat

e.   Ophthalmology

3.   Outline the basic techniques of evaluation and resuscitation of trauma patients using the American College of Surgeons (ACS) Advanced Trauma Life Support (ATLS) protocol.

4.   Specify the trauma services needed for initial evaluation and resuscitation in the hospital setting. Categorize appropriate pre-hospital or emergency medicine system levels of care.

5.   Discuss wound care management in the emergency department and other settings. Outline the management of the following drains and tubes: nasogastric tube (NGT), urinary bladder catheter, chest tube (CT), central venous line (CVL), arterial line (AL).

6.   Explain the characteristics of basic surgical skill, including:

a.   Sterile technique

b.   Incisions

c.   Wound closures

d.   Knot tying

e.   Handling of tissues

f.   Selection/use of operating instruments

g.   Universal precautions

7.   Discuss the management of trauma involving the musculoskeletal system, including the need for casts, splints, and traction.

8.   Summarize basic critical care management principles.

9.   Analyze pharmacological support for trauma, resuscitation, and intensive care unit patients.

10.   Identify the management principles for a trauma patient in the intensive care unit.

11.   Outline the factors associated with rehabilitation as they apply to initial and early patient care.

12. Discuss the indications for, and the provision of, nutritional support for elderly patients sustaining trauma.

13. Outline the indications for such basic surgical procedures as:

    a. Laparotomy

    b. Debridement of injured tissues

    c. Ultrasound

    d. Medical antishock trousers (MAST)

    e. HARE traction splint

    f. Splinting

    g. Diagnostic peritoneal lavage (DPL)

    h. Thoracotomy/thoracostomy

    i. Hemorrhage control

14. Discuss the primary causes/mechanisms of injury in the following list that contribute to making trauma the fifth leading cause of death in those aged 65 and older:

    a. Falls

    b. Motor vehicle crashes

    c. Pedestrian injuries

    d. Burns

    e. Domestic abuse

15. Concept of low energy, high energy transfer injury

16. Mechanisms of injury and possible consequences, e.g. GSW, stabbing, seat belt injuries

17. Indications for use of uncrossmatched blood

Senior Level:

1. Explain trauma preventive measures, both medical and legal (e.g., the use of helmets and seat belts).

2. Describe and explain the mechanics/ballistics associated with various wounding agents.

3. Discuss the management of associated medical conditions seen in the trauma patient such as diabetes, chronic obstructive pulmonary disease, hypertension, coronary artery disease, and HIV.

4. Identify the indications for emergency operative procedures such as burr holes, Cricothyrotomy, insertion of cardiopulmonary assist devices, and resuscitative thoracotomy.

5. Formulate a plan for rehabilitation to return the trauma patient to full functional life.

6. Define abdominal compartment syndrome. Describe how to measure intra-abdominal pressures and develop a treatment plan to treat abdominal compartment syndrome.

7. Define "Damage Control Surgery." Describe the sequence of damage control surgery in the treatment of the traumatized patient.

8. Analyze the transfer of a patient to an appropriate facility utilizing air medical services.

9. Discuss the availability and use of institutional and community support services for trauma patients such as social work, home health care, and vocation rehabilitation (physical and occupational therapy).

10. Discuss the management of a trauma service, including the training of its members in emergency medicine services, emergency department, operating room, intensive care, and rehabilitation.

11. Outline the economic impact of the following aspects of patient care:

    a. Vocational rehabilitation

    b. Nursing homes

    c. Insurance

    d. Diagnostic-related groups (DRG's) associated with management of trauma

    e. Billing and coding

    f. Managed care

Patient Care that is compassionate, appropriate, and effective for the treatment of health problems and the promotion of health.

Junior Level:

1. Complete an ACS ATLS course as a provider.
2. Participate in trauma evaluation, resuscitation, operative management, and intensive care unit (ICU) supervision of a multiply-injured patient.
3. Evaluate the patient to determine quality of emergency medical service (EMS) care.
4. Insert a variety of tubes:

a.	Endotracheal	d.	Intra-arterial
b.	Thoracostomy	e.	Diagnostic peritoneal lavage (DPL)
c.	Intravenous	f.	Urinary bladder catheter
g.	Nasogastric tube		

5. Apply and remove all types of dressings and splints, including the vacuum pack dressing.
6. Make and close a variety of incisions and tie knots using sterile technique.
7. Evaluate critical care parameters and make decisions, under direct supervision, regarding change in care.
8. Direct the evaluation of an acutely-injured patient to include resuscitation and the decision for operation.
9. Assess nutritional needs and institute necessary nutritional support.
10. Formulate rehabilitation plans for trauma patients.
11. Monitor the trauma patient in the intensive care unit, suggesting changes in management as indicated.
12. Manage pharmacologic treatment plans for patients during resuscitation and in the critical care unit.
13. Perform basic surgical procedures such as:
    a. Laparotomy
    b. Wound debridement
    c. Application of traction devices for both head and extremities
    d. Recognize and treat sucking chest wound
    e. Blunt and penetrating soft tissue and skeletal injury
    f. Assessment and initial management of multiply injured patient
    g. Arrest of hemorrhage by pressure and tourniquet

h.   Appropriate immobilization during assessment

i.   Recognition of major vascular trauma

j.   Assessment of ischemic limb

k.   Chest drain insertion

l.   Diagnostic peritoneal lavage

m.   Technical Skills and Procedures

     (1)   Laparotomy- trauma

     (2)   Liver trauma-debridement/packing

     (3)   Pancreatectomy-distal

     (4)   Splenectomy

     (5)   Splenic repair

     (6)   Management of hollow organ injury

Senior Level:

1.   Coordinate EMS activities for initial trauma management to include instructional programs.

2.   Manage penetrating wounds through understanding the injury potential of wounding mechanisms.

3.   Provide management for pre-existing disease states in injured patients with appropriate consultation.

4.   Perform all operative and management procedures for trauma to the chest, abdomen, extremities, and head with direct supervision.

5.   Supervise central line placement, cricothyrotomy, CT, DPL, and ultrasound by junior house staff.

6.   Direct rehabilitation plans with appropriate consultation.

7.   Organize hospital resources to provide services for trauma patients and direct patient flow in the emergency department, the operating room, and the intensive care unit.

8.   Provide appropriate referrals for vocation rehabilitation, nursing home services, and physical rehabilitation.

9.   Triage multiple trauma victims.

10.   Practice the principles of damage control surgery in severely-injured patients.

Practice-Based Learning and Improvement that involves investigation and evaluation of their own patient care, appraisal and assimilation of scientific evidence, and improvements in patient care.

INFORMATION TECHNOLOGY AND POPULATION COMPARISONS REFERENCES

Barton R. Wound care. In: Trunkey DD, Lewis FR (eds). Current Therapy of Trauma (4th ed). St.Louis, MO: Mosby, 1999;53-58.

Cameron JL (ed). Trauma and emergency care. Current Surgical Therapy (7th ed). St. Louis : Mosby, 2001.

Cheatham ML. Intra-abdominal hypertension and abdominal compartment syndrome. In: Nelson LD (ed). New Horizons: New Advances in the Care of Critically Injured Patients. Hagerstown , MD : Lippincott Williams & Wilkins, Spring 1999;96-115.

Cullinane DC , Nunn GR, Morris JA. Geriatric trauma. In: Trunkey DD, Lewis FR (eds). Current Therapy of Trauma (4th ed). St.Louis, MO: Mosby, 1999;92-96.

Hoyt DB, Potenza BM, Cryer HG, et al. Trauma. In: Greenfield LJ, Mulholland M, Oldham KT, Zelenock GB, Lillemoe KD (eds), Surgery: Scientific Principles and Practice (2nd ed). Philadelphia : Lippincott-Raven, 1997;267-422.

Knudson MM. Definitive care phase: geriatric trauma. In: Greenfield LJ, Mulholland M, Oldham KT, Zelenock GB, Lillemoe KD (eds), Surgery: Scientific Principles and Practice (2nd ed). Philadelphia : Lippincott-Raven, 1997;386-390.

MacKersie RC, Campbell AR , Cammarano WB. Principles of critical care. In: Feliciano DV, Moore EE, Mattox KL. Trauma (4th ed). CT : Appleton and Lange, 2000;1231-1266.

Rotondo MF, Zonies DH. The damage control sequence and underlying logic. In: Hirshberg A, Mattox KL (eds). Damage Control Surgery. Surg Clin of N Amer 1997;77:761-778.

Rozycki GS, Ballard RB. Ultrasound in initial trauma evaluation. In: Trunkey DD, Lewis FR (eds). Current Therapy of Trauma (4th ed). St.Louis, MO: Mosby, 1999;144-150.

Sanders AB. (ed). Emergency Care of the Elder Person. St. Louis : Beverly Cracom Publications, 1996.

Sheridan RL, Tompkins RG. Burns. In: Greenfield LJ, Mulholland M, Oldham KT, Zelenock GB, Lillemoe KD (eds), Surgery: Scientific Principles and Practice (2nd ed). Philadelphia : Lippincott-Raven, 1997;422-438.

10.2A GERIATRIC TRAUMA

The Geriatric Trauma unit was revised by Scott G. Sagraves, MD, from the Curriculum, third edition, by Lori J. Morgan, MD, Lucy A. Wibbenmeyer, MD, and G. Patrick Kealey, MD.

UNIT OBJECTIVES:

Demonstrate an understanding of the epidemiology and pathophysiology of injury in elderly patients.

Demonstrate an ability to utilize these concepts for improved assessment and management of the elderly trauma patient.

Medical Knowledge about established and evolving biomedical, clinical, and cognate (e.g. epidemiological and social-behavioral) sciences and the application of this knowledge to patient care.

Epidemiology of Elderly Patient Trauma

The resident will know the:

1.   Demographics of the elderly population in the total population of the United States

2.   Leading cause of injury death in the elderly population

3.   Other major causes of injury death in the elderly population

4.   Risk factors for trauma in older people

5.   Increase in injury mortality in elderly people compared to younger cohorts

6.   The cost of trauma care for elderly patients

Pathophysiology of Elderly Trauma Patients

The resident will be prepared to explain the:

1.   Need for obtaining an accurate medical history

2.   Impact of comorbidities on outcomes

3.   Effects of various common medications on the elderly trauma patient

4.   Concept of cerebral atrophy and possible delays in diagnosis of closed head injury (CHI)

5.   Poor outcomes in severe CHI in elderly patients

6. Decreased pulmonary reserve in elderly people and the need for aggressive pulmonary care

7. Decreased cardiovascular reserve and the need for early and aggressive monitoring of the elderly trauma patient

8. Decreased renal function and the need for adjusting medication doses and volume resuscitation for this

9. Loss of bone mass in elderly people and the risk of severe injury with only minor impacts

10. High incidence of complications in the elderly trauma patients

11. Need for a thorough evaluation of the context of the injury and the pre-morbid condition of the patient

12. Rehabilitation of elderly trauma patients.

Practice-Based Learning and Improvement that involves investigation and evaluation of their own patient care, appraisal and assimilation of scientific evidence, and improvements in patient care.

INFORMATION TECHNOLOGY AND POPULATION COMPARISONS REFERENCES

Abrams WB, Beers MH, Berkow R (eds). Falls and gait disorders. The Merck Manual of Geriatrics (2nd ed). Whitehouse Station , NJ : Merck Research Laboratories, Merck & Co., Inc., 1995;65-78.

Aucar JA, Mattox KL. Trauma. In: Adkins RB, Jr., Scott HW, Jr. (eds), Surgical Care for the Elderly (2nd ed). Philadelphia : Lippincott-Raven Publishers, 1998;427-438.

De Maria E, Kenney P, Merriam, et al. Survival after trauma in geriatric patients. Ann Surg 1987;206(6):738-43.

Ferrara PC. Geriatric trauma: outcomes of elderly patients discharged from the ED. Am J Emerg Med 1999;17(7):629-632.

Ferrara PC, Bartfield JM, D'Andrea CC. Outcomes of admitted geriatric trauma victims. Am J Emerg Med 2000;18(5):575-580.

Gubler K, Davis R, Koepsell T, et al. Long-term survival of elderly trauma patients. Arch Surg 1997;132:1010-1014.

Gubler K, Maier R, Davis R, et al. Trauma recidivism in the elderly. J Trauma 1996;41(6):952-956.

Harrington DT, Pruitt BA, Jr. Thermal injuries. In: Adkins RB, Jr., Scott HW, Jr. (eds), Surgical Care for the Elderly (2nd ed). Philadelphia : Lippincott-Raven Publishers, 1998;439-456.

Kilaru S, Garb J, Emhoff T, et al. Long-term functional status and mortality of elderly patients with severe closed head injuries. J Trauma 1996;41(6):957-963.

Mandavia D, Newton K. Geriatric trauma: contemporary issue in trauma. Emerg Med Clin of N Amer 1998;16(1):257-274.

Milzman DP. Resuscitation of the geriatric patient. Emerg Med Clin of N Amer 1991;14(1):233-244.

National Center for Health Statistics. Health, United States, 1996-97 and Injury Chartbook. Hyattsville , MD : 1997.

National Center for Injury Prevention and Control. Unintentional injury fact sheet: fall and hip fractures among the elderly. Atlanta : Center for Disease Control, 1998.

National Highway Traffic Safety Administration. Older population traffic safety facts. US Department of Transportation, 1996.

National Safety Council. Accident Facts: 1997 Edition. Chicago : 1997.

Oreskovich M, Howard J, Copass M, et al. Geriatric trauma: injury patterns and outcome. J Trauma 1984;24(7):565-572.

Phillips S, Rond P, Kelly S, et al. The failure of triage criteria to identify geriatric patients with trauma; results from the Florida Trauma Triage Study. J Trauma 1996;40(2):278-283.

Schiller W, Knox R, Chleborad W. A five-year experience with severe injuries in elderly patients. Accid Ana and Prev 1995;27(2):167-174.

Schwab CW, Kauder D. Trauma in the geriatric patient. Arch Surg 1992;127:701-706.

Schwab C, Young G, et al. DRG reimbursement for trauma: the demise of the trauma center (the use of ISS grouping as an early predictor of total hospital cost). J Trauma 1988;28(7):939-946.

Zeitlow S, Capizzi P, Bannon M, et al. Multisystem geriatric trauma. J Trauma 1994;37(6):985-988.

SECTION 11.3   BURN INJURY

UNIT OBJECTIVES:

Demonstrate an understanding of the concepts of burn injury and its pathophysiology.

Demonstrate the ability to apply these concepts to the evaluation, resuscitation, clinical management, and rehabilitation of the burned patient.

Medical Knowledge about established and evolving biomedical, clinical, and cognate (e.g. epidemiological and social-behavioral) sciences and the application of this knowledge to patient care.

1.   Review the epidemiology, prevention, and socioeconomic and psychologic effects of burns.

2.   Describe the histologic and functional anatomy of the skin, adnexa, and subcutaneous tissues.

3.   Outline the physics and dynamics of thermal injury and the progression of tissue damage.

4.   Assess the appearance of the burn wound in relation to its depth, bacteriologic condition, healing potential, and requirement for intervention.

5.   Review the criteria for adequate evaluation of a burned patient, including historical aspects of the type of burn and subjective physical findings.

6.   Discuss an initial treatment plan for stabilization and fluid resuscitation of a burned patient based on the above evaluation.

7.   Describe the clinical factors necessitating immediate intervention to preserve life, limb, and function (PS of compartment syndrome).

8.   Outline the principles of burn shock, immunologic alteration, and bacteriologic pathology of burned skin.

9.   Define the "Rule of Nines" as it relates to total body surface area of the burn.

10.   Describe the relationship between burn depth and the degree of the burn.

11.   Review the basic principles and controversies concerning the management of the burn wound, and describe a clinical plan for its care.

12. Analyze the principles of systemic and local antibacterial agents in the burn wound.

13. Explain the special circumstances created by electrical, chemical, and inhalation burn injury, and apply their relation to the management.

14. Describe the pathology and management of inhalation injury, noting its relation to mortality, morbidity, and time course of patient recovery.

15. Explain the etiology and treatment of carbon monoxide poisoning.

16. Discuss the physics and pathology of the electrical burn and its relation to associated organ injury, including:

    a. Current   d. Neurological injury

    b. Entrance and exit wounds   e. Vascular problems

    c. Deep tissue involvement   f. Rhabdomyolysis

17. Review the indications for and contributions of physical and occupational therapy.

18. Describe the anatomy of the hand in relation to the specialized requirements of management and rehabilitation of the burned hand.

19. Describe the indications, techniques for harvest, application, immobilization, and care of split- and full- thickness skin grafts.

20. Explain the principles of wound contracture, and report desirable and harmful effects of contracture on:

    a. Initial management of the burn victim

    b. Closure of the burn wound

    c. Rehabilitation of the burn patient

21. Describe and explain the following terms:

    a. Compartment syndromes

    b. Burn eschar contraction

    c. Fasciotomy and escharotomy incisions and techniques

22. Summarize the treatment of chemical burns to include pathology, sources, decontamination, and management.

23. Review and analyze the special circumstances, management, and rehabilitation of burns in the pediatric patient.

24. Describe the indications for, and basic techniques of, plastic and reconstructive intervention in the burn wound to alleviate:

   a. Scar contracture

   b. Underlying joint contracture

   c. Hypertrophic scar

25. Summarize the activities of a specialized burn team or unit in the overall management of the burn patient to include the following:

   a. Physical therapy   d. Recreational therapy

   b. Occupational therapy   e. Burn nursing

   c. Psychological counseling   f. Cosmetics

Patient Care that is compassionate, appropriate, and effective for the treatment of health problems and the promotion of health.

1. Provide emergency burn patient evaluation and monitoring.

2. Determine the level of care and need for transfer to a burn facility.

3. Estimate the depth and percent body surface area of burns.

4. Implement fluid resuscitation protocols for children and adults.

5. Select and apply appropriate dressings and topical antibacterials.

6. Manage systemic effects of the burn wound in the critically injured surgical patient, considering:

   a. Sepsis

   b. Gastrointestinal (GI) effects

   c. Immunologic problems

   d. Cardio-respiratory effects

   e. Abdominal compartment syndrome

7. Manage treatment of inhalation injury:

   a. Flexible laryngotracheoscopy

      b.   Ventilator management

8.   Manage carbon monoxide poisoning.

9.   Manage wound therapy, including:

      a.   Eschar formation and slough

      b.   Re-epithelization

      c.   Tangential and fascial excision

      d.   Debridement of deep tissues

      e.   Skin graft harvest and application

10.   Evaluate electrical burns, including:

      a.   Entrance and exit wound

      b.   Cardiac, vascular, neurologic, ophthalmologic effects

      c.   Deep tissue destruction

      d.   Rhabdomyolysis

11.   Institute treatment of chemical burns, including:

      a.   Identification of types and sources

      b.   Management by dilution or neutralization

      c.   Treatment of systemic effects of local chemicals

12.   Manage eschar contracture and edema control:

      a.   Techniques of escharotomy

      b.   Techniques of fasciotomy

13.   Manage the treatment of the burned child, including initial therapy, systemic support, and special care needs with input from the pediatric intensive care team, including child abuse.

14.   Direct clinical management and supervision of the burn team.

Practice-Based Learning and Improvement that involves investigation and evaluation of their own patient care, appraisal and assimilation of scientific evidence, and improvements in patient care.

INFORMATION TECHNOLOGY AND POPULATION COMPARISONS REFERENCES

Cheatham ML. Intra-abdominal hypertension and abdominal compartment syndrome. In: Nelson LD (ed). New Horizons: New Advances in the Care of Critically Injured Patients. Hagerstown , MD : Lippincott Williams & Wilkins, Spring 1999;96-115.

Chung KC, Wilkins EG, Rees RS, et al. Skin and subcutaneous tissue review in general surgery. In: O'Leary JP (ed). The Physiologic Basis of Surgery (2nd ed). Baltimore : Williams and Wilkins, 1996;561-580.

Goodwin CW, Finkelstein JL, Madden MR. Burns. In: Schwartz SI (ed)., Principles of Surgery (6th ed). New York : McGraw-Hill, Inc., 1994;225-278.

Jordan BS, Harrington DT. Management of the burn wound, burn management. Nursing Clin of N Amer 1997;32(2):251-273.

Kokoska ER, Wainwright DI, Parks DH. Pathophysiology of thermal injury. In: Miller TA (ed), Modern Surgical Care: Physiologic Foundations and Clinical Applications (2nd ed). St. Louis : Quality Medical Publishing, Inc., 1998;1313-1336.

Ramzy PI, Barret JP, Herndon DN. Thermal injury. Crit Care Clin 1999;15(2):333-352.
Sheridan RL, Tompkins RG. Burns. In: Greenfield LJ, Mulholland M, Oldham KT, Zelenock GB, Lillemoe KD (eds), Surgery: Scientific Principles and Practice (2nd ed). Philadelphia : Lippincott-Raven, 1997;422-438.
http://www.ameriburn.org

Yowler W, Fratianne RB. Current status of burn resuscitation. Clin Plast Surg 2000;27(1):1-10.

11.3A GERIATRIC BURNS

UNIT OBJECTIVES:

Demonstrate an understanding of the epidemiology and pathophysiology of burn injury in the elderly patient.

Demonstrate the ability to apply these concepts to the evaluation and therapeutic management of the elderly burn patient.

Medical Knowledge about established and evolving biomedical, clinical, and cognate (e.g. epidemiological and social-behavioral) sciences and the application of this knowledge to patient care.

1.   Describe the age-related changes in the anatomy and functional characteristics of the skin and adnexa.
2.   Define the extent and depth of thermal injury as a percent of the body surface injured, and use specific anatomical terms to describe the depth of injury.
3.   Discuss the fluid resuscitation and clinical stabilization of the elderly burn patient as a function of the above description of the burn wound.
4.   Define and describe fluid shifts and physiologic derangements associated with the burn injury as a function of age.
5.   Describe the management of the burn wound including the use of topical antimicrobial agents, biologic dressings, and skin grafts in the elderly burn patient.
6.   Review the special problems of electrical, chemical, and drug- related injury to the skin.
7.   Describe the morbidity and mortality rates in elderly burn patients and the impact of inhalation injury on these rates.
8.   Review the epidemiology and socioeconomic factors associated with burn injuries in the elderly patient.
9.   Describe the prevention of burn injuries in elderly patients.
10.   Describe the physiologic changes and limitations that occur as aging progresses.
11.   Describe the role of the multidisciplinary team in the support and rehabilitation of the elderly burn patient.

12. Describe the techniques and indications for skin grafting using spit and full thickness grafts from elderly and atrophic skin.

13. Outline the factors in withholding or withdrawing care in geriatric burn patients.

Practice-Based Learning and Improvement that involves investigation and evaluation of their own patient care, appraisal and assimilation of scientific evidence, and improvements in patient care.

INFORMATION TECHNOLOGY AND POPULATION COMPARISONS REFERENCES

Cadier MA, Shakespeare PG. Burns in octogenarians. Burns 1995;21:200-204.

Deitch ES. A policy of early excision and grafting in elderly burn patients shortens the hospital stay and improves survival. Burns 1985;12:109-114.

Harrington DT, Pruitt BA, Jr. Thermal injuries. In: Adkins RB, Jr., Scott HW, Jr. (eds), Surgical Care for the Elderly (2nd ed). Philadelphia : Lippincott-Raven Publishers, 1998;439-456.

Lewandowski R, Pegg S, Fortier K, Skimmings A. Burn injuries in the elderly. Burns 1993;19:513-515.

Matsumura H, Sugamata A. Aggressive wound closure for elderly patients with burns. J Burn Care Rehabil 1994; 15:18 -23.

Saffle JR, Davis B, Williams P, et al. Recent outcomes in the treatment of burn injury in the US : a report from the American Burn Assn patient registry. J Burn Care Rehabil 1995;16:219-232.

Saffle JR, Larson CM, Sullivan J, Shelby J. The continuing challenge of burn care in the elderly. Surgery 1990;108:534-543.

SECTION 11.4   MINIMAL ACCESS SURGERY

UNIT OBJECTIVES:

Demonstrate an understanding of the applications and risks of minimal access surgery (MAS).

Demonstrate an understanding of the technical and physiologic principles of minimal access surgical techniques.

Develop specific technical skills and demonstrate proficiency in performance of basic laparoscopy, laparoscopic cholecystectomy, and other minimal access procedures.

Synthesize the principles of minimal access surgery into a practice philosophy conducive to the development and evaluation of future surgical techniques.

Medical Knowledge about established and evolving biomedical, clinical, and cognate (e.g. epidemiological and social-behavioral) sciences and the application of this knowledge to patient care.

Section One: Overview

1.   Differentiate between conventional open and scope-assisted surgery, including:

   a.   Anesthetic considerations

   b.   Effects of pneumoperitoneum

   c.   Cardiovascular stability

   d.   Need for team participation

   e.   Differences in patient outcome

2.   Discuss the physical limitations imposed on the user participating in minimal access surgery, including:

   a.   Surgeon fatigue and diminished proficiency over time

   b.   Two-dimensional perspective

   c.   Visual limitations of scope and monitoring equipment

   d.   Crucial importance of patient position and cannula position for optimum exposure

3.   Understand strategies to offset the difficulties suggested in #2 above, including:

   a.   Proper alignment of eye-camera-instrument axes

b.   Efficient biomechanics

c.   Effective use of assistants

d.   Appropriate use of other advanced technologies such as endoscopic ultrasound

4.   Analyze the factors affecting the decision to select a minimal access approach (as opposed to an open surgical approach) for a particular clinical problem.

5.   Explain the concept of the learning curve, and discuss the need for quality control in the education and evaluation of surgical house staff in developing proficiency in minimal access surgery.

6.   Explain the mechanics and principles for safe and effective use of the following equipment/procedures:

a.   Cautery (monopolar and bipolar)

b.   Ultrasonic shears

c.   Laser

d.   Telescopic direction (straight and angled laparoscope)

e.   Insulation technique and hazards

f.   Maintaining visualization of operative field

g.   Dissecting and knot tying

7.   Discuss appropriate anesthetic management for minimal access (MA) techniques for surgery involving the abdomen, thorax, and joints and soft tissue spaces.

8.   Summarize areas of current investigation in MAS, including:

a.   Virtual reality

b.   Use of robots/robotics

c.   Three-dimensional imaging systems

d.   Dissection techniques for soft tissues

9.   Summarize protocols for appropriate cleaning, sterilization, maintenance, and handling of MA equipment.

10.   Discuss the potential economic impact of increased utilization of operating room time, advanced equipment, and disposable instruments on health care costs.

Section Two: Basic Laparoscopic Skills

1. Discuss techniques for gaining access to the abdomen, including:

    a. Veress needle

    b. Open (Hassan cannula)

    c. Direct visualization trocars

2. Describe the sequence of steps involved in establishing a pneumoperitoneum, including:

    a. Selection of first puncture site

    b. Initial entry via Veress needle or Hassan cannula

    c. Tests to confirm entry into peritoneum

    d. Initial insufflation

    e. Initial exploration of abdomen

    f. Placement of additional trocars

3. Discuss indications for and limitations of diagnostic laparoscopy, as well as pros and cons of this diagnostic technique compared with other diagnostic modalities such as CT scan or ultrasound.

4. Discuss recognition and management of complications, including major vascular injury, massive Carbon dioxide embolus, or visceral injury.

5. List contraindications for laparoscopic surgery, and be able to explain why these conditions are considered relative or absolute contraindications.

Section Three: Laparoscopic Cholecystectomy (LC)

1. Discuss the indications and contraindications for laparoscopic cholecystectomy.

2. Describe the technical aspects of preparing for and operating on a patient undergoing LC.

3. Identify major considerations for the decisions involved in converting from laparoscopic to open cholecystectomy, including:

    a. Difficulty identifying anatomy (i.e., common duct)

    b. Poor visibility

    c. Hemorrhage control

4. Select management options for handling bile duct injuries, including immediate and delayed diagnosis and treatment.

5. Specify the indications and technique for percutaneous cholangiography, endoscopic ultrasound, and common bile duct exploration (CBDE), including use of choledochoscopy.

6. Discuss management of the patient with common duct stones, including:

   a. Choice of approach (open common duct exploration, versus laparoscopic CBDE, versus LC followed by/preceded by endoscopic stone extraction)

   b. Timing of surgery

   c. Safety and cost-effectiveness of each approach

Section Four: Additional Laparoscopic Procedures

1. Describe current theories, including advantages and disadvantages, regarding the use of laparoscopic anti-reflux procedures and myotomies.

   a. Discuss advantages and limitations of thoracoscopic versus laparoscopic approach for esophagomyotomy.

   b. Discuss indications and contraindications for addition of partial fundoplication to esophagomyotomy.

   c. Describe management of paraesophageal hernia.

2. Outline the potential benefits and limitations to:

   a. Laparoscopy-assisted colectomy

   b. Pre- and trans- peritoneal groin hernia repairs

   c. Laparoscopic ventral hernia repair

   d. Appendectomy

3. Summarize other intra-abdominal laparoscopic procedures currently being performed, including:

   a. Adrenalectomy

   b. Gastrectomy

     c.   Splenectomy

     d.   Donor nephrectomy

Section Five: Thoracoscopic Procedures

1. Identify the potential applications of thoracoscopic surgery, including:

     a.   Pulmonary resection

     b.   Lung biopsy

     c.   Pleurectomy/decortication

     d.   Esophageal surgery

     e.   Sympathectomy

2. Discuss anesthetic management of a patient undergoing thoracoscopy.
3. Discuss pros and cons of thoracoscopic versus open surgery for pulmonary disease.

Patient Care that is compassionate, appropriate, and effective for the treatment of health problems and the promotion of health.

Junior Level:

1. Provide assistance in laparoscopic surgery (e.g., manage camera, first assist).
2. Demonstrate familiarity with laparoscopic equipment, including setup and trouble-shooting:

     a.   Insufflator

     b.   Camera

     c.   Video equipment

3. Demonstrate understanding of basic principles of patient positioning and room setup for diagnostic laparoscopy and LC.
4. Perform entry of body cavities using open (Hassan cannula) and closed (Veress needle) access techniques.

5. Recognize when satisfactory pneumoperitoneum has been achieved. Demonstrate familiarity with danger signs (e.g., hypotension, hypercarbia) and appropriate action when patient does not tolerate pneumoperitoneum.

6. Perform MAS procedures of increasing complexity under supervision, including:
    a. Diagnostic laparoscopy
    b. LC
    c. Laparoscopic appendectomy
    d. Other procedures not requiring suturing or other advanced techniques

7. Demonstrate facility with laparoscopic suturing and knot-tying using a box trainer or other simulator.

8. Demonstrate the ability to convert from an MA to an open approach in a variety of surgical settings.

9. Perform appropriate preoperative work-up, and supervise postoperative care of patients undergoing laparoscopic procedures.

Senior Level:

1. List equipment needed for complex procedures, select instruments needed, set up room (including patient position) and equipment, troubleshoot equipment when malfunction occurs.

2. Demonstrate facility in endoscopic knot-tying, stapling, and suturing, either in a box-trainer, an animal model, or the operating room.

3. Participate in increasingly complex procedures under supervision, such as:
    a. Laparoscopic hiatal hernia repair
    b. Laparoscopic surgery for achalasia
    c. Laparoscopic splenectomy
    d. Laparoscopic inguinal hernia repair

4. Demonstrate understanding of uses of endoscopic ultrasound and other intraoperative adjuncts.

5. Complete additional MAS training as necessary through specialized courses at the home or outside institution to certify one's proficiency in performing currently practiced and widely accepted procedures.

Practice-Based Learning and Improvement that involves investigation and evaluation of their own patient care, appraisal and assimilation of scientific evidence, and improvements in patient care.

INFORMATION TECHNOLOGY AND POPULATION COMPARISONS REFERENCES

Arregui ME, Fitzgibbons RJ, Jr, Kathourda N, et al. Principles of Laparoscopic Surgery: Basic and Advanced Techniques. New York: Springer-Verlag, 1995.

Brunt LM, Soper NJ. Laparoscopic surgery. In: Zinner MJ, Schwartz SI, Ellis H (eds), Maingot's Abdominal Operations (10th ed). CT: Appleton & Lange 1997;239-285.

Cameron JL (ed). Minimally invasive surgery. Current Surgical Therapy (6th ed). St. Louis: Mosby, 1998;1159-1250.

Ogunbiyi OA, Fleshman JW. Colorectal cancer and laparoscopic colorectal surgery in the elderly patient. In: Zenilman ME, Soper NJ (eds), Gastrointestinal surgery in the elderly. Problems in General Surgery 1996;13(3):154-162.

SAGES. Curriculum Guide for Resident Education in Surgical Endoscopy. Santa Monica, CA: Society American Gastrointestinal Endoscopic Surgeons, 1998:1-25.

Scott-Conner CEH. Minimal access surgery (Parts I and II). Surg Cl of N Amer August and October, 2000.

Scott-Conner CEH (ed). The SAGES Manual: Fundamentals of Laparoscopy and GI Endoscopy. New York: Springer Verlag, 1998.

Zucker KA (ed). Surgical Laparoscopy (2nd ed). Philadelphia: Lippincott Williams & Wilkins, 2001.

http://www.bgsm.edu/surg-sci/atlas/atlas.html

http://www.laparoscopy.com

http://www.laparoscopy.net

SECTION 11.5   ORGAN TRANSPLANTATION

UNIT OBJECTIVES:

Demonstrate an understanding of the history of clinical transplantation and interpret the guidelines for preparing patients for organ transplantation.

Demonstrate a working understanding of the fundamental immunologic principles governing organ transplantation and immunosuppression.

Demonstrate understanding of the potential metabolic, physiologic, and malignant side effects of immunosuppressants.

Medical Knowledge about established and evolving biomedical, clinical, and cognate (e.g. epidemiological and social-behavioral) sciences and the application of this knowledge to patient care.

Section One: Background/Preparation

1.   Demonstrate a working knowledge of the history and evolution of clinical transplantation, including:

     a.   Early vascular surgery

     b.   Concept of tolerance

     c.   First successful organ transplants

     d.   Introduction of immunosuppressive agents

2.   Describe the anatomic and biologic terms associated with organ transplantation, donor and recipient relationships, and grafting between species.

3.   Explain the human leukocyte antigen (HLA) complex, including its genetic location and composition, pattern of inheritance, and the difference between Class I and II antigens of the major histocompatibility complex (MHC). Consider these aspects:

     a.   Serological determination HLA

     b.   Molecular methods of HLA

     c.   Cross matching

4. Discuss the role of tissue typing in the identification and preparation of patients for organ transplantation to include:

    a. Natural, pre-formed antibodies

    b. Acquired antibodies

    c. The role of panel reactive antibody (PRA) (sensitization)

    d. The effect of tissue typing compatibility on graft survival

5. Discuss advanced age as a <u>positive</u> consideration in solid organ transplantation by considering the importance of:

    a. Physiologic status vs. absolute age in years

    b. Rates of organ rejection and its severity among the elderly

    c. Elderly compliance with medical regimens

    d. Extended life expectancy

6. Compare the 5-year survival for patients aged 60 and older receiving a renal transplant with those undergoing dialysis.

7. Define the criteria for organ and tissue donation; apply these criteria to critically ill patients.

8. Explain the clinical definition of brain death, including a discussion of the available laboratory and radiologic studies to support the clinical criteria.

9. Analyze and formulate a plan for management of the organ donor.

10. Outline the development of organ preserving solutions and techniques, and describe the currently practiced methods for handling and storing vascularized organs.

<u>Section Two: Clinical Transplantation</u>

1. Discuss the current method for the allocation of organs for transplantation, including consideration of the need, availability, and philosophical biases surrounding organ donation. (Be prepared to utilize the algorithm for assigning organs based on the results of HLA typing, PRA, blood type, age, and time-waiting.)

2. Explain the united organ sharing (UNOS) method for assigning organs to potential recipients. Discuss how local procurement agencies function to optimize the donor organ pool and facilitate coordination of organ harvesting and their subsequent distribution.

3. Analyze and outline the indications for kidney, pancreas, heart, and lung transplant; relate the relative frequency of these operations as well as rates of patient and graft survival.

4. Specify the various drug schemes for induction, maintenance, and rejection therapy, including new "rescue" therapies.

5. Describe the mechanism of action, dosing schedule, and side effects of the following immunosuppressive drugs:

   a. Azathioprine

   b. Prednisone

   c. Anti-lymphocyte globulin

   d. Cyclosporine

   e. Anti-T3 monoclonal antibody

   f. Tacrolimus (FK506)

   g. Anti IL-2R Moab

   h. Mycophenolate mofetil

   i. Rapamycin

6. Analyze the short- and long- term risks of chronic immunosuppression:

   a. Opportunistic infections   d. Lymphoproliferative disease

   b. Cardiovascular problems   e. Rejection

   c. Autoimmune diseases

7. Evaluate the diagnostic maneuvers to detect hyperacute, acute and chronic organ rejection.

8. Acute and chronic renal failure:
   Causes

   a. Pathophysiology

   b. Treatment options

   c. Complications

9.   Indications and contraindications for: Kidney transplantation

Cadaveric and live kidney donation

     e.   Anatomy

     f.   Kidney anatomy and anomalies

     g.   Implantation site

     h.   Immunology

     i.   HLA matchings

     j.   Cytotoxic cross match

     k.   Rejection

     l.   Immunosuppression

     m.   Principles of pre-op preparation and post-op management

Patient Care that is compassionate, appropriate, and effective for the treatment of health problems and the promotion of health.

1.   Evaluate potential candidates for living-related and cadaveric vascularized organ transplantation, including:

     a.   Clinical suitability

     b.   Strength of social support

     c.   Expected graft and patient survival

2.   Participate in the pre- and post- operative surgical management of patients after vascularized organ transplant.

3.   Assist/perform kidney, pancreas, and heart transplantation.

4.   Participate in the perioperative management of immunosuppressive drug therapy, including monitoring drug levels and treating potential toxicities.

5.   Participate in the evaluation of patients suspected of organ rejection to include:

     a.   Laboratory and radiologic testing

     b.   Administration of immunosuppressive (IS) agents

     c.   Following patients for potential acute and chronic side effects

6. Participate in the preparation and handling of multiple organ harvest in the brain dead patient.

7. Define suitability characteristics of organs for transplantation.

8. Formulate a response to these ethical questions:

    a. Should an individual with renal disease, who is 70-75 years old, have access to the scarce resource of cadaver kidneys?

    b. Should the surgeon reasonably consider renal transplantation in older recipients when the nephrologist contends that dialysis is the preferred method of treatment?

9. Manage postoperative surgical complications, including wound infection, anastomotic stenoses and leaks, and lymphocele formation.

10. Manage post-op care

    a. Investigations

        (1) Fluid management

        (2) Drug therapy

        (3) Renal biopsy

    b. Identify and treat post-op complications

        (1) Vascular complications

        (2) Ureteric complications

        (3) Rejection

        (4) Infection

        (5) Drug side effects

11. Technical Skills and Procedures

    a. Kidney transplant-donor operation-cadaver

    b. Kidney transplant-donor operation-live donor

    c. Kidney transplant-complete operation

Practice-Based Learning and Improvement that involves investigation and evaluation of their own patient care, appraisal and assimilation of scientific evidence, and improvements in patient care.

INFORMATION TECHNOLOGY AND POPULATION COMPARISONS
REFERENCES

Albrechtsen D, Leivestad T, Sodal G, et al. Kidney transplantation in patients older than 70 years of age. Transplant Proc 1995;27:986-988.

Bromberg JS, Punch JD, Merion RM, et al. Transplantation and immunology. In: Greenfield LJ, Mulholland M, Oldham KT, Zelenock GB, Lillemoe KD (eds), Surgery: Scientific Principles and Practice (2nd ed). Philadelphia : Lippincott-Raven, 1997;527-632.

Cecka JM, Terasaka PI. Optimal use of older donor kidneys: older recipients. Transplant Proc 1995;27:801-802.

Diethelm AG, Deierhoi MH, Barber WH, et al. Organ transplantation in clinical surgery. In: Davis JH, Sheldon GF (eds), Clinical Surgery (2nd ed). St. Louis : Mosby/Multimedia, 1995:880-914.

Faubert PF, Porush JG. Renal Disease in the Elderly (2nd ed). New York : Marcel Dekkar, Inc., 1998;1-488.

Flye MW. Atlas of Organ Transplantation. Philadelphia : WB Saunders Co., 1994.

Ghobrial RM, Kahan BD. Physiologic basis of transplantation. In: Miller TA (ed), Modern Surgical Care: Physiologic Foundations and Clinical Applications (2nd ed). St. Louis : Quality Medical Publishing, Inc., 1998;110-148.

Greenfield LJ, Mulholland M, Oldham KT, Zelenock GB, Lillemoe KD (eds). Transplantation and immunology. Surgery: Scientific Principles and Practice (3rd ed). Philadelphia : Lippincott-Raven, 2001:518-632

Haisch CE, Verbanac KM. Immunity and the immunocompromised patient. In: Miller TA (ed), Modern Surgical Care: Physiologic Foundations and Clinical Applications (2nd ed). St. Louis : Quality Medical Publishing, Inc., 1998;83-109.

Janeway CA , Travers P, Walport M, Shlomchik M (eds). Immunobiology. New York : Garland Publishing, 2001.

Kahan BD, Ponticelli C. Principles and Practice of Renal Transplantation. Malden , MA : Blackwell Science, 2000.

Morris PJ. Kidney Transplantation: Principles and Practice (5th ed). Philadelphia : WB Saunders Co., 2001.

Norman DJ, Turka LA. Primer on Transplantation. Mt. Laurel , NJ : American Society of Transplantation, 2001.

Richie RE, Pierson RN, III, Fox M, et al. Solid organ transplantation. In: Adkins RB, Jr., Scott HW, Jr. (eds), Surgical Care for the Elderly (2nd ed). Philadelphia : Lippincott-Raven Publishers, 1998;477-490.

Rohrer RJ. Basic immunology for surgeons. In: O'Leary JP (ed), The Physiologic Basis of Surgery (2nd ed). Baltimore : Williams and Wilkins, 1996;141-152.

Schaubel D, Desmeules M, Mao Y, et al. Survival experience among elderly end-stage renal disease patients—a controlled comparison of transplantation and dialysis. Transplantation 1995;60:1389-1394.

Vivas CA, Hickey DP, Jordan ML, et al. Renal transplantation in patients 65 years old or older. J Urol 1992;147:990-993.

http://www.unos.org

SECTION 11.6   SURGICAL ONCOLOGY

UNIT OBJECTIVES:

Demonstrate understanding of the biology, pathology, diagnosis, treatment, and prognosis of neoplastic diseases.

Demonstrate proficiency in diagnosis, preparation, operative treatment, and total management of the cancer patient, including long-term follow-up care.

Understand surgical options of curative and palliative care for cancer patients.

Understand the network of community resources and their functions, available to patients at end of life.

Knowledge of general surgical support needed in the management of conditions affecting the reticulo-endothelial and haemopoetic systems.

Lymphatic conditions: Knowledge of the general surgical support needed in the management of conditions affecting the Lymphatic system. Simple lymph node biopsy.

Conditions involving the spleen: Knowledge of the general surgical support needed in the management of conditions affecting the spleen.

Medical Knowledge about established and evolving biomedical, clinical, and cognate (e.g. epidemiological and social-behavioral) sciences and the application of this knowledge to patient care.

<u>Junior Level</u>:

1.   Discuss frequency/death rates of the top five benign and malignant neoplasms in men, women, and children in the United States.

2.   Describe trends of increasing, decreasing, and high incidence for certain solid neoplasms.

3.   Explain the implications of the heterogeneous cellular makeup of most solid neoplasms with reference to clinical behavior and response to adjuvant treatment.

4.   Discuss the mechanisms of cellular apoptosis and the potential feasibility for therapeutic applications.

5.   Identify genetic factors associated with neoplastic disease in regard to known proto-oncogenes.

6.   Define current theories of carcinogenesis.

7. Summarize the tenets of tumor biology, including the biochemical events of invasion and metastasis; describe the natural history of these lesions.

8. Identify and differentiate between the diagnostic features of benign versus malignant neoplasms (gross and microscopic).

9. Predict patterns of presentation of malignant neoplasms.

10. Describe the characteristics of the various staging systems and explain their use in evaluating malignant neoplasms.

11. Outline the appropriate usage of tumor markers, tumor excretory metabolites, and diagnostic cytologic techniques.

12. Describe the principles of surgical technique for operative procedures designed for cure of malignant diseases and their application to endoscopic operative techniques.

13. Summarize the nutritional requirements for cancer patients, and describe how they differ from those recommended for a healthy patient.

14. Describe indications for curative versus palliative treatment, and formulate therapeutic plans for each approach.

15. Outline the status of the current predominant investigative work in cancer immunotherapy.

16. Explain the rationale for the use of heat shock proteins in conjunction with immunology.

17. Summarize current techniques of genetic screening for cancer.

18. Describe the biologic rationale, mechanisms, and current status of gene therapy for malignancy.

19. Describe the enzymatic determinants of prognosis for epithelial derived cancers and their biologic sources.

20. Discuss the economic and psychosocial issues associated with malignant disease, and analyze how they affect the management of patients with cancer, including:
    a. Ethics of cancer management
    b. Rehabilitation
    c. Home care resources
    d. Patient support groups
    e. Family support groups
    f. Enterostomal therapy

g.   Cost containment

h.   Pre-admission procedures and authorization

i.   Conservation of in-patient resources

j.   Special problems of the elderly

k.   Tumor registry data

21.   Identify available social service and community agency resources to address the issues
        listed in #20 above.

22.   Lymphatic conditions:

a.   Non-Hodgkin's Lymphoma

b.   Lymphadenopathy

c.   Hodgkin's disease

d.   Staging classifications

23.   Conditions involving the spleen: Indications for elective splenectomy-hemolytic anemia,
        ITP

a.   Thrombocytopenia, myeloproliferative disorders

b.   Indications for emergency splenectomy

c.   Sequelae of splenectomy

d.   Splenic conditions

e.   Thrombophilia

Senior Level:

1.   Apply clinical screening for common malignancies. Recognize typical presentations and
        clinical manifestations for different types of neoplasms.

2.   Describe the stimuli for and the biologic events in angiogenesis and the potential
        therapeutic implications thereof.

3.   Discuss the known facts relative to tumor suppressive genes and the implications of
        mutations.

4. Stage specific neoplasms both clinically and pathologically, including the tumor, nodes, and metastasis system (TNM).

5. Relate tumor staging to prognosis.

6. Describe differences in presentation, treatment, and outcomes for malignancy in older patients.

7. Compare each applicable treatment modality to the prognosis for tumors within the scope of general surgery.

8. Apply post-treatment screening/surveillance for common malignancies.

9. Discuss the known facts relative to tumor recurrence after local resection of a primary lesion of the breast and colon with regard to survival.

10. Identify margins of resection and how this relates to local recurrence.

11. Describe the indications for and actions of pharmacologic support in the postoperative state.

12. Describe the indications and means for implementing nutritional support in the pre- and post- operative cancer patient.

13. Explain the fundamental principles of radiation oncology and detail its application as a primary therapy for the treatment of selected benign and malignant lesions.

14. Summarize the indications and appropriate modalities for adjuvant therapy within the scope of general surgery, including chemotherapy, radiation therapy, immunotherapy, and gene therapy.

15. Describe radioimmunoguided surgery (RIGS) and its clinical applications.

16. Explain the rationale and methodology employed in lymphatic mapping and sentinel node biopsies along with the expected level of positive findings.

17. Understand the surgical options for venous access and oncologic care, and their risks/complications.

18. Describe the criteria and necessary procedures for intraoperative monitoring of cardiovascular and pulmonary functions of the cancer patient.

19. Analyze and explain a holistic approach to the treatment of patients with cancer.

20. Analyze the medical preparation of patients for cancer surgery to include the correction of metabolic and nutritional deficits.

21. Indicate the potential alterations in pulmonary function in the elderly patient which may affect preoperative preparation and postoperative management.

22. Identify the indications of anticipated need in elderly patients for:

    a. Postoperative urinary tract decompression

    b. Nutritional support

    c. Thromboembolism prophylaxis

23. Define and apply the criteria for palliative versus curative treatment plans.

24. Analyze and explain the rationale for combined adjuvant modalities in the prevention and treatment of cancer recurrence.

25. Apply proper clinical and demographic data to the tumor registry.

26. Outline the indications for and initiate requests for appropriate consultation.

27. Demonstrate a working knowledge of prior research milestones, current research efforts, and cancer research methodology.

Patient Care that is compassionate, appropriate, and effective for the treatment of health problems and the promotion of health.

Junior Level:

1. Perform a complete history and physical examination on patients with cancer.

2. Formulate an appropriate differential cancer diagnosis, and record an independent, written diagnosis for each cancer patient assigned.

3. Excise benign lesions of skin, dermal appendages, and breast. Demonstrate proper wound care and follow-up management.

4. Excise skin cancers, demonstrating proper wound margins and appropriate wound closure and follow-up management.

5. Close wounds following major resections.

6. Manage colostomies and ileostomies.

7. Design an appropriate nutritional support program for a cancer patient both pre- and post-operatively.

8. First assist on colostomies, ileostomies, and wedge resections of lung and liver.

9. Perform lymph node biopsies, breast biopsies, and procedures of similar magnitude.

10. Cut en bloc gross surgical specimens.

11. Interpret frozen section slides with supervision.

12. Perform nutritional assessments and plan nutritional support programs.

13. Perform feeding gastrostomies and tube jejunostomies.

14. Record clinical and pathological correlations by presenting the clinical picture and operative findings on each assigned cancer patient.

15. Perform all varieties of endoscopy (upper and lower gastrointestinal) and bronchoscopy.

16. Lymphatic conditions:

    Planning appropriate diagnostic tests

17. Conditions involving the spleen:

    a. Planning appropriate treatment schedule in consultation with hematologist

    b. Technical Skills and Procedures

Senior Level:

1. Demonstrate the capability for independent function in all aspects of cancer patient management, including palliative care planning.

2. Prepare and defend the preoperative assessment plan for the elderly patient in preparation for:

    a. Gastric resection

    b. Colon resection

    c. Pancreatic resection (Whipple Procedure)

    d. Mastectomy

3. Stage specific neoplasms clinically and pathologically using the TNM system.

4. Prepare patients medically for cancer surgery, including correction of nutritional and metabolic deficits.

5. Specify and prepare management plans for nutritional support in the elderly patient. Indicate differences to be expected in requirements compared to patients less than 50 years of age.

6.   Assess the need and institute appropriate monitoring both pre- and post- operatively.

7.   Use appropriate support from pharmacologic agents.

8.   Prepare an operative plan for treatment of malignant disease.

9.   Perform colostomies, colostomy closures, and bowel anastomoses of all types.

10.   Demonstrate proficiency in the use and interpretation of operative and endoscopic ultrasonography.

11.   Demonstrate proficiency in fine-needle and core biopsies of the breast.

12.   Demonstrate proficiency in endoscopic ultrasonography for detection of hepatic metastases and depth of invasion of colorectal lesions.

13.   Demonstrate proficiency in gamma probe-directed or dye-directed sentinel lymph node biopsy for breast cancer and melanoma.

14.   Assume responsibility for managing the psychosocial aspects of neoplastic disease.

15.   Perform, with appropriate supervision, major resections in neck, chest, abdomen, breast, and extremity, including complex operative procedures (e.g., Whipple procedures, construction of ileal loop bladder, major neck dissections, segmental and lobar hepatic resections).

16.   Utilize appropriate social agencies and support groups in cancer patient management.

17.   Assume teaching responsibilities for junior residents as assigned.

18.   Use laser therapy, photodynamic therapy, and cryotherapy when indicated, observing proper precautions.

19.   Participate in a multidisciplinary tumor board.

Practice-Based Learning and Improvement that involves investigation and evaluation of their own patient care, appraisal and assimilation of scientific evidence, and improvements in patient care.

INFORMATION TECHNOLOGY AND POPULATION COMPARISONS
REFERENCES

Ackerman RJ, Vogel RL, Johnson LA, et al. Morbidity, mortality, and functional outcome. J Fam Pract 1995;40:129-135.

Baile W, Lenzi R, Kudelka A, et al. Communicating bad news: outcome of a workshop for oncologists. J Cancer Educ 1997;12:166-173.

Balducci L (ed). Geriatric Oncology. Philadelphia: JB Lippincott, 1992;1-409.

Buckman R. What You Really Need to Know About Cancer—A Comprehensive Guide for Patients and Their Families. Baltimore: Johns Hopkins University Press, 1997.

Cameron JL (ed). Current Surgical Therapy (7^h ed). St. Louis: Mosby, 2001.

Clement DG, Retchin SM, Brown RS, et al. Access and outcomes of elderly patients enrolled in managed care. JAMA 1994;271:1487-1492.

Eilber FC, Eilber FR. Soft tissue sarcoma. In: Cameron JL (ed). Current Surgical Therapy (7^h ed). St. Louis: Mosby, 2001;1213-1217.

Girgis A, Sanson-Fisher W. Breaking bad news: consensus guidelines for medical practitioners. J Clin Oncol 1997;13:2449-2456.

Krag DN. Minimal access surgery for staging regional lymph nodes: the sentinel-node concept. Current Problems in Surgery 1998;35(11):953-1016.

Lange JR. Melanoma. In: Cameron JL (ed). Current Surgical Therapy (7th ed). St. Louis: Mosby, 2001;1208-1212.

McMasters KM, Wong SL, Edwards MJ, et al. Factors that predict the presence of sentinel lymph node metastasis in patients with melanoma. Surgery 2001;130:151-156.

Mulholland MW, Longo WE, Vernava AM, III. Neoplastic disorders of the gastrointestinal tract. In: Miller TA (ed), Modern Surgical Care: Physiologic Foundations and Clinical Applications (2nd ed). St. Louis: Quality Medical Publishing, Inc., 1998;668-687.

Niederhuber JE, Crooks D. Neoplastic disease: pathophysiology and rationale for treatment. In: Miller TA (ed), Modern Surgical Care: Physiologic Foundations and Clinical Applications (2nd ed). St. Louis: Quality Medical Publishing, Inc., 1998;220-249.

Nyhus LM, Baker RJ, Fischer JE (eds). Mastery of Surgery (3rd ed). Boston: Little, Brown and Co., 1997.

Obrand DI, Gordon PH. Results of local for rectal carcinoma. Can J Surg 1996;39:463-468.

Quirt CF, McKillop WJ, Ginsberg AD, et al. Do doctors know when their patients don't? Survey of doctor/patient communication in lung cancer. Lung Cancer 1997;18:1-20.

Reinhold RB, Doherty FJ, Mele FM, et al. Selected technologies and general surgery. In: O'Leary JP (ed), The Physiologic Basis of Surgery (2nd ed). Baltimore: Williams and Wilkins, 1996;618-644.

Roberts CS, Cox CE, Reintgen DS, et al. Influence of physician communication on newly diagnosed breast patients' psychologic adjustment and decision-making. Cancer 1994;74:336-341.

Suzuki K, Dozois RR, Devine RM, et al. Curative reoperation for locally recurrent rectal carcinoma. Dis Colon Rectum 1996; 39:730-736.

Townsend CM, Jr., Beauchamp RD, Evers BM, Mattox KL (eds). Sabiston Textbook of Surgery (16th ed). Philadelphia: WB Saunders Company, 2001.

Velanovich V. Preoperative screening based on age, gender, and concomitant medical diseases. Surgery 1994;115:56-61.

Watters JM, Kirkpatrick SM, Hopbach D, et al. Aging exaggerates the blood glucose response to total parental nutrition. Can J Surg 1996;39:481-485.

Watters JM, Moulton SB, Clancy SM, et al. Aging exaggerates glucose intolerance following injury. Trauma 1994;37:786-791.

Weidner N, Folkman J, Pozza F, et al. Tumor angiogenesis: a new significant and independent prognostic indicator in early-stage breast carcinoma. J Natl Cancer Inst 1992;84:1875-1887.

Woltering EA, Holder WD, Jr, Edney JA, et al. Oncology. In: O'Leary JP (ed), The Physiologic Basis of Surgery (2nd ed). Baltimore: Williams and Wilkins, 1996;153-183.

http://www.cancer.gov/cancer_information

http://www.cancer.org

http://www.surgonc.org

SECTION 11.7　　　**BREAST SURGERY**

UNIT OBJECTIVES:

Demonstrate knowledge of the anatomy, physiology, and pathophysiology of the breast.

Demonstrate the ability to surgically manage diseases of the breast.

Understand the advancements of minimally invasive and conservative breast surgeries.

Assess and manage breast abscess and mastitis.

Medical Knowledge about established and evolving biomedical, clinical, and cognate (e.g. epidemiological and social-behavioral) sciences and the application of this knowledge to patient care.

Junior Level:

1.　　Describe the anatomy of the breast.

2.　　Explain the hormonal regulation of the breast.

3.　　Summarize the incidence, epidemiology, and risk factors associated with breast cancer.

4.　　Distinguish between these common entities in the differential diagnosis of breast masses:

a.	Fibroadenomas	d.	Fibrocystic disease
b.	Cysts	e.	Fat necrosis
c.	Abscesses	f.	Cancer

5.　　Explain the general indications, uses, and limitations of mammography. Define the importance and impact of screening mammography.

6.　　Discuss the principles and historic context of the basic options available for the treatment of breast cancer such as:

a.　　Radical mastectomy

b.　　Modified mastectomy

c.　　Lumpectomy and axillary dissection

7.　　Outline the genetic and environmental factors associated with carcinoma of the breast.

8.　　Describe the following pathological types of breast cancer, including the biology, natural history, and prognosis of each:

　　　　　255

a.   Infiltrating ductal carcinoma

b.   Ductal carcinoma in situ (DCIS)

c.   Infiltrating lobular carcinoma

d.   Lobular carcinoma in situ

9.   Describe the presentation, natural history, pathology, and treatment of the following benign breast diseases:

      a.   Lactational breast abscess

      b.   Chronic recurring subareolar abscess

      c.   Intraductal papilloma

      d.   Atypical epithelial hyperplasia

      e.   Fibroadenoma

10.   Explain the steps in the clinical decision tree that are involved in the work-up of a breast mass.

11.   Discuss the role of mammography, needle aspiration, fine-needle biopsy, open biopsy, and mammographic needle localization and biopsy.

12.   Explain the mechanics and potential value of the stereotactic needle biopsy.

13.   Outline the diagnostic work-up and the differential diagnosis of various forms of nipple discharge.

14.   Explain the use of tumor, nodes, and metastases (TNM) staging in the treatment of breast cancer.

15.   Summarize the rationale for using a team approach to facilitate the complex discussions and explanation of options for the newly diagnosed breast cancer patient prior to definitive treatment (e.g., team of oncologist, surgeon, plastic surgeon, and radiation therapist).

16.   Explain the role of reduction and augmentation mammoplasty.

17.   Discuss several causes of gynecomastia and outline an appropriate work-up.

18.   Effects of pregnancy and lactation

19.   Imaging and role of conservative treatment

20.   Bacteriology of breast infection

Senior Level:

1.   Describe the characteristics, diagnosis, and therapy of less common lesions of the breast
        such as:

        a.   Inflammatory carcinoma   e.   Cystosarcoma phylloides
        b.   Paget's Disease   f.   Bilateral breast carcinoma
        c.   Lactiferous duct fistula   g.   Male breast carcinoma
        d.   Mondor's Disease

2.   Understand the methodologies and results of landmark breast cancer trials: B-04, B-06,
        B-17, B-24 (NSABP)
3.   Define appropriate breast conservation therapies, their benefits, and comparative
        outcomes, and compare them with modified radical mastectomy.
4.   Summarize the role of adjuvant chemotherapy and radiation therapy for the treatment of
        primary breast carcinoma.
5.   Outline the importance of estrogen and progesterone receptors in the prognosis and
        treatment of breast cancer.
6.   Describe the basic issues in the staging and treatment of metastatic breast cancer,
        including the role of:

        a.   Chemotherapy
        b.   Radiation therapy
        c.   Hormonal therapy

7.   Summarize the physiologic changes associated with pregnancy, including breast
        problems peculiar to pregnancy. Theorize appropriate management of breast cancer
        diagnosed during pregnancy.
8.   Formulate plans for basic patient care, including pre-, intra-, and post- operative care.
9.   Summarize the major considerations for post-mastectomy breast reconstruction.
10.   Identify and analyze the data addressing controversial areas of breast disease, such as:

a.   Current concepts in the management of cancer

b.   Cancer prevention techniques, such as tamoxifen and raloxifene

c.   Role of various adjuvant therapy programs.

d.   Biological behavior of lesions such as lobular carcinoma in situ

e.   Benefit and frequency of screening mammograms

f.   Relationship of mammographic parenchymal patterns to the risk of subsequent malignancy

11.   Review and evaluate the following areas of research in breast disease:

a.   Role of breast cancer susceptibility genes

b.   Monoclonal antibodies

c.   Other breast markers, including Her-2/neu, cathepsin D, and flow cytometry with chromosomal analysis

12.   Explain the role of sentinel lymph node biopsy for breast cancer

a.   Sensitivity and specificity

b.   Indication and contraindications

c.   Technique

d.   Treatment plan based on findings

Patient Care that is compassionate, appropriate, and effective for the treatment of health problems and the promotion of health.

<u>Junior Level</u>:

1.   Take an appropriate history to evaluate breast patients to include:

a.   Pertinent risk factors

b.   Previous history of breast problems

c.   Current breast symptoms

2.   Demonstrate an increasing level of skill in the physical examination of the breast, including recognition of the range of variation in the normal breast.

3. Perform simple procedures such as:

    a.   Diagnostic fine-needle aspiration of cysts

    b.   Drainage of simple breast abscesses

    c.   Core needle biopsy of breast masses

    d.   Open biopsy of superficial masses

4. Identify common lesions such as fibroadenomas, cysts, mastitis, and cancer.

5. Interpret signs suspicious for malignancy on mammogram such as stellate masses or suspicious microcalcifications.

6. Perform open breast biopsies and other operative procedures such as simple mastectomy and excision of intraductal papillomas, under direct supervision.

7. Demonstrate the ability to satisfactorily orient the surgical specimen for pathologic examination.

8. Determine the indications and special requirements for tissue processing for estrogen and progesterone receptors.

9. Educate patients to perform breast self-examination.

10. Demonstrate familiarity with male breast problems, including gynecomastia and male breast cancer.

    a.   Discuss risk factors

    b.   Outline appropriate work-up and management

Senior Level:

1. Independently evaluate a new breast patient through history and physical examination, ordering appropriate and cost-effective tests such as mammogram, ultrasound, or fine-needle aspiration (FNA).

2. Formulate a diagnostic work-up and treatment plan for most common breast problems, including the common types of breast carcinomas.

3. Consult and interact with other members of the professional cancer team in explaining options to the newly diagnosed breast cancer patient.

4. Perform, under direct supervision, more advanced procedures on the breast such as:

a. Radical mastectomy

b. Modified mastectomy

c. Lumpectomy and axillary dissection

d. Sentinel lymph node biopsy

e. Excision of lactiferous duct fistula

f. Needle-localized breast biopsy

g. Simple mastectomy for gynecomastia

5. Acquire basic experience with breast reconstruction and cosmetic surgical techniques.

6. Evaluate the physical status of patients who report for evaluation of augmentation and reduction mammoplasties.

7. Prescribe various types of adjuvant therapy such as:

a. Chemotherapy

b. Hormonal therapy

c. Radiation therapy

d. Biologic response modifiers

8. Manage unusual breast diseases such as:

a. Inflammatory carcinoma

b. Paget's Disease

c. Lactiferous duct fistula

d. Mondor's Disease

e. Bilateral breast cancer

f. Male breast cancer

g. Cystosarcoma phylloides

9. Describe the evolving role of bone marrow transplantation in the management of selected breast cancer patients.

10. Outline an appropriate follow-up schedule for patients who have undergone:

a. Treatment of breast cancer with curative intent

b. Treatment of DCIS

c. Biopsy which revealed Fibroadenoma, benign epithelial hyperplasia, or fibrocystic disease with atypia

Practice-Based Learning and Improvement that involves investigation and evaluation of their own patient care, appraisal and assimilation of scientific evidence, and improvements in patient care.

INFORMATION TECHNOLOGY AND POPULATION COMPARISONS
REFERENCES

Bland KI, Copeland EM, III (eds). The Breast: Comprehensive Management of Benign and Malignant Diseases (2nd ed). Philadelphia: WB Saunders Col, 1998.

Donegan WL, Redlich PN. Breast cancer in men. Surg Clin North Amer 1996;76:343-366.

Harris JR, Lippman ME, Morrow M, et al. (eds). Diseases of the Breast. Philadelphia: Lippincott-Raven, 1996.

Hecht JR, Winchester DJ. Male breast cancer. Amer J Clin Pathol 1994;102:S25-30.

Heimann R, Powers C, Halpem HJ, et al. Breast preservation in stage I and II carcinoma of the breast: the University of Chicago experience. Cancer 1996;78:1722-1730.

McCarthy EP, Burns RB, Freund KM, et al. Mammography use, breast cancer stage at diagnosis, and survival among older women. J Am Geriatr Soc 2000;48:1226-1233.

McGreevy JM, Bland KI. The breast. In: O'Leary JP (ed), The Physiologic Basis of Surgery (2nd ed). Baltimore: Williams and Wilkins, 1996;285-311.

Schnitt SJ, Hayman J, Gelman, et al. A prospective study of conservative surgery alone in the treatment of selected patients with stage I breast cancer. Cancer 1996;77:1094-1100.

Silen W, Matory WE, Jr, Love SM. Atlas of Techniques in Breast Surgery. Philadelphia: Lippincott-Raven Publishers, 1996.

Silverstein MJ (ed). Ductal Carcinoma In Situ of the Breast. Baltimore: Williams & Wilkins, 1997.

Winchester DP, Cox JD. Standards for diagnosis and management of invasive breast carcinoma. (Amer College of Radiology, Amer College of Surgeons, College of Amer Pathologists, Soc of Surgical Oncology), CA: A Cancer Journal for Clinicians 1998;48:83-107.

Winchester DP, Strom EA. Standards for diagnosis and management of ductal carcinoma in situ (DCIS) of the breast. (Amer College of Radiology, Amer College of Surgeons, College of Amer Pathologists, Soc of Surgical Oncology), CA: A Cancer Journal for Clinicians 1998;48:108-128.

11.7A BREAST DISEASE IN THE ELDERLY PATIENT

Medical Knowledge about established and evolving biomedical, clinical, and cognate (e.g. epidemiological and social-behavioral) sciences and the application of this knowledge to patient care.

The resident should be able to:

1. Articulate currently accepted guidelines for breast cancer screening in the elderly patient.
2. Describe the demographics of breast cancer in the elderly
3. Describe currently accepted surgical treatment.
4. Discuss the use of adjuvant chemotherapy.
5. Describe the barriers that prevent adequate treatment in some elderly women.
6. Discuss appropriate modification of cancer therapy in the frail elderly woman.
7. Discuss the diagnostic evaluation of an elderly male with a breast lump.
8. Discuss the treatment of male breast cancer.
9. Discuss the role of hormonal therapy in older patients.

Practice-Based Learning and Improvement that involves investigation and evaluation of their own patient care, appraisal and assimilation of scientific evidence, and improvements in patient care.

INFORMATION TECHNOLOGY AND POPULATION COMPARISONS REFERENCES

Benhaim DI, Lopchinsky R, Tartter PI. Lumpectomy with tamoxifen as primary treatment for elderly women with early-stage breast cancer. Am J Surg 2000;180(3):162-166.

Bergman L, Van Dongen JA, van Ooijen B, et al. Could tamoxifen be a primary treatment choice for elderly breast cancer patients with locoregional disease? Breast Cancer Res Treat 1995;1:77-83.

Busch E, Kemeny M, Fremgen A, et al. Patterns of breast cancer care in the elderly. Cancer 1996;78:101-111.

Doherty GM. Management of breast cancer in the elderly. Prob Gen Surg 1996;13:110-113.

Gajdos C, Tartter PI, Bleiweiss IJ, et al. The consequence of undertreating breast cancer in the elderly. JACS 2001;192(6):698-707.

Given B, Given C, Azzouz F, Stommel M. Physical functioning of elderly cancer patients prior to diagnosis and following initial treatment. Nurs Research 2001;50(4):222-232.

Grady KE, Lemkau JP, Mc Vay JM, et al. The importance of physician encouragement in breast cancer screening of older women. Prevent Med 1992;21:766-780.

Grube BJ, Hansen NM, Ye W. et al. Surgical management of breast cancer in the elderly patient. Am J Surg 2001;182(4):359-364.

Hebert-Croteau N. Brisson J, Latreille J, et al. Compliance with consensus recommendations for the treatment of early stage breast carcinoma in elderly women. Cancer 1999;85(5):1104-1113.

Law TM, Hesketh PJ, Porter KA, et al. Breast cancer in elderly women: presentation, survival, and treatment options. Surg Clin North Am 1996;76:289-308.

McCarthy EP, Burns RB, Freund KM, et al. Mammography use, breast cancer stage at diagnosis, and survival among older women. J Am Geriatr Soc 2000;48:1226-1233.

Michalski TA, Nattinger AB. The influence of black race and socioeconomic status on the use of breast-conserving surgery for Medicare beneficiaries. Cancer 1997;79:314-319.

Mincey BA, Moraghan TJ, Perez EA. Prevention and treatment of osteoporosis in women with breast cancer. Mayo Clin Proc 2000;75(8):821-829.

Muss HB. Breast cancer in older women. Semin Oncol 1996;23:82-88.

Newschaffer CJ, Penberthy L, Desch CE, et al. The effect of age and comorbidity in the treatment of elderly women with nonmetastatic breast cancer. Arch Intern Med 1996;156:85-90.

O'Hanlon DM, Kent P, Kerin MJ, et al. Unilateral breast masses in men over 40: a diagnostic dilemma. Amer J Surg 1995;170:24-26.

Plowman PN. Adjuvant therapy in breast cancer: optimal use in the elderly. Drugs Aging 1996;9:185-190.

Repetto L, Costantini M, Campora E, et al. A retrospective comparison of detection and treatment of breast cancer in young and elderly patients. Breast Cancer Res Treat 1997;43:27-31.

Rozenberg S, Ham H, Liebens F. Screening mammography in elderly women. Research on Breast Cancer in Older Women Consortium. JAMA 2000;283(24):3203-2304.

Sandison AJ, Gold DM, Wright P, et al. Breast conservation or mastectomy: treatment choice of women aged 70 years and older. Br J Surg 1996;83:994-996.

Secreto G, Venturelli E, Bucci A, et al. Intra-tumour amount of sex steroids in elderly breast cancer patients. (An approach to the biological characterization of mammary tumours in the elderly.) J Steroid Biochem Mol Biol 1996;58:557-561.

Solin LJ, Schultz DJ, Fowble BL. Ten-year results of the treatment of early-stage breast carcinoma in elderly women using breast-conserving surgery and definitive breast irradiation. Int J Radiat Oncol Biol Phys 1995;33:45-51.

Vlastos G, Mirza NQ, Meric F, et al. Breast conservation therapy as a treatment option for the elderly. The MD Anderson experience. Cancer 2001;92(5):1092-1100.

Voogd AC, Repelaer B, van Driel OJ, et al. Changing attitudes toward breast-conserving treatment of early breast cancer in the southeastern Netherlands: results of a survey among surgeons and a registry-based analysis of patterns of care. Eur J Surg Oncol 1997;23:134-138.

Wanebo HJ, Cole B, Chung M, et al. Is surgical management compromised in elderly patients with breast cancer: Ann Surg 1997;225:579-586.

Williams JC, Helvie MA. Recommendations for mammographic screening of elderly women. AJR 2000;175(4):1182-1183.

Zenilman ME, Bender JS, Magnuson TH, et al. General surgical care in the nursing home patient: results of a dedicated geriatric surgery consult service. J Am Coll Surg 1996;183:361-370.

Zhang Y, Kiel DP, Freger BE, et al. Bone mass and the risk of breast cancer among postmenopausal women. N Engl J Med 1997;336:611-617.

SECTION 11.8   ENDOCRINE SURGERY

UNIT OBJECTIVES:

Demonstrate knowledge of endocrine anatomy and physiology, both normal and pathological.

Demonstrate the ability to apply this knowledge to the surgical care of patients.

Identify, investigate and manage surgical patients with common metabolic disorders.

Thyrotoxicosis: Identify, investigate and manage surgical patients with thyrotoxicosis.

Hypothyroidism: Identify, investigate and manage surgical patients with hypothyroidism.

Hypercalcaemia: Identify, investigate and manage surgical patients with Hypercalcaemia.

Cortico-steroid therapy: Knowledge of the significance of corticosteroid therapy in patient care.

Diabetes Mellitus: Identify, investigate and manage surgical patients with diabetes mellitus.

Hyponatremia: Identify, investigate and manage surgical patients with hyponatremia

Assessment of neck swellings.

Medical Knowledge about established and evolving biomedical, clinical, and cognate (e.g. epidemiological and social-behavioral) sciences and the application of this knowledge to patient care.

1.   Describe the normal anatomy, histology, physiology, and pertinent biochemistry of the following organs:

    a.   Thyroid gland

    b.   Parathyroid gland

    c.   Hypothalamus

    d.   Pituitary gland

    e.   Endocrine pancreas

    f.   Adrenal glands

    g.   Gastrointestinal tract as an endocrine organ

    h.   Gonads as endocrine organs

2.   Discuss fully the secretion and the control thereof of the following:

    a.   Thyroxin and thyroid stimulating hormone

b. Parathyroid hormone

c. Adrenocorticotropic hormone (ACTH)/cortisol

d. Insulin/glucagon

e. Catecholamines (epinephrine, norepinephrine, dopamine)

f. Gastrin/secretin/cholecystokinin

g. Serotonin/histamine

h. Estrogen/progesterone/testosterone (and their releasing factors)

i. Oxytocin/vasopressin

j. Growth hormone

k. Melanocyte stimulating hormone

l. Prolactin

m. Motilin/gastric inhibitory peptide/enteroglucagon/vasoactive intestinal peptide

n. Somatostatin

3. Summarize the following aspects of endocrine pathology:

a. The criteria for the diagnosis of malignancy

b. Chromosomal abnormalities as a screening/diagnostic tool

c. The unique characteristics about the clinical epidemiology of patients with sporadic versus familial disease

d. Define and differentiate multiple endocrine neoplasia (MEN) type I, MEN II, and familial non-MEN syndromes

e. Fine-needle aspiration biopsy

f. DNA ploidy

4. Explain the integrated concept of clinical neuroendocrinology, the cells and organs of the amine precursor uptake decarboxylase (APUD) system, and the known clinical endocrine syndromes.

5. Outline the approach to the surgical management of diseases of the endocrine systems:

a. Is the treatment of each disease primarily surgical or medical?

b. Is surgical treatment different for benign versus malignant disease?

c. Is surgical treatment curative or palliative?

d. Is surgical treatment directed at the target organ or primary organ?

e. What role does lesion localization play in endocrine disorders?

6. Discuss the pathophysiology, clinical presentation, work-up, and treatment of the following diseases:

a. A solitary thyroid nodule

b. A multinodular thyroid gland

c. Thyrotoxicosis

d. Primary, secondary, and tertiary hyperparathyroidism

e. Insulinoma/glucagonoma/vipoma

f. Zollinger-Ellison syndrome

g. Gastrointestinal carcinoid tumors

h. Endogenous hypercortisolism (Cushing's syndrome vs. Cushing's disease; secondary to pituitary, adrenal, and ectopic causes)

i. Pheochromocytoma

j. Primary hyperaldosteronism

l. The incidentally discovered adrenal mass

m. Galactorrhea

n. Gigantism/dwarfism

7. Discuss the preoperative preparation/management of the following:

a. Hypercalcemic crisis

b. Thyroid "storm"

c. Grave's disease/Hashimoto's disease

d. Pheochromocytoma

e. Hyperaldosteronism

f. Endogenous hypercortisolism

g. Insulinoma/gastrinoma

h. Carcinoid syndrome

i. Adrenal insufficiency crisis

8.   Outline the differential diagnosis of:

    a.   Hypercalcemia

    b.   Hypoglycemia

    c.   Hypergastrinemia

    d.   Elevated serum thyroxin level

    e.   A decreased sensitive thyroid stimulating hormone (TSH) level

    f.   Elevated ACTH levels

9.   Discuss corticosteroid administration for elderly patients for diseases more common in that population. Explain the following disease entities as they relate to problems in the elderly patient:

    a.   Cushing's syndrome

    b.   Exogenous hypercortisolism

    c.   Chronic alcohol abuse

    d.   Chronic intake of self-administered "arthritis pills"

10.   Discuss the surgical approaches to:

    a.   The left adrenal gland

    b.   The right adrenal gland

    c.   The anterior pituitary gland

    d.   The head of the pancreas

    e.   The body/tail of the pancreas

    f.   The inferior parathyroid glands

    g.   The superior parathyroid glands

    h.   A retrosternal goiter

11.   Identify and discuss areas of endocrine surgery in which patient management is controversial and areas in which change is taking place, including:

    a.   Zollinger-Ellison syndrome

    b.   Thyrotoxicosis

    c.   Genetic screening for neuroendocrine syndromes

d.   Minimally invasive parathyroidectomy

12.   Summarize key physiologic alterations of the neuroendocrine system that occur with normal aging. Include explanation of these alterations that can occur with advancing age:

    a.   Plasma noradrenaline concentrations increase

    b.   Steady decrease in aldosterone secretion

    c.   Plasma renin activity declines

    d.   Plasma cortisol levels significantly increase

13.   Summarize significant issues in the management of anesthesia in endocrine surgery, including:

    a.   Airway management during neck surgery

    b.   Cardiovascular manipulation during thyroid and pheochromocytoma operations

    c.   Special attention to electrolyte management

14.   Critique the role of the following developments in the surgical management of endocrine problems:

    a.   Localizing modalities (e.g., metaiodobenzylguanine [MIBG], sestamibi, selective venous sampling, intraoperative tumor localization, rapid parathyroid hormone [PTH] assays)

    b.   Diagnostic assays (e.g., sensitive TSH, C-peptide, fine needle aspiration)

15.   Causes of enlargement of salivary glands / thyroid gland incl. thyroglossal cyst / lymph nodes / other (vascular, skin & soft tissue incl. branchial cyst)

Patient Care that is compassionate, appropriate, and effective for the treatment of health problems and the promotion of health.

Junior Level:

1.   Complete a preliminary evaluation of patients suspected of having endocrine disease to include:

a. Focused history

b. Family history

c. Physical examination

d. Appropriate relevant diagnostic studies

2. Participate in the pre- and post- operative care of patients undergoing endocrine surgery.

3. Observe endocrine surgery cases.

4. Perform a detailed evaluation of patients with suspected endocrine disease.

5. Manage the pre- and post- operative care of patients with endocrine disease, under supervision.

6. Observe and assist in surgery of the thyroid, parathyroid and adrenal glands, as well as those of the pancreas.

7. Spend quality time working under the direct supervision of a cytopathologist in the surgical pathology laboratory.

8. Investigation of neck swellings including diagnostic imaging, ENT assessment, pathology and biochemistry.

9. Biopsy-FNA : Lymph node biopsy-cervical

Senior Level:

1. Develop a comprehensive plan for the surgical management of endocrine disease.

2. Perform or assist in the performance of adrenal, pancreas, thyroid, and parathyroid surgery.

3. Evaluate patients with complex endocrine disease and present a differential diagnosis.

4. Perform surgery on the adrenals, pancreas, thyroid, and parathyroids.

5. Independently manage the diagnosis, pre- and post- operative care, and surgery for a variety of endocrine surgery cases.

6. Understand the indications for minimally invasive parathyroidectomy.

Practice-Based Learning and Improvement that involves investigation and evaluation of their own patient care, appraisal and assimilation of scientific evidence, and improvements in patient care.

INFORMATION TECHNOLOGY AND POPULATION COMPARISONS

REFERENCES

Brunt LM, Halverson JD. The endocrine system. In: O'Leary JP (ed), The Physiologic Basis of Surgery (2nd ed). Baltimore: Williams and Wilkins, 1996;312-348.

Cameron JL (ed). Endocrine glands. Current Surgical Therapy (7th ed). St. Louis: Mosby, 2001;620-677.

Clark OH. Endocrine Surgery of the Thyroid and Parathyroid Glands. St. Louis: CV Mosby Company, 1985.

Costello D, Norman J. Minimally invasive radioguided parathyroidectomy. Surg Oncol Clin N Amer 1999;8(3):555-564.

Edis AJ, Grant CS, Egdahl RH. Manual of Endocrine Surgery (2nd ed). New York: Springer-Verlag, 1984.

Greenfield LJ, Mulholland M, Oldham KT, Zelenock GB, Lillemoe KD (eds). Surgical endocrinology. Surgery: Scientific Principles and Practice (2nd ed). Philadelphia: Lippincott-Raven, 1997;1283-1415.

Miller TA (ed). The endocrine system. Modern Surgical Care: Physiologic Foundations and Clinical Applications (2nd ed). St. Louis: Quality Medical Publishing, Inc., 1998;1089-1236.

Van Heerden JA, Grant CS. Diseases of the adrenal glands: surgical aspects. In: Adkins RB, Jr., Scott HW, Jr. (eds), Surgical Care for the Elderly (2nd ed). Philadelphia: Lippincott-Raven Publishers, 1998;411-426.

Van Heerden JA, Young WF Jr, Grant CS, et al. Adrenal surgery for hypercortisolism: surgical aspects. Surgery 1995;117:466-472.

Whitman ED, Norton JA. Endocrine surgical diseases of elderly patients. In: Zenilman ME, Roslyn JJ (eds), Surgery in the elderly patient, Surg Cl of N Amer 1994;74(1):127-144.

http://www.aace.org

http://www.endocrinology.org

SECTION 11.9   ABDOMINAL SURGERY

UNIT OBJECTIVES:

Demonstrate an understanding of the anatomy, physiology, pathophysiology, and presentation of diseases of the abdominal cavity and pelvis.

Demonstrate the ability to formulate and implement a diagnostic and treatment plan for diseases of the abdomen and pelvis that are amenable to surgical intervention.

Can safely recognize acute appendicitis as a cause of the acute abdomen.

Diagnosis and management of abdominal wall hernia, including operative management of primary inguinal hernia.

Recognize and initiate treatment for most strangulated hernia, operation with assistance.

Strangulated inguinal hernia: Recognize and treat strangulated inguinal hernia, including operation for a straightforward case.

Strangulated femoral hernia: Recognize and initiate treatment for strangulated femoral hernia.

Strangulated incisional hernia: Recognize and initiate treatment of strangulated incisional hernia

Diagnosis and treatment of abdominal wall masses.

Medical Knowledge about established and evolving biomedical, clinical, and cognate (e.g. epidemiological and social-behavioral) sciences and the application of this knowledge to patient care.

<u>Junior Level</u>:

1.   Describe the embryological development of the peritoneal cavity and the positioning of the abdominal viscera.

2.   Diagram the anatomy of the abdomen including its viscera and anatomic spaces:

    a.   Musculoskeletal envelope

    b.   Lesser sac

    c.   Subphrenic spaces

    d.   Morrison's pouch

    e.   Foramen of Winslow

    f.   Pouch of Douglas

    g.   True pelvis

275

h.   Lateral gutters

i.   Contents of the retroperitoneum

j.   Major lymph node groups and their drainage

3.   Surgical outcome is dependent on coexistent disease. Describe changes in the following organ systems that result from the aging process:

a.   Heart   d.   Brain

b.   Lung   e.   Hematopoietic system

c.   Kidney   f.   Gastrointestinal tract

4.   Explain absorption and secretory functions of the peritoneal surfaces and the diaphragm.

5.   Describe the anatomy of the omentum and its role in responding to inflammatory processes.

6.   Assess the following signs associated with the acute abdomen and describe their pathophysiology:

a.   Referred pain   c.   Guarding

b.   Rebound tenderness   d.   Rigidity

7.   Specify characteristics of the history, physical examination findings, and mechanism of visceral and somatic pain for the following processes:

a.   Acute appendicitis   d.   Ureteral colic

b.   Bowel obstruction   e.   Diffuse peritonitis

c.   Perforated ulcer   f.   Biliary colic

8.   List possible distinctions in the presentation and examination of the elderly patient with the following causes of acute abdomen:

a.   Perforated viscus

b.   Cholecystitis

9.   Discuss the differences in the physiologic response to stress in the geriatric patient.

10.   Explain the mechanism of referred pain in:

a.	Ruptured spleen	d.	Renal colic
b.	Biliary colic	e.	Pancreatitis
c.	Basilar pneumonia	f.	Inguinal hernia

11. Discuss the following causes of paralytic ileus:

   a. Postoperative electrolyte imbalance

   b. Retroperitoneal pathology

   c. Trauma

   d. Extraperitoneal disease (central nervous system, lung)

12. Illustrate use of the following diagnostic studies in the work-up of each process in #7 and #10 above:

   a. Laboratory evaluation

   b. Urinalysis

   c. Plain x-rays

   d. Contrast gastrointestinal (GI) studies

   e. Ultrasound

   f. Computed axial tomography (CAT)

   g. Biliary studies

   h. Renal studies

13. When considering the possibility of wound complications:

   a. What are the risk factors for abdominal wound infection?

   b. What are the contributing factors for abdominal wound dehiscence and evisceration?

   c. What are the usual clinical presentations and timing?

   d. What is the incidence of wound infection in surgeries involving the biliary tree, upper GI tract, and colon?

   e. List wound complications that are more problematic in the elderly patient.

14. Identify the anatomic locations for the following intra-abdominal abscesses; name disease process(es) associated with each:

    a. Left subphrenic space   f. Pelvis

    b. Right subphrenic space   g. Left paracolic gutter

    c. Subhepatic space   h. Right paracolic gutter

    d. Lesser sac   i. Psoas muscle

    e. Interloop

15. Differentiate between the conditions favoring percutaneous drainage versus operative drainage for each of the abscesses in #14. Describe the safest and most effective approach using each technique

16. Differentiate between the following intestinal fistulas and the organs to which they most often communicate:

    a. Esophageal   c. Enteric (including duodenal)

    b. Gastric   d. Colonic

17. Explain the formation of fistulas in each of the following disease processes or factors:

    a. Operative complications (bowel injury with abscess formation)

    b. Inflammatory bowel disease

    c. Acute pancreatitis

    d. Foreign body or prosthetic material

    e. Malignancy

18. Explain the role of a fistulogram in the diagnosis of intra-abdominal fistulas and abscesses.

19. List the factors that prevent healing of a fistula.

20. Summarize the conditions favoring operative versus non-operative treatment for fistulas listed in #16.

21. Describe the anatomy, clinical presentation, and complications of non-operative management for these hernias:

    a. Direct and indirect inguinal, femoral, and obturator

b.   Sliding hiatal

c.   Paraesophageal

d.   Ventral

e.   Umbilical

f.   Spigelian

g.   Paraduodenal

h.   Richter's

i.   Lumbar and Petit

j.   Parastomal

k.   Diaphragmatic

      (1)   Posterolateral (Bochdalek)

      (2)   Anterior (Morgagni)

      (3)   Traumatic

l.   Internal

22.   Name the hernia types that are most common in elderly patients, and explain how they may become problematic.

23.   Define a Richter's hernia and describe its clinical presentation.

24.   Define a sliding hernia and describe its repair.

25.   Differentiate between incarceration and strangulation.

26.   Strangulated inguinal hernia: Anatomy of inguinal region including inguinal canal, femoral canal, abdominal wall and related structures e.g. adjacent retroperitoneum and soft tissues

27.   Pathophysiology of strangulated hernia

28.   Postoperative complications of repair of strangulated hernia

29.   Strangulated femoral hernia:

30.   Pathology of the acute and chronic conditions; Hematoma, Sarcoma, Desmoid Tumors

31.   Principles of management of Desmoid tumors and sarcomas

32.   Treatment options

Current methods of operative repair including open mesh, laparoscopic mesh and posterior wall plication, to include the underlying principles, operative steps, risks, benefits, complications and process of each

Senior Level:

1. Summarize the surgical procedures available for repair of the hernias listed in #21 above.

2. Outline the uses of prosthetic material and management of infection for incisional or recurrent hernias involving prosthetic material.

3. Construct a plan for the diagnosis and potential for surgical repair of the following congenital abdominal wall defects:

   a. Gastroschisis   c. Diastasis Recti

   b. Omphalocele

4. Discuss the management of umbilical hernia in infants.

5. Describe the indications for contralateral exploration in the repair of an inguinal hernia in an infant.

6. Explain the operative approaches for each of the following, including laparoscopic:

   a. Abdominal cavity: liver/biliary tract, spleen, small bowel, large bowel, and pelvis

   b. Retroperitoneal organs: kidneys, pancreas, adrenal glands, abdominal aorta

   c. Thoracoabdominal aorta

   d. Pericardial sac

7. Outline the techniques for wound closure (including type of suture material) for each of the incisions named in #6 immediately above.

8. Describe the use and method of placement of retention sutures.

9. Explain the rationale for and mechanics of techniques of peritoneal dialysis in:

   a. Renal failure

   b. Management of peritoneal infections or pancreatitis

10. Assess the treatment of secondary peritoneal infections due to peritoneal dialysis catheters.

11.	Describe the pathophysiology and treatment of ascites in:

    a.	Malignancy

    b.	Hepatic disease: cirrhosis, Budd Chiari Syndrome

    c.	Chylous leak

    d.	Pancreatic leak

    e.	Cardiac disease

    f.	Renal disease

    g.	Bile leak

12.	Explain the indications for use and complications of peritoneo-venous shunts.

13.	Describe the etiology, manifestations, and treatment of:

    a.	Desmoid tumors

    b.	Rectus sheath hematoma

    c.	Retroperitoneal fibrosis

14.	Describe the more common retroperitoneal tumors, sarcomas, and liposarcomas. (What are their clinical presentations, treatments, and prognoses?)

Patient Care that is compassionate, appropriate, and effective for the treatment of health problems and the promotion of health.

<u>Junior Level</u>:

1.	Perform, record, and report complete patient evaluation and assessment.

2.	Evaluate and diagnose the acute abdomen.

3.	Assist with hernia repairs in the groin or umbilicus, demonstrating a basic understanding of the anatomy and surgical repair.

4.	Interpret the following in coordination with attending radiologists and staff:

    a.	Acute abdominal series (identify free air, small bowel obstruction, ileus, colonic pseudo-obstruction, volvulus; the presence of ascites, atelectasis vs. pneumonia)

    b.	Upper GI series

    c.	Barium enema (identify neoplasms, signs of ischemia)

  d. Abdominal ultrasound and CT scans

5. Evaluate and institute management of abdominal wound problems, including:

  a. Infection

  b. Evisceration

  c. Fasciitis

  d. Dehiscence

6. Coordinate pre- and post- operative care for the patient with the acute abdomen.

7. Institute drainage for abdominal wall fistula and protection of surrounding structures, especially skin.

8. Assist in closure of abdominal incisions; exhibit competency in suture technique.

9. Natural history of appendicitis

10. Pathophysiology of appendicitis

11. Effects of overwhelming sepsis and its management

12. Strangulated inguinal hernia:

13. History and examination to identify strangulated hernia

14. Resuscitation

15. investigation of possible strangulated inguinal hernia

16. Operative strategy for strangulated inguinal hernia

17. Postoperative management

18. Strangulated femoral hernia:

  a. History and examination to identify strangulated hernia

  b. Resuscitations

  c. Investigation of possible strangulated femoral hernia

19. Operative strategy for strangulated femoral hernia

  Postoperative management

20. Strangulated incisional hernia:

  a. History and examination

  b. Resuscitation

  c. Investigation of possible strangulated incisional hernia

21. Operative strategy

  Postoperative management

22. Technical Skills and Procedures

  a. Hernia repair-epigastric

  b. Hernia repair-femoral

  c. Hernia repair-incisional

  d. Hernia repair-incisional recurrent

  e. Hernia repair-inguinal

  f. Hernia repair-inguinal recurrent

  g. Hernia repair-umbilical/paraumbilical

<u>Senior Level</u>:

1. Open and close abdominal incisions of all varieties.

2. Treat wound complications such as infections and evisceration. Use retention sutures appropriately.

3. Assist with thoracoabdominal and retroperitoneal exposures for access to kidneys, pancreas, aorta, iliac arteries.

4. Perform laparotomy for acute abdomen, demonstrating a systematic approach for determination of the etiology of the process via a systematic abdominal exploration and appropriate measures for its management (e.g., acute appendicitis, small bowel obstruction, perforated peptic ulcer [the 5th year resident should be able to guide the more junior resident through the case]).

5. Perform more complex laparotomies involving diffuse peritonitis in the septic patient (e.g., a gangrenous or severely inflamed gallbladder or perforated diverticulitis requiring resection).

6. Coach a junior resident through the repair of simple hernia (indirect inguinal or umbilical). (The chief resident should be able to perform repair of any of the hernias mentioned earlier in the text.)

7.   Provide appropriate surgical drainage for any intra-abdominal abscess.

8.   Serve as an effective surgical team leader.

Practice-Based Learning and Improvement that involves investigation and evaluation of their

own patient care, appraisal and assimilation of scientific evidence, and improvements in

patient care.

INFORMATION TECHNOLOGY AND POPULATION COMPARISONS REFERENCES

Adkins RB, Jr., Marshall BA. Anatomic and physiologic aspects of aging. In: Adkins RB, Jr., Scott HW, Jr. (eds), Surgical Care for the Elderly (2nd ed). Philadelphia: Lippincott-Raven Publishers, 1998;11-24.

Cameron JL (ed). Small bowel. Large bowel. Current Surgical Therapy (7th ed). St. Louis: Mosby, 2001;122-327.

Frantz MG, Norman J, Fabri PJ. Increased morbidity of appendicitis with advancing age. Amer Surg 1995;61:40-44.

Greenfield LJ, Mulholland M, Oldham KT, Zelenock GB, Lillemoe KD (eds), Small intestine. Colon, rectum, and anus. Hernia, mesentery, and retroperitoneum. Surgery: Scientific Principles and Practice (2nd ed). Philadelphia: Lippincott-Raven, 1997;805-855, 1033-1205, 1207-1281.

Maddern GJ, Hiatt JR, Phillips EH (eds). Hernia Repair: Open Vs Laparoscopic Approaches. New York: Churchill Livingstone, 1997.

Miettinen P, Pasanen P, Salonen A, et al. The outcome of elderly patients after operation for acute abdomen. Ann Chir Gynaecol 1996;85:11-15.

Miller TA (ed). Small and large intestine. Modern Surgical Care: Physiologic Foundations and Clinical Applications (2nd ed). St. Louis: Quality Medical Publishing, Inc., 1998;410-490.

Myers SI, Miller TA. Acute abdominal pain: physiology of the acute abdomen. In: Miller TA (ed), Modern Surgical Care: Physiologic Foundations and Clinical Applications (2nd ed). St. Louis: Quality Medical Publishing, Inc., 1998;641-667.

Nyhus LM, Baker RJ, Fischer JE (eds). Mastery of Surgery (3rd ed). Boston: Little, Brown and Co., 1997.

Nyhus LM, Condon RE (eds). Hernia (3rd ed). Philadelphia: Lippincott, 1989.

Nyhus LM, Vitello JM, Condon RE (eds), Abdominal Pain: A Guide to Rapid Diagnosis. Norwalk, Conn: Appleton & Lange, 1995.

Pollak R, Nyhus LM. Diagnosis and management of intestinal obstruction and herniae. In: Adkins RB, Jr., Scott HW, Jr. (eds), Surgical Care for the Elderly (2nd ed). Philadelphia: Lippincott-Raven Publishers, 1998;335-344.

Rosenthal RA. Small-bowel disorders and abdominal wall hernia in the elderly patient. In: Zenilman ME, Roslyn JJ (eds), Surgery in the elderly patient, Surg Cl of N Amer 1994;74(2):261-291.

Rosenthal RA, Schrieber ML. Small bowel and appendix. In: Zenilman ME, Soper NJ (eds), Gastrointestinal surgery in the elderly. Problems in General Surgery 1996;13(3):121-132.

Shoji BT, Becker JM. Colorectal disease in the elderly patient. In: Zenilman ME, Roslyn JJ (eds), Surgery in the elderly patient, Surg Cl of N Amer 1994;74(2):293-316.

Silen W (ed). Cope's Early Diagnosis of the Acute Abdomen (19th ed). New York: Oxford University Press, 1996.

Skandalakis JE, Gray SW (eds). Hernia: Surgical Anatomy and Technique. New York: McGraw-Hill, Inc., 1989.

Suzuki K, Dozois RR, Devine RM, et al. Curative reoperation for locally recurrent rectal carcinoma. Dis Colon Rectum 1996; 39:730-736.

Townsend CM, Jr. (ed). Sabiston Textbook of Surgery: the Biological Basis of Modern Surgical Practice (16th ed). Philadelphia: WB Saunders Co., 2001.

Zinner MJ, Schwartz SI, Ellis H (eds). Maingot's Abdominal Operations (10th ed). CT: Appleton & Lange 1997; vols I-II.

SECTION 11.10   ALIMENTARY TRACT AND DIGESTIVE SYSTEM

UNIT OBJECTIVES:

Demonstrate an understanding of the anatomy, physiology, and pathophysiology of the alimentary tract and digestive system.

Demonstrate the ability to manage problems of the alimentary tract and digestive system that are amenable to surgical intervention.

Recognize and manage acute intestinal obstruction, including supervised laparotomy in straightforward cases

Initial assessment of patients with GI bleeding and the basics of their ongoing care.

Blood loss and Hypotension: Understanding of the pathophysiology of blood loss and its emergency management.

Recognition of cause of gastrointestinal bleeding: Ability to assess the likely cause of GI bleeding and arrange investigation.

Treatment: Initial treatment and arranging investigations for GI bleeding.

Postoperative care: Supervised postoperative care of patients who have had surgery for GI bleeding.

Complications: Knowledge of complications of GI bleeding and recognition of rebleeding.

Diagnosis and management of simple perforated peptic ulcer, including operation.

Diagnosis and preop management: Diagnosis of perforated peptic ulcer.

Operative and Postoperative management: Operation for simple perforated peptic ulcer cases

Basic knowledge of the management of stomas in consultation with stoma care nurses.

Indications for stomas: Understanding of the indications for stomas.

Preoperative Evaluation for stomas: Competency in the preoperative care of a patient requiring a stoma.

Stoma creation and closure: Some experience in construction of an ileostomy and a colostomy.

Postoperative Care: Basic postoperative care of patients after stoma formation.

Complications: Knowledge of some complications of stoma formation.

Stoma Management: Usual management of stomas in consultation with stoma care nurses.

Stoma Physiology: Knowledge of the physiology of different stomas.

Patient Education and Counselling: Knowledge of the effect of a stoma on medication absorption.

Basic understanding of the diagnosis and the emergency surgical treatment of inflammatory bowel disease.

Inflammatory Bowel Disease-Etiology: Knowledge of the Etiology of inflammatory bowel disease.

Inflammatory Bowel Disease-Epidemiology: Knowledge of the epidemiology of inflammatory bowel disease.

Inflammatory Bowel disease-Clinical manifestations: Recognition of the clinical manifestations of inflammatory bowel disease.

Inflammatory Bowel Disease-Differential diagnosis: Understanding of the means of diagnosing inflammatory bowel disease.

Ulcerative colitis-Medical management: Basic medical management of ulcerative colitis in consultation with gastroenterology.

Ulcerative colitis- surgical management: Knowledge of the indications for emergency surgical treatment of ulcerative colitis.

Crohn's disease-medical management: Basic medical management of Crohn's disease in consultation with gastroenterology.

Crohn's disease-complications: Knowledge of the complications of Crohn's disease which might require emergency surgery.

Crohn's disease -surgical management: Basic knowledge of the commonest surgical procedures for Crohn's disease

Crohn's Disease-anorectal: Emergency management of anorectal Crohn's disease.

Other inflammatory conditions-ischemic colitis: Understanding of the Etiology and management of ischemic colitis.

Other inflammatory conditions-radiation bowel disease: Awareness of radiation bowel disease.

Other inflammatory conditions-infectious colitis: Diagnosis and management of infectious colitis in consultation with infectious disease physicians.

Fecal Incontinence- Epidemiology: Understanding of the epidemiology of fecal incontinence.

Fecal Incontinence-Evaluation: Ability to make an initial suggestion of the type of incontinence after history and examination.

Fecal Incontinence- Non-operative Management: Simple conservative management of fecal incontinence.

Rectal Prolapse: Knowledge of the epidemiology and incidence of rectal prolapse.

Constipation-General Consideration: Understanding of causes and treatment of simple constipation.

Constipation-Specific Conditions- Motility Disorders: Basic management of colonic pseudo-obstruction.

Irritable Bowel Syndrome: Competency in the management of irritable bowel syndrome.

Diverticular Disease: Diagnosis of diverticular disease, elective medical management and initial emergency management of complications.

Volvulus: Diagnosis of possible colonic volvulus

Rectal bleeding: Ability to appropriately investigate rectal bleeding

Massive lower GI bleeding: Resuscitation and initial management of massive lower GI tract bleeding

Colon Trauma: Diagnosis of colon trauma

Rectal Trauma: Recognition of possible rectal trauma

Foreign Bodies: Evaluation of patients with rectal foreign bodies.

Epidemiology of Colorectal Cancer and Polyps: Knowledge of the epidemiology of colorectal cancer and polyps.

Etiology: Knowledge of the Etiology of colorectal neoplasia.

Colorectal Cancer Screening: Knowledge of the principles of colorectal cancer screening.

Clinical Presentation: Recognize the symptoms and signs of colorectal cancer at different sites.

Staging and Prognostic Factors: Understanding of staging and prognostic factors for colorectal cancer.

Management of Colon Cancer: Knowledge of the principles of management of colon cancer.

The Detection and Treatment of Recurrent and Metachronous Colon: Knowledge of the risks and patterns of recurrent colorectal cancer and basic palliative care.

Miscellaneous Malignant Lesions of the Colon and rectum: Diagnosis and surgical treatment of the more common manifestations of carcinoid tumor.

Anal Neoplasia: Knowledge of the pathophysiology of anal neoplasia.

Competency in the diagnosis and some medical and surgical treatments of common benign anorectal disease.

Hemorrhoids: Diagnosis and the outpatient treatment of hemorrhoids.

Anal Fissure: Diagnosis and the medical treatment of anal fissure.

Abscess and fistula: Diagnosis and management of simple perineal abscess.

Hidradenitis Suppurativa: Diagnosis of hidadrenitis suppuritiva.

Pilonidal Disease: Diagnosis and the medical and surgical treatment of pilonidal disease.

Anal Stenosis: Knowledge of the Etiology of anal stenosis.

Pruritus Ani: Diagnosis and the medical management of pruritis ani.

Sexually Transmitted Diseases: Diagnosis and the medical and surgical treatment of condylomata acuminata.

Medical Knowledge about established and evolving biomedical, clinical, and cognate (e.g. epidemiological and social-behavioral) sciences and the application of this knowledge to patient care.

<u>Junior Level:</u>

1. Define the basic scientific principles of the alimentary tract and digestive system diseases to include:

    a. Anatomy, embryology, and biochemistry of the gastrointestinal (GI) tract

        (1) Embryologic development of primitive foregut and hindgut and its appendages, including normal rotation and fixation

        (2) Histology of alimentary tract, including differentiation of cell types

        (3) Anatomy of alimentary tract from esophagus to anus with emphasis on systemic blood supply, portal venous drainage, neural-endocrine axis, and lymphatic drainage

        (4) Abdominal anatomy, explaining its relationship to lower thorax, retroperitoneum, and pelvic floor

(5)

        (5)   Mucosal transport, including mechanism of absorption of nutrients and water

        (6)   Sites of electrolyte and acid-base regulation

  b.   GI physiology

        (1)   Physiology of deglutition and phases of digestion

        (2)   Neuroendocrine control of GI secretion and motility

        (3)   Regional controls of mucosal secretion and absorption (neural and hormonal)

        (4)   Enterohepatic circulation

        (5)   Neuromuscular control of defecation

        (6)   Digestion of sugars, fats, proteins, vitamins, and cofactors

        (7)   Rates of mucosal turnover

        (8)   Nutritional needs of surgical patients

        (9)   Normal secretory rates for the stomach, small bowel, biliary tree, and pancreas

  c.   Normal bacterial flora and their concentrations in the upper and lower GI tract

  d.   Immunologic properties of the GI tract and how this barrier is affected by: trauma, sepsis, burns, malnutrition, and chronic disease.

  e.   Principles of intestinal healing

        (1)   Normal GI tissue integrity and strength and how this relates to healing of anastomoses

        (2)   Effects of suturing and stapling techniques of the gut

2.   Explain and give examples for the following aspects of gastrointestinal diseases:

  a.   Infections inside and outside the GI tract from esophagus to anus, including the peritoneum

  b.   Embryologic abnormalities of the GI tract, including:

(1)	Strictures	(4)	Atresias
(2)	Stenoses	(5)	Duplications
(3)	Webs	(6)	Malrotations

  c.   Congenital and acquired abnormalities of gut motility

d. Neoplasia of the GI tract

e. Ulceration of the proximal and distal GI tract

f. Causes of GI obstruction

g. Causes of paralytic ileus

h. Causes of GI hemorrhage

i. Causes of GI perforation

j. Causes of abdominal abscess formation or secondary peritonitis

k. Short gut and malabsorptive conditions

l. Acute and chronic mesenteric ischemia

m. Portal hypertension and venous thrombosis

n. Inflammatory bowel diseases

o. Causes of an acute abdomen

p. Management of intestinal ostomies

q. Traumatic injury to abdominal viscera

r. Ischemic bowel

3. Discuss some of the more common diseases of the esophagus in elderly patients, to include:

a. Motility disorders   d. Inflammatory disease

b. Esophageal injuries   e. Gastroesophageal reflux

c. Diverticular disease   f. Tumors (benign and malignant)

4. Outline the essential characteristics of routine and highly specialized diagnostic evaluation of the alimentary tract, including:

a. History

    (1) Pain   (4) Prior episodes

    (2) Nausea/emesis   (5) Past surgical history

    (3) Bowel function

b. Physical examination:

    (1) Inspection   (3) Percussion

    (2) Auscultation   (4) Palpation

c.   Radiologic examinations, including:

      (1)   Barium swallow

      (2)   Upper GI Series with small bowel follow-through

      (3)   Enteroclysis

      (4)   Ultrasound

      (5)   Transesophageal echo

      (6)   Computerized Tomography

      (7)   Magnetic Resonance Imaging

      (8)   Barium enema

      (9)   Angiograms

      (10)   Nuclear scans for bleeding or to evaluate for Meckle's diverticulum

d.   Fiberoptic endoscopy

e.   Rigid anoscopy and sigmoidoscopy

f.   Tests of GI function including:

      (1)   Manometry

      (2)   pH measurement

      (3)   Gastric analysis (basal and stimulated)

      (4)   Radioisotope clearance studies

           (a)   Technetium 99m

           (b)   Technetium HIDA (hepatic 2,6-dimethyliminodiacetic acid) dynamic biliary imaging

      (5)   Gastric emptying studies

      (6)   Transit times

      (7)   Hormonal determinations

      (8)   Absorption

5.   Summarize current medical management and its potential limitations; explain the role of surgical intervention when management fails in the following:

a.   Peptic ulcer disease   d.   Gastroparesis

b.   Esophageal varices   e.   Inflammatory bowel disease

c.   Upper and lower GI bleeding   f.   Diverticulitis

6.   Etiology of intestinal obstruction

7.   Recognition of cause of gastrointestinal bleeding:

   a.   All causes of GI bleeding

   b.   Treatment options

   c.   Indications for operations

   d.   Role of endoscopic procedures and interventional radiology

8.   Postoperative care:

   a.   Fluid balance

   b.   Complications:

9   Gastro/duodenum-perforated PU closure

10.   Indications for stomas:

   a.   Indications for colostomy

   b.   Indications for ileostomy

   c.   Complications: High-output ileostomy

11.   Stoma Management:

   a.   Stoma appliances, and appropriate selection

   b.   Stoma Physiology

12.   Patient Education and Counselling:

   The possible effects that a stoma may have on medication dosage and absorption

13.   Inflammatory Bowel Disease-Etiology:

   The contribution of genetics and immune function to the development of inflammatory
   bowel disease (IBD)

14.   The possible influence of infectious agents, psychological issues and environmental
   factors Inflammatory Bowel Disease-Epidemiology

15.   The epidemiologic features of Crohn's disease and ulcerative colitis
   Inflammatory Bowel Disease-Differential diagnosis: The endoscopic, radiographic, and
   laboratory findings of ulcerative colitis and Crohn's disease

16. The distinguishing histologic characteristics of ulcerative colitis and Crohn's disease

17. The differential diagnosis of Inflammatory Bowel Disease

18. Ulcerative colitis-Medical management:

    The mechanism of action, indication, appropriate dosage, side effects, and toxicity of the   drugs used for the treatment of ulcerative colitis: aminosalicylates, corticosteroids, antibiotics

19. Ulcerative colitis- Surgical management: Be able to identify the indications for surgery for ulcerative colitis including: severe acute colitis, toxic megacolon, hemorrhage

20. Crohn's disease-medical management: The mechanism of action, indication, appropriate dosage, side effects, and toxicity of the drugs used for the treatment of Crohn's disease: aminosalicylates, corticosteroids, antibiotics

21. Other inflammatory conditions-ischemic colitis:

    a. Vascular anatomy of the colon

    b. The Etiology of acute colonic ischemia

22. Other inflammatory conditions-radiation bowel disease:
    Vascular anatomy of the colon

23. Other inflammatory conditions-infectious colitis:

    a. Epidemiology, Etiology, pathogenesis, laboratory and endoscopic evaluation, medical management and indications for surgery for clostridium difficile colitis

    b. In suspected infectious colitis understand relevance of travel history, role of stool culture, testing for ova, cysts and parasites and hot stool sample for amoebiasis, role of lower GI endoscopy with biopsy for histological evaluation and culture, role of rectal and perineal swabs, role of serology in the detection of amoebiasis and strongyloidiasis, infectious colitis as a precipitating factor for inflammatory bowel disease

24. Management of diarrhea in the immunocompromised patient including HIV

25. Fecal Incontinence-Epidemiology: Classification of the various types of incontinence, their incidence and their pathophysiology

26. Rectal Prolapse: The incidence, pathophysiology and epidemiology of rectal prolapse

27. Constipation-General Consideration:

    a. Normal colonic physiology (including gut hormones and peptides) and the process of defecation

    b. Definition of constipation and its epidemiology

    c. Classification of types and causes of constipation differential diagnosis in a patient with constipation

    d. Different types of laxatives and describe the indications, contraindications, modes of action, and complications of each: stimulant, osmotic, bulk-forming, lubricant Constipation-Specific Conditions:

    e. Common causative factors for colonic pseudo-obstruction

28. Diverticular Disease: Etiology of colonic diverticular disease

    a Incidence and epidemiology of colonic diverticular disease

    b. Complications and classification of diverticular disease including: bleeding, perforation, abscess, fistula, and stricture

29. Volvulus:

    a. Etiology of volvulus of the colon

    b. Incidence and epidemiology of volvulus of the colon

    c. Complications of colonic volvulus including obstruction, ischemia, perforation

30. Rectal bleeding:

    a. Etiology of lower GI bleeding

    b. Massive lower GI bleeding:

31. Colon Trauma:

    a. Uses and limitations of the following imaging and diagnostic tests in the evaluation of blunt abdominal trauma

        (1) Plain abdominal films

        (2) Computed tomography scan

(3) Ultrasound

(4) Peritoneal lavage

32. Rectal Trauma:

Identify clinical situations requiring evaluation for rectal trauma

33. Epidemiology of Colorectal Cancer and Polyps:

    a. Epidemiology of colorectal cancer and polyps including incidence and prevalence, influence of socio-economic, racial and geographic factors

    b. Etiological factors in colorectal neoplasia: Diet: fat, fiber, calcium, selenium, vitamins (antioxidants), dietary inhibitors, alcohol and smoking, prostaglandin inhibitors

34. Adenoma-carcinoma sequence:

    a. evidence, categorize adenomas into low risk, intermediate and high risk and discuss screening procedures, significance of metaplastic polyps

    b. Susceptibility to colorectal cancer (CRC): family history, Personal Past History (CRC, Polyps, Other Cancers), groups at risk

    c. Hereditary non-polyposis colorectal cancer (HNPCC): clinical features Familial adenomatous polyposis: clinical definition, extracolonic lesions, cancer risk

    d. Colorectal Cancer Screening: Current screening strategies for the following:

        (1) The general population

        (2) Persons at moderate risk

        (3) Persons at high risk

35. Distribution of CRC within the colon

    a. Staging and Prognostic Factors:

    b. Current staging systems (Dukes, TNM)

    c. Clinical prognostic factors: age, mode of presentation, clinical stage, blood. transfusion

    d. Histologic/biochemical features: histological grade, mucin secretion, signet-cell histology, venous invasion

e. The significance of extent of disease including patterns of spread: direct continuity, intramural, transmural, distal margins, circumferential margins, transperitoneal, lymphatic, Hematogenous implantation

36. Management of Colon Cancer:

   a. The indications and contraindications for surgical treatment

   b. Pre and post op care

   c. Operative technique

   d. Outcomes and complications of colon cancer

37. The Detection and Treatment of Recurrent and Metachronous Colon:

   a. Patterns of recurrence

   b. Risks and detection of metachronous lesions

38. Anal Neoplasia:

   a. Anatomical, Etiology, and epidemiologic features: The significance of the anatomical distinction between the anal margin and the anal canal tumors

   b. The differential lymphatic drainage of the anal canal and margin

   c. The histological transition of the anal canal

39. Hemorrhoids:

   a. Etiology of internal and external hemorrhoids

   b. Anatomical distinctions between internal and external hemorrhoids

   c. Classifications for internal hemorrhoids

   d. Modifications of therapy with: Inflammatory bowel disease (IBD), Pregnancy, HIV, Coagulopathies

40. Anal Fissure:

   a. Etiology of anal fissure

   b. Anatomical location of a classic anal fissure

41. Abscess and fistula:

    a. The origin of cryptoglandular abscess and fistula

    b. Classification of anorectal cryptoglandular abscess-based on anatomical spaces

    c. Parks classification of anal fistula

    d. The natural history of surgically-treated anal abscess, including the risk of fistula

    e. Operative strategy for anal fistula based on sphincter involvement/location

    f. Complications resulting from abscess/fistula surgery: recurrence, incontinence

42. Pilonidal Disease: Pathophysiology of pilonidal disease

43. Anal Stenosis: Etiology

44. Pruritus Ani: Etiology and clinical presentation of pruritus ani

45. Sexually Transmitted Diseases: Etiology of condylomata acuminata

<u>Senior Level</u>:

1. Specify the pathophysiology of multisystem problems of the alimentary tract and digestive system, including neurohumoral and hormonal interactions.

2. Explain the physiologic rationale for the following gastrointestinal operations:

    a. Vagotomy

    b. Pyloroplasty

    c. Gastric resection for ulcer disease and reconstructive techniques

    d. Small bowel resection with anastomosis

    e. Ostomy formation

    f. Resection of GI tract segments with nodes for tumors

    g. Bypass of GI tract segments for resectable tumors

    h. Drainage of pancreatic cysts (internal vs. external)

    i. Drainage of abdominal and retroperitoneal abscesses (percutaneous vs. operative)

3. Detail the standard intraoperative techniques and alternatives associated with each of the above operations.

4. Explain the indications and contraindications for diagnostic and therapeutic endoscopy of the alimentary tract.

5. Assess alternatives to surgical intervention in the management of complex diseases of the alimentary tract and digestive system such as:

   a. Short gut syndrome

   b. Achalasia

   c. Barrett's esophagus

   d. Intestinal polyposis

   e. Inflammatory bowel disease

   f. Seropositive status for H. pylori

   g. Multifocal atrophic gastritis in the elderly

6. Discuss the surgical ramifications of the following statement: "The expectation of more frequent vague gastrointestinal complaints by the elderly patient may delay presentation with significant illness and diagnosis."

7. Summarize the preoperative, intraoperative, and postoperative management of complex diseases of the alimentary tract and digestive system, including:

   a. Re-operative abdomen

   b. Failed peptic ulcer and reflux operation

   c. Management of post-gastrectomy syndromes

   d. High output GI fistulas

   e. Inflammatory bowel disease with strictures, pouches, ostomies, and perineal fistulas

   f. Recurrent colon malignancy

   g. Carcinomatosis

Patient Care that is compassionate, appropriate, and effective for the treatment of health problems and the promotion of health.

<u>Junior Level</u>:

1. Evaluate emergency department or clinic patients who present with problems referable to the GI tract.

2. Serve as assistant to the primary surgeon during operations of the esophagus, stomach, small intestine, colon, and anorectum.

3. Perform less complicated surgical procedures such as:

    a. Gastrostomy

    b. Meckel's diverticulectomy

    c. Appendectomy

    d. Hemorrhoidectomy

    e. Anal fissurectomy and fistulectomy

    f. Incision and drainage of perirectal abscesses

4. Accept responsibility for (under the guidance of the chief resident and attending surgeon) the postoperative management of:

    a. Nasogastric tubes

    b. Intestinal tubes

    c. Intra-abdominal drains

    d. Intestinal fistulas

    e. Abdominal incisions (simple and complicated)

5. Evaluate and manage nutritional needs (enteral and parenteral) of surgical patients until normal GI function returns.

6. Provide follow-up care to the surgical patient in the outpatient clinic or surgical office.

7. Laparotomy and division of adhesions

8. Perform stoma construction and closure

9. Postoperative Care:

    a. Appreciate the normal postoperative course for colostomy and ileostomy function

    b. Recognize the signs, symptoms and management for the following complicationa that occur in the immediate postoperative period: ischemia, mucocutaneous separation

10. Recognize and manage high-output ileostomy

11. Recognize ileostomy food obstruction

12. Stoma Management:

    a. Early postoperative management of conventional stoma

    b. Advise on various skin barriers and accessory products available for the management of stomas

    c. Advise on dietary considerations for patients with an ileostomy or a colostomy, including impact of diet on stoma output, flatus, odor, bolus obstruction

13. Stoma Physiology:

Appropriately manage fluid and electrolyte abnormalities

14. Stoma creation and closure:

    a. Ileostomy-construction

    b. Colostomy-construction

    c. Ileostomy-closure

    d. Colostomy-closure

    e. Hartmann's procedure

    f. Hartmann's reversal

15. Inflammatory Bowel disease-Clinical manifestations: Recognize and compare the clinical pattern, presenting symptoms, physical findings and natural history of ulcerative colitis and Crohn's disease.

16. The extraintestinal manifestations of IBD

17. Ulcerative colitis-Medical management: Recognize the presentation and manage proctitis, left-sided colitis, extensive colitis, severe acute colitis, toxic megacolon, Joint management of a patient unresponsive to initial treatment

18. Crohn's disease-medical management:

    a. Initial treatment specific to the site of involvement in a patient with Crohn's disease

    b. Crohn's disease-complication:

    c. Management of the following complications of Crohn's disease:

obstruction/stenosis, fistula, abscess, perforation, hemorrhage, toxic megacolon, severe acute colitis

    d.   Crohn's disease -surgical management:

    e.   Indications and contraindications, operative technique, postoperative care, functional results, risk of recurrence, and complications of operations for Crohn's disease

    f.   Crohn's Disease-anorectal: Management of the following manifestations of anorectal Crohn's disease: abscess

19.   Other inflammatory conditions- ischemic colitis:

    a.   Clinical presentation of ischemic colitis

    b.   Natural history, diagnosis, and be able to manage ischemic colitis

20.   Technical Skills and Procedures: Crohn's disease -surgical management

    a.   Colectomy - right

    b.   Ileocaecectomy for Crohn's

21.   Fecal Incontinence-Evaluation:

    a.   Take a directed history to differentiate types of incontinence

    b.   Perform a physical examination to differentiate types of incontinence

    c.   Fecal Incontinence-Non-operative Management:

    d.   Outline a non-operative bowel management plan incorporating : dietary measures

22.   Rectal Prolapse:

Clinical presentation and findings in rectal prolapse

23.   Constipation-General Consideration:

    a.   Take a directed history for a patient with constipation and perform a directed. physical examination

    b.   Constipation-Specific Conditions:

24.   Evaluate a patient with suspected colonic pseudo-obstruction

25. Irritable Bowel Syndrome: Diagnose irritable bowel syndrome and outline a medical treatment program that may include the following: diet, fibre, laxatives, prokinetic medications, enemas, suppositories, psychological support

26. Diverticular Disease:

   a. Recognize the clinical patterns (including right sided diverticular disease) presenting symptoms, physical findings and natural history of colonic diverticular disease

   b. Arrange appropriate diagnostic studies in suitable sequence in the evaluation of both acute and chronic colonic diverticular disease

   c. Medical and dietary management of colonic diverticular disease

   d. Medical management for acute diverticulitis

   e. Preoperative assessment including awareness of the indications for surgery, surgical procedures, and complications for acute diverticulitis

   f. Perioperative care for surgical procedures

27. Volvulus:

   a. Recognize the clinical patterns, presenting symptoms, physical findings, and natural history of colonic volvulus based upon its site

   b. Arrange diagnostic studies in appropriate sequence

28. Rectal bleeding:

   a. Arrange appropriate evaluation of the patient based on age and other medical conditions

   b. Assess hemodynamic stability and outline a resuscitation plan

   c. Outline an algorithm for the evaluation of lower GI bleeding including exclusion of coagulopathy, gastroscopy, colonoscopy

29. Colon Trauma:

   a. Manage the patient with penetrating abdominal trauma with understanding of the criteria for exploratory laparotomy, wound exploration, peritoneal lavage

   b. Rectal Trauma:

    c.   Diagnosis of rectal trauma and associated injuries

    d.   Foreign Bodies:

    f.   Evaluate patients with rectal foreign bodies

30.   Recognize the clinical signs and symptoms of patients presenting with colorectal cancer

    a.   The Detection and Treatment of Recurrent and Metachronous Colon:

    b.   Methods for detection of recurrence: CEA, colonoscopy, imaging

    c.   Palliative care

    d.   Miscellaneous Malignant Lesions of the Colon and rectum: Recognize the clinical presentation, assess prognostic factors, and manage carcinoid - Ileal, appendiceal, carcinoid syndrome

31.   Hemorrhoids:

    a.   Assessment of the signs and symptoms of the following: thrombosed external hemorrhoids, internal hemorrhoids by stage, skin tags

    b.   Management of hemorrhoids including the indications and contraindications for: rubber-band ligation, injection sclerotherapy, infrared coagulation, operative hemorrhoidectomy

    c.   Perform two of the OPD techniques

    d.   Manage the complications resulting from OPD management: bleeding, pain, sepsis

32.   Anal Fissure:

    a.   Assessment of the signs and symptoms of anal fissure

    b.   Arrange the nonoperative management of anal fissure, including indications, contraindications, and complications of stool modifications/softeners, topical anesthetics, topical pharmacology

    c.   Indications, contraindications, and complications of the following: lateral internal sphincterotomy, anal stretch

33. Abscess and fistula: Differentiate cryptoglandular abscess and fistula from other causes

    a. Assessment of abscess/fistula by techniques designed to elucidate pathological anatomy: Goodsall's rule and digital examination

    b. Management of anorectal abscess including preoperative and postoperative care and the appropriate procedure based on anatomical spaces

    c. Modify therapy for: Fournier's gangrene, necrotizing fasciitis

    d. Assess rectovaginal fistula in terms of Etiology and location

34. Hidradenitis Suppurativa: Assess the symptoms and signs of hidradrenitis suppurativa

35. Pilonidal Disease:

    a. Assess the symptoms and signs of pilonidal disease: abscess, sinus

    b. Perform surgical management of pilonidal disease

36. Pruritus Ani: Arrange medical management and surgical management of pruritus ani with attention to: hygiene, diet, anatomical (obesity, deep anal cleft), coexisting anal pathology, systemic disease, gynecologic-associated, infections, post antibiotic syndrome, contact dermatitis, dermatology, radiation, neoplasm, idiopathic pruritis ani

37. Sexually Transmitted Diseases:

Diagnosis of condylomata acuminate

38. Technical Skills and Procedures Hemorrhoids

    a. Hemorrhoids-OP treatment (injection, banding or infrared coagulation)

    b. Hemorrhoidectomy-operative

    c. Abscess and fistula:

    d. Abscess-drainage through perineal region

    e. Pilonidal Disease:

    f. Pilonidal sinus-lay open

    g. Pilonidal sinus-excision and suture

    h. Sexually Transmitted Diseases:

    i. Anal skin tags/warts-excision (topical chemicals) and surgical treatment options j. for condylomata acuminata

Senior Level:

1. Perform initial consultation for inpatients with problems of the GI tract; develop differential diagnosis and initiate treatment plan.

2. Assist the chief resident and attending staff with complex digestive system cases.

3. Perform, under appropriate supervision, GI operations, including:

   a. Vagotomy

   b. Pyloroplasty

   c. Gastric resection and reconstructive techniques

   d. Small bowel resection with anastomosis

   e. Drainage of pancreatic cysts

   f. Drainage of abdominal and retroperitoneal abscesses

   g. Lysis of adhesions

   h. Repair of enterotomies

   i. Colon resection

   j. Creation of ostomies

4. Develop diagnostic and therapeutic endoscopy skills such as:

   a. Diagnostic esophagogastroduodenoscopy

   b. Endoscopic control of GI bleeding

   c. Percutaneous endoscopic gastroscopy

   d. Dilation of intestinal strictures

   e. Assist with endoscopic retrograde cholangiopancreatography (ERCP)

   f. Diagnostic colonoscopy

   g. Polypectomy

5. Select and interpret appropriate pre- and post- operative diagnostic studies.

6. Assist junior residents in the diagnosis, surgical management, and follow-up care of patients with diseases of the alimentary tract and digestive system.

7. Coordinate intervention of multiple specialties that may be involved in management of complex GI problems such as:

   a. Variceal hemorrhage

b.   Biliary obstruction

   c.   Chronic varices

   d.   Inflammatory bowel disease

   e.   Chronic abdominal pain

   f.   Chronic constipation

   g.   Localized and advanced malignancies

8.   Perform appropriate re-operative laparotomy for a variety of gastrointestinal problems.

9.   Supervise postoperative care of GI and digestive tract surgical patients.

Practice-Based Learning and Improvement that involves investigation and evaluation of their own patient care, appraisal and assimilation of scientific evidence, and improvements in patient care.

INFORMATION TECHNOLOGY AND POPULATION COMPARISONS REFERENCES

Dunn JCY, Ashley SW. Surgery for esophageal disease in the elderly patient. In: Zenilman ME, Soper NJ (eds), Gastrointestinal surgery in the elderly. Problems in General Surgery 1996;13(3):44-54.

Fischer JE. Surgical Basic Science. St. Louis: Mosby/Multimedia, 1993.

Gorman RC, Morris JB, Kaiser LR. Esophageal disease in the elderly patient. In: Zenilman ME, Roslyn JJ (eds), Surgery in the elderly patient, Surg Cl of N Amer 1994;74(1):93-112.

Greenfield LJ, Mulholland M, Oldham KT, Zelenock GB, Lillemoe KD (eds). Esophagus. Stomach and duodenum. Small intestine. Surgery: Scientific Principles and Practice (2nd ed). Philadelphia: Lippincott-Raven, 1997;653-744. 745-804. 805-856.

Jaffe BM, Mason GR, Kahrilas PJ, et al. The digestive system. In: O'Leary JP (ed), The Physiologic Basis of Surgery (2nd ed). Baltimore: Williams and Wilkins, 1996;406-440.

Levine BA, Ashikari A. Malignancies of the stomach and duodenum in the elderly. In: Zenilman ME, Soper NJ (eds), Gastrointestinal surgery in the elderly. Problems in General Surgery 1996;13(3):67-74.

McFadden DW, Zinner MJ. Gastroduodenal disease in the elderly patient. In: Zenilman ME, Roslyn JJ (eds), Surgery in the elderly patient, Surg Cl of N Amer 1994;74(1):113-126.

Miller TA (ed). The alimentary tract. Modern Surgical Care: Physiologic Foundations and Clinical Applications (2nd ed). St. Louis: Quality Medical Publishing, Inc., 1998;319-727.

Peeler BB, Adkins RB, Jr, Scott HW, Jr. Diseases of the stomach and duodenum. In: Adkins RB, Jr., Scott HW, Jr. (eds), Surgical Care for the Elderly (2nd ed). Philadelphia: Lippincott-Raven Publishers, 1998;277-290.

Schaefer DC, Cheskin LJ. The older gut: surgical implications. In: Zenilman ME, Soper NJ (eds), Gastrointestinal surgery in the elderly. Problems in General Surgery 1996;13(3):8-13.

Schwartz SI (ed). Principles of Surgery (6th ed). New York: McGraw-Hill, Inc., 1994.

Silen W (ed). Cope's Early Diagnosis of the Acute Abdomen (19th ed). New York: Oxford University Press, 1996.

Sleisenger MH, Fordtran JS. Gastrointestinal Disease: Pathophysiology, Diagnosis, Management. (5th ed). Philadelphia: WB Saunders Co., 1993.

Townsend CM, Jr., Beauchamp RD, Evers BM, Mattox KL (eds). Sabiston Textbook of Surgery (16th ed). Philadelphia: WB Saunders Company, 2001.

Youngblood RW. Surgical diseases of the esophagus. In: Adkins RB, Jr., Scott HW, Jr. (eds), Surgical Care for the Elderly (2nd ed). Philadelphia: Lippincott-Raven Publishers, 1998;269-276.

Zinner MJ, Schwartz SI, Ellis H (eds). Maingot's Abdominal Operations (10th ed).
CT: Appleton & Lange 1997; vols I-II.

Zollinger RM, Zollinger RM, Jr. Atlas of Surgical Operations (7th ed). New York: McGraw-Hill, 1993.

Zuidema GD (ed). Shackleford's Surgery of the Alimentary Tract (4th ed). Philadelphia: WB Saunders Company, 1996; vols. I-V.

http://www.acg.gi.org

http://www.fascrs.org

http://www.gastro.org

http://www.ssat.com

SECTION 11.11   LIVER, BILIARY TRACT AND PANCREAS

UNIT OBJECTIVES:

Demonstrate knowledge of the anatomy, physiology, and pathophysiology of the liver, biliary tract, and pancreas.

Demonstrate the ability to manage disease and injury of the liver, biliary tract, and pancreas amenable to surgical intervention.

Diagnose and early management of acute gallstone disease, including acute cholecystitis, empyema, acute biliary colic and cholangitis.

Awareness of the possibility and initial management of injuries to biliary tract, including iatrogenic

Diagnosis and early management of acute pancreatitis.

Basic investigation and management of liver metastases.

Medical Knowledge about established and evolving biomedical, clinical, and cognate (e.g. epidemiological and social-behavioral) sciences and the application of this knowledge to patient care.

Junior Level:

Liver and Biliary Tract

1.   Describe the anatomy of the liver and biliary system, including commonly found variations.

2.   Describe the physiology and function of liver and biliary system to include:

a.	Glucose metabolism	d.	Drug metabolism
b.	Protein synthesis	e.	Reticuloendothelial system
c.	Coagulation	f.	Function of bile in fat
g.	metabolism		

3.   Explain the formation of bile, its composition, and its function in digestion. Describe the pathophysiology of gallstone formation.

4.   Correlate bile formation and composition with disease states affecting the biliary system such as gallstone formation and biliary obstruction.

5. Discuss the enterohepatic circulation of bile.

6. Outline the work-up and differential diagnosis of the jaundiced patient.

7. Identify the most significant determinants of mortality in elderly patients following cholecystectomy.

8. Discuss various types of liver cysts (echinococcal or hydatid, nonparasitic) and the appropriate management of each.

9. Discuss the principal characteristics of and the treatment for the following:

   a. Metastatic lesions to the liver

   b. Primary malignancies of liver and biliary tree

   c. Benign tumors of the liver

10. Summarize the etiologies and management of pyogenic and amebic hepatic abscesses.

11. Explain types of infectious hepatitis (A, B, C) with:

   a. Modes of transmission

   b. Diagnosis

   c. Time course for serologic conversion

   d. Natural course

12. Outline the pathophysiology, evaluation, and management of the following:

a.	Choledochal cysts	h.	Gallstone pancreatitis
b.	Caroli's disease	i.	Benign biliary strictures
c.	Sclerosing cholangitis	j.	Acute cholecystitis
d.	Primary biliary cirrhosis	k.	Symptomatic gallstones
e.	Secondary biliary cirrhosis	l.	Acalculous cholecystitis
f.	Cholangitis	m.	Biliary dyskinesia
g.	Gallstone ileus	n.	Congenital biliary atresia

13. History & examination

   a. Investigation

   b. Resuscitation

   c. Decision making re conservative v. surgical treatment and early v. delayed operation

    d.   Non-operative treatment including ERCP, cholecystostomy

    e.   Operative options

    f.   Postoperative management

14.   Complications

    a.   Postoperative problems

    b.   Methods of bile duct repair - primary repair over a T-tube; hepaticojejunostomy with Roux-en-Y reconstruction

15.   Anatomy of liver and segments

    a.   Physiology of liver and liver function

    b.   Understanding of metastatic process

    c.   Pathology of primary colorectal cancer and liver metastases

    d.   Prognostic factors

    e.   Diagnostic techniques including modern imaging

    f.   Role of tumor markers in early diagnosis

    e.   Screening and surveillance following surgery for colorectal cancer

    g.   Modern chemotherapy, both intrahepatic and systemic for liver metastases

    h.   Different forms of in-situ ablative techniques, including radiofrequency ablation

    i.   Full knowledge of factors influencing surgical outcome following resection

Pancreas

1.   Describe the anatomy of the pancreas, including regional vascular anatomy.

2.   Summarize changes that occur in the anatomy of the pancreas with aging by considering:

    a.   Duodenal C loop   c.   Atrophy of pancreas

    b.   Head of the pancreas   d.   Pancreatic ductal anatomy

3.   Discuss the physiology of the pancreas, including endocrine and exocrine function and hormonal regulation.

    a.   Endocrine-islet cells

   (1) Alpha (Glucagon)

   (2) Beta (Insulin)

   (3) Delta (Somatostatin)

   (4) Non-Beta (pancreatic polypeptide)

  b. Exocrine--acinar cells

   (1) Lipase

   (2) Amylase

  c. Hormonal regulation

   (1) Secretin--bicarbonate secretion

   (2) Cholecystokinin--enzyme secretion

4. Explain the pathophysiology of pancreatitis to include:

  a. Common etiologies such as:

   (1) Gallstones

   (2) Alcohol related

   (3) Trauma

   (4) Medications

   (5) Postoperative

   (6) Post endoscopic retrograde cholangiopancreatography (ERCP)

   (7) Idiopathic

  b. Diagnosis, evaluation, and medical management

  c. Role of peritoneal lavage

  d. Complications of pancreatitis, such as:

   (1) Adult respiratory distress syndrome (ARDS; Acute lung injury-ALI also used)

   (2) Hypovolemia

   (3) Pseudocyst

   (4) Abscess

   (5) Sterile pancreatic necrosis

   (6) Infected pancreatic necrosis

  e. Indications for operative management of pancreatitis

f.   Management of gallstone pancreatitis with timing of surgery

g.   Methods of prognostic assessment

5.   Describe the incidence of these diseases in the elderly patient:

      a.   Cholelithiasis

      b.   Acute gallstone pancreatitis

      c.   Pancreatic carcinoma

6.   Explain the pathophysiology of carcinoma of the pancreas to include:

      a.   Typical history and presentation

      b.   Diagnostic evaluation using:

            (1)   Computed axial tomography

            (2)   Ultrasound

            (3)   ERCP

            (4)   Percutaneous transhepatic cholangiography (PTC)

            (5)   Arteriography

            (6)   Laparoscopy/laparotomy

      c.   Indications for:

            (1)   Operative versus nonoperative biliary drainage

            (2)   Percutaneous versus endoscopic stenting

            (3)   Resection

            (4)   Concomitant gastrojejunostomy with operative biliary bypass

7.   Discuss presentation, evaluation, and management of pancreatic pseudocysts with attention to:

      a.   Complications of pseudocysts (hemorrhage, infection, rupture)

      b.   Timing of drainage

      c.   Percutaneous versus surgical drainage

      d.   Indications for external versus internal drainage

      e.   Choice of internal drainage procedure

8.   Explain the diagnosis and management of pancreatic ascites.

a.   Etiology

b.   Clinical features

c.   Scoring system - recognition of severity

d.   Pathophysiology

e.   Complications

f.   Investigations CRP, US, CT

g.   Treatment options

h.   Role of systemic antibiotics

i.   Management of pancreatic necrosis

j.   ERCP, MRCP

Senior Level:

Liver and Biliary Tract

1.   Analyze alternatives to surgery in the management of gallstones, such as:

a.   Oral dissolution with ursodeoxycholic acid

b.   Extracorporeal shock wave lithotripsy

c.   Endoscopic sphincterotomy

2.   Compare laparoscopic versus open cholecystectomy.

3.   Analyze the potential significance of finding a filling defect on ultrasonography or liver scan in an elderly patient. Discuss:

a.   Frequency of metastatic cancer vs. primary tumors in liver

b.   Correlation between incidence of gastrointestinal malignancy and increasing age

4.   Assess management alternatives for common bile duct stones:

a.   Open versus laparoscopic common bile duct exploration

b.   ERCP

5. Since acute cholecystitis is becoming one of the more common indications for emergency admissions of elderly patients to a surgical service, specify factors contributing to its being a more complex disease in elderly vs. young patients by considering:

    a. Incidence of comorbid disease such as diabetes

    b. Atypical clinical presentation (right upper quadrant pain, fever, leukocytosis)

    c. Signs of sepsis or septic shock

    d. Jaundice

    e. Altered mental status

6. Discuss the pathophysiology of hepatic cirrhosis and portal hypertension to include:

    a. Various etiologies of cirrhosis (alcohol and hepatitis)

    b. Differential diagnosis of portal hypertension (prehepatic, hepatic, posthepatic)

    c. Medical management of ascites, encephalopathy, and other complications of cirrhosis

    d. Child's classification of cirrhosis and its relationship to prognosis and surgical mortality

    e. Perioperative management of the cirrhotic patient

    f. Medical management of bleeding esophageal varices using Vasopressin, Sengstaken-Blakemore tube, sclerotherapy, and transjugular intrahepatic portosystemic shunts (TIPS)

    g. Surgical management of bleeding esophageal varices to include:

        (1) Selection of operative candidates

        (2) Appropriate selection of procedures such as:

            (a) Selective and nonselective shunts

            (b) Devascularization procedures

            (c) Esophageal transection

    h. Surgical management of ascites with peritoneovenous shunts to include patient selection and complications

7. Discuss Budd-Chiari Syndrome (pathophysiology and management).

8. Outline indications and contraindications for liver transplantation in adults and children.

9. Explain factors important to the choice of treatment options for the elderly patient with hepatobiliary disease, including:

    a. Cardiovascular disease

    b. Cerebrovascular disease

    c. Renal insufficiency

    d. Systemic hypoperfusion

    e. Curative/palliative procedure

    f. Quality of life issues

Pancreas

1. Describe the etiology, pathophysiology, and management of chronic pancreatitis to include:

    a. Indications for operative management

    b. Selection of appropriate operative procedure such as:

        (1) Longitudinal pancreaticojejunostomy (Puestow-Gillesby Procedure)

        (2) Caudal pancreaticojejunostomy (Duval Procedure)

        (3) Subtotal pancreatectomy

        (4) Pancreatoduodenectomy

    c. Role of celiac ganglion ablation (chemical splanchnicectomy) in pain control

2. Summarize the common sequelae of chronic pancreatitis to include pain, fat malabsorption, and diabetes.

3. Discuss diagnosis, evaluation, and surgical management of cystic neoplasms of the pancreas (mucinous and serous cystadenomas; cystadenocarcinoma).

4. Compare the probabilities of coexisting intra-abdominal pathology in elderly vs. younger patients. Consider:

    a. Acute pancreatitis

    b. Mesenteric ischemia

    c. Gangrenous cholecystitis

    d. Perforated viscus

5. Describe the diagnosis, evaluation, and surgical management of the following islet cell tumors of the pancreas:

    a. Gastrinoma (Zollinger-Ellison Syndrome)

    b. Glucagonoma

    c. Somatostatinoma

     d.   Insulinoma

     e.   VIPoma (Verner-Morrison Syndrome, WDHA Syndrome)

6.   Describe the diagnosis and management of pancreas divisum.

Chief Level:

Liver and Biliary Tract

1.   Detail the appropriate surgical management of any selected disorder of the liver or biliary tract.

2.   Analyze the technical details of each surgical procedure and options that may be available with pros and cons of each.

3.   Summarize the common complications associated with surgical management of liver and biliary tract disease.

4.   Summarize the principles of perioperative management of liver and biliary tract disease.

Pancreas

1.   Outline the appropriate surgical management of disorders of the pancreas to include:

     a.   Pancreatoduodenectomy (Whipple Procedure)

     b.   Distal pancreatectomy

     c.   Total pancreatectomy

     d.   Subtotal (distal 95%) pancreatectomy

     e.   Longitudinal pancreaticojejunostomy (Puestow Procedure)

     f.   Internal drainage of pseudocysts (cystogastrostomy, cystoduodenostomy, Roux-en-Y cystojejunostomy)

2.   Explain the technical details of the above procedures, including the options available and the pros and cons of each.

3.   Describe the common complications associated with surgical management of diseases of the pancreas.

4.   Summarize the principles of perioperative management of diseases of the pancreas.

Patient Care that is compassionate, appropriate, and effective for the treatment of health problems and the promotion of health.

<u>Junior Level:</u>

<u>Liver and Biliary Tract</u>

1. Perform history and physical examination specifically focused on liver and biliary system.

2. Select and interpret appropriate laboratory and radiologic evaluations in the work-up of the jaundiced patient to include:

    a. Alkaline phosphatase, serum glutamic oxaloacetic transaminase (SGOT), serum . glutamic pyruvic transaminase (SGPT), direct and indirect bilirubin, Prothrombin time (PT) and partial thromboplastin time (PTT)

    b. Endoscopic retrograde cholangiopancreatography (ERCP)

    c. Percutaneous transhepatic cholangiography (PTC)

    d. Liver-spleen scan

    e. Hepatobiliary nuclear scan (HIDA)

    f. Oral cholecystogram (OCG)

    g. Ultrasound

    h. Computed axial tomography

    i. Arteriography

3. Assist in the perioperative management of patients undergoing hepatobiliary surgery.

4. Assist in management of patients with bleeding esophageal varices including the use of:

    a. Vasopressin

    b. Sengstaken-Blakemore tube

    c. Sclerotherapy

5. Perform uncomplicated hepatobiliary surgery under supervision, such as cholecystectomy, both laparoscopic and open, with operative cholangiography.

6. Assist in more advanced hepatobiliary operations.

7. Technical Skills and Procedures

    a. Cholecystectomy-laparoscopic

    b. Cholecystectomy-open

    c. Biliary-CBD-exploration

    d. Cholecystostomy

    e. Laparotomy for biliary peritonitis with placement of drains

    f. Biliary-bile duct injury repair

    g. Biliary-Hepaticojejunostomy

    h. Techniques of liver biopsy

    i. Postoperative management of major liver resection

    j. Management of liver failure

Pancreas

1. Perform history and physical examination focused on the pancreas.

2. Select and interpret appropriate laboratory and radiologic examinations in evaluation of pancreatic disease, including:

    a. Serum amylase and lipase

    b. Urinary amylase

    c. Computed axial tomography

    d. Ultrasound

    e. Endoscopic retrograde cholangiopancreatography (ERCP)

    f. Arteriography

3. Assist in management of patient with acute pancreatitis.

4. Assist in perioperative management of patients undergoing pancreatic surgery.

5. Perform minor pancreatic procedures under supervision such as external drainage of pseudocyst or internal drainage via cystgastrostomy.

    a. Pancreatectomy-distal

    b. Pancreatic debridement

    c. Pancreatic pseudocyst drainage

Senior Level:

Liver and Biliary Tract

1. Perform detailed evaluation of patients with liver and biliary disease and plan appropriate management and operative approach.

2. Perform, under supervision, increasingly complex hepatobiliary surgery:

    a.   Laparoscopic cholecystectomy with cholangiography

    b.   Common bile duct exploration with choledochoscopy

    c.   Biliary drainage procedures, such as:

        (1)   Choledochoduodenostomy

        (2)   Roux-en-Y and loop choledochojejunostomy

        (3)   Cholecystojejunostomy

        (4)   Sphincteroplasty

    d.   Drainage of liver abscess

    e.   Peritoneovenous shunts

    f.   Complicated cholecystectomy--acute, gangrenous

    g.   Simple liver resection

Pancreas

1. Perform detailed evaluation of patients with pancreatic disease and plan appropriate medical or surgical management.

2. Perform increasingly complex pancreatic surgery such as:

    a.   Internal drainage of pseudocysts with Roux-en-Y cystojejunostomy

    b.   Longitudinal pancreaticojejunostomy (Puestow Procedure)

    c.   Distal pancreatectomy

    d.   Biliary bypass for carcinoma

Chief Level:

Liver and Biliary Tract

1. Coordinate overall care of patients with hepatobiliary disease including:

    a.   Initial evaluation

    b.   Appropriate diagnostic studies

      c.   Indicated consultations

      d.   Operative management

2.   Perform complex hepatic and biliary surgery:

      a.   Anatomic liver resection

      b.   Portosystemic shunts:

            (1)   Portocaval, end-to-side and side-to-side

            (2)   Mesocaval

            (3)   Distal splenorenal (Warren)

            (4)   Central splenorenal

      c.   Complicated procedures on extrahepatic bile ducts for:

            (1)   Cholangiocarcinoma

            (2)   Choledochal cyst

            (3)   Benign biliary stricture

      d.   Liver transplant

      e.   Kasai procedure (hepatoportoenterostomy)

3.   Supervise and instruct junior house staff in minor hepatobiliary procedures.

Pancreas

1.   Coordinate overall care of patients with complex pancreatic disease, including initial evaluation, appropriate diagnostic studies, and operative management of:

      a.   Pancreatic abscess and infected pancreatic necrosis

      b.   Cystadenomas

      c.   Periampullary carcinoma

      d.   Endocrine tumors of the pancreas

2.   Perform complex pancreatic procedures such as:

      a.   Whipple resection

      b.   Total or subtotal pancreatectomy

      c. Operative debridement and drainage of pancreatic abscess or infected necrosis d.	Surgical exploration for islet cell tumors of the pancreas

e.	Local resection for ampullary tumors

3.	Supervise and instruct junior house staff in minor pancreatic procedures.

Practice-Based Learning and Improvement that involves investigation and evaluation of their own patient care, appraisal and assimilation of scientific evidence, and improvements in patient care.

INFORMATION TECHNOLOGY AND POPULATION COMPARISONS REFERENCES

Cameron JL (ed). Atlas of Surgery: Gallbladder and Biliary Tract, the Liver, Portasystemic Shunts, the Pancreas. Vol I. Philadelphia: BC Decker, Inc., 1990.

Cameron JL (ed). The liver. Portal hypertension. Gallbladder and biliary tree. Pancreas. Current Surgical Therapy (7th ed). St. Louis: Mosby, 2001;328-586.

Frey CF, Suzuki M, Isaju S, et al. Pancreatic resection for chronic pancreatitis. Surg Clin North Am 1989;69(3):499-528.

Ger R. Surgical anatomy of the liver. Surg Clin North Am 1989;69(2):179-192.

Glassman JA. Biliary Tract Surgery: Tactics and Techniques. New York: Macmillan Publishing Co. Inc., 1989.

Greenfield LJ, Mulholland M, Oldham KT, Zelenock GB, Lillemoe KD (eds). Pancreas. Liver and portal venous system. Gallbladder and biliary tract. Surgery: Scientific Principles and Practice (2nd ed). Philadelphia: Lippincott-Raven, 1997;857-1081.

Kahng KU, Roslyn JJ. Surgical issues for the elderly patient with hepatobiliary disease. In: Zenilman ME, Roslyn JJ (eds), Surgery in the elderly patient, Surg Cl of N Amer 1994;74(2):345-373.

Kahng KU, Roslyn JJ. Liver, gallbladder, and biliary tract disease. In: Adkins RB, Jr., Scott HW, Jr. (eds), Surgical Care for the Elderly (2nd ed). Philadelphia: Lippincott-Raven Publishers, 1998;291-304.

Klein AS, Yeo CJ, Lillemoe K, et al. Liver, biliary tract, and pancreas. In: O'Leary JP (ed), The Physiologic Basis of Surgery (2nd ed). Baltimore: Williams and Wilkins, 1996;441-478.

Lillemoe KD. Pancreatic and periampullary carcinoma in the elderly. In: Zenilman ME, Soper NJ (eds), Gastrointestinal surgery in the elderly. Problems in General Surgery 1996;13(3):108-120.

Lillemoe KD. Pancreatic disease in the elderly patient. In: Zenilman ME, Roslyn JJ (eds), Surgery in the elderly patient, Surg Cl of N Amer 1994;74(2):317-344.

Lillemoe KD, Cameron JL. Surgical management of pancreatic disease. In: Adkins RB, Jr., Scott HW, Jr. (eds), Surgical Care for the Elderly (2nd ed). Philadelphia: Lippincott-Raven Publishers, 1998;305-326.

Magnuson TH. Surgery of the biliary tree in the aging patient. In: Zenilman ME, Soper NJ (eds), Gastrointestinal surgery in the elderly. Problems in General Surgery 1996;13(3):75-82.

Mayer KL, Frey CF. Benign diseases of the pancreas in the elderly. In: Zenilman ME, Soper NJ (eds), Gastrointestinal surgery in the elderly. Problems in General Surgery 1996;13(3):91-107.

Miller TA (ed). Liver, biliary tract, pancreas, and spleen. Modern Surgical Care: Physiologic Foundations and Clinical Applications (2nd ed). St. Louis: Quality Medical Publishing, Inc., 1998;491-622.

Sitzmann JV. Surgical treatment of liver disease in the elderly. In: Zenilman ME, Soper NJ (eds), Gastrointestinal surgery in the elderly. Problems in General Surgery 1996;13(3):83-90.

Skandalakis LJ, Rowe JS, Jr., Gray SW, et al. Surgical embryology and anatomy of the pancreas. Surg Cl of N Amer 1993;73(4):661-697.

Skandalakis LJ, Rowe JS, Jr., Gray SW, et al. Surgical embryology and anatomy of the pancreas. Surg Cl of N Amer 1993;73(4):661-697.

Trede M, Carter DC (eds). Surgery of the Pancreas (2nd ed). New York: Churchill Livingstone, 1996;1-709.

Zenilman ME, Soper NJ (eds). Gastrointestinal surgery in the elderly. Problems in General Surgery 1996;13(3):1-164.

Zinner MJ, Schwartz SI, Ellis H (eds). Maingot's Abdominal Operations (10th ed). CT: Appleton & Lange 1997; vols I-II.

SECTION 11.12   VASCULAR SURGERY

UNIT OBJECTIVES:

Demonstrate knowledge of the anatomy, physiology, and pathophysiology of the vascular system, including congenital and acquired diseases.

Demonstrate the ability to surgically manage the preoperative, operative, and postoperative care of patients with arterial, venous, and lymphatic disease.

Ability to identify the chronically ischemic limb and perform femoral exploration and anastomosis under supervision.

Atherosclerosis: Knowledge of the basic pathophysiology of chronic lower limb ischemia

Chronic Lower Limb Ischemia - Assessment: Diagnosis and principles of investigation of chronic lower limb ischemia.

Chronic lower limb ischemia - Surgery: Basic knowledge of possible surgical intervention for chronic limb ischemia

Chronic lower limb ischemia - Conservative Management: Ability to arrange suitable conservative management of chronic lower limb ischemia.

Amputation: Recognize indications for amputation and know how to perform common amputations with assistance for less common procedures

The diagnosis of ruptured aortic aneurysm

   a.   The assessment and preoperative management of most patients with ruptured aortic aneurysm

   b.   To assist at surgery for ruptured aortic aneurysm

   c.   Have knowledge of the principles of postoperative management of ruptured aortic aneurysm

   d.   The recognition of complications following surgery for ruptured aneurysm.

Primary varicose veins: Ability to assess and manage primary varicose veins.

The ability to recognize acute limb ischemia and initiate emergency management.

   a.   To recognize and initiate emergency treatment for acute limb ischemia

b.   To recognize some of the complications of treatment of acute limb ischemia

c.   The understanding of the management of thrombolysis

Medical Knowledge about established and evolving biomedical, clinical, and cognate (e.g. epidemiological and social-behavioral) sciences and the application of this knowledge to patient care.

Junior Level:

1.   Describe human arterial and venous anatomy.

2.   Describe basic arterial and venous hemodynamics.

3.   Discuss the anatomy, pathology, and pathophysiology of the arterial wall.

4.   Review and describe the basic clinical manifestations of the following vascular disorders:

    a.   Obstructive arterial disease

    b.   Aneurysmal arterial disease

    c.   Thromboembolic disease--arterial and venous

    d.   Chronic venous insufficiency and lymphatic obstruction

    e.   Portal hypertension

    f.   Congenital vascular disease

5.   Assess patients' vascular systems using appropriate skills in history-taking and clinical examination.

6.   Describe the relationship of the following disorders/practices to atherosclerotic vascular disease:

    a.   Diabetes mellitus   d.   Congestive heart failure

    b.   Hypertension   e.   Hyperlipidemia

    c.   Renal failure   f.   Smoking

7.   Describe life-threatening signs of vascular disease and indicate when immediate intervention is required.

8.   Differentiate between the following diagnostic tools available for assessing vascular disease and explain the relative contribution of each:

    a.   Angiography

b.   Computed axial tomographic (CAT) scanning

c.   Magnetic resonance imaging (MRI) and magnetic resonance angiography (MRA)

d.   Duplex scanning (ultrasonography)

9.   Analyze and be prepared to explain the following concept: vascular disease, and specifically arterial disease may be diffuse and clinically silent, but it still represents a major threat to the patient.

10.   Summarize the etiology and therapeutic options of specific categories of vascular disease:

a.   Venous disease

(1)   Varicose vein disease

(2)   Post-phlebitic syndrome

(3)   Thromboembolic disease

(4)   Pulmonary embolism

(5)   Portal hypertension

b.   Lymphatic disease

(1)   Anatomy of lymphatic system and lymphatic return

(2)   Congenital lymphatic anomalies

(3)   Acquired lymphatic disease

(4)   Operative procedures for correction of lymphatic disease

c.   Arterial disease

(1)   Atherosclerosis and its related disorders

(2)   Aortic and other vascular aneurysms

(3)   Inflammatory vascular disease

(4)   Atherosclerotic vascular disease

(5)   Arterial embolic disease

(6)   Arteriovenous fistulas or malformations

(7)   Extracranial cerebrovascular disease

(8)   Neurovascular compression syndromes (thoracic outlet syndrome)

(9)   Visceral ischemic syndromes

(10)   Renovascular hypertension

(11)   Degenerative arterial disease

(12)   Trauma

(13)   Interactions of cardiovascular and pulmonary systems

d. Pathophysiology of peripheral vascular disease

    (1) Arterial stenosis

    (2) Aneurysmal disease

    (3) Arteriovenous fistulas (local and cardiac hemodynamic effects)

    (4) Venous thrombosis

e. Interaction of cardiovascular and pulmonary systems

f. Miscellaneous

    (1) Tumors

    (2) Sympathetic nervous system

    (3) Congenital vascular syndromes

11. Outline the principles of non-invasive laboratory diagnosis; include a description of the role and limitations of the vascular laboratory.

12. Discuss basic principles of Doppler ultrasound in preparation for performing bedside arterial and venous Doppler testing.

13. Outline the principles of care for ischemic limbs.

14. Describe the natural history of medically treated vascular disease in the following categories:

a. Carotid arterial stenosis

b. Abdominal aortic aneurysm

c. Chronic femoral artery occlusion

15. Summarize principles for the preoperative assessment and postoperative care of patients undergoing major vascular surgical procedures.

16. Outline the fundamental elements of nonoperative care of the vascular patient, including the role of risk assessment and preventive measures.

17. Indicate the role of anticoagulant agents, including antiplatelet agents, in the management of patients with vascular disease.

18. Analyze the role of the endothelium in atherosclerosis, thrombosis, and thrombolysis.

19. Describe the hemodynamics and pathophysiology of:

a. Claudication

b.   Transient ischemic attack (TIA)

c.   Stroke

d.   Mesenteric angina

e.   Angina pectoris

f.   Renovascular hypertension

g.   Arteriovenous (AV) fistula

20.   Explain the concept of critical arterial stenosis.

21.   Differentiate between acute arterial and acute deep venous occlusion.

22.   Discuss the principles of angiography to include the following considerations:

a.   Indications and complications (including contrast-induced renal failure)

b.   Principles and techniques of intraoperative angiography

c.   Principles and techniques of emergency room angiography

23.   Discuss the principles of and contraindications for anticoagulation and thrombolytic therapy.

24.   Describe the surgically correctable causes of hypertension and their diagnostic modalities.

25.   Explain the risk: reward ratios of surgical care for patients with vascular disease.

26.   Discuss the mechanics of action and the therapeutic role of the following pharmacologic types of agents:

a.   Vasopressors

b.   Vasodilators

c.   Adrenergic blocking agents

d.   Anticoagulants

e.   Antiplatelet agents

f.   Thrombolytics

27.   Illustrate the general principles of vascular surgical technique including:

a.   Vascular control and suturing

b.   Endarterectomy

c. Angioplasty

d. Bypass grafting

28. Determine a plan for assessment of operative risk in these categories:

a. Cardiac

b. Pulmonary

c. Renal

d. Metabolic

e Levels of anesthetic risk

29. Discuss clotting factors and how they interact (coagulation cascade).

30. Discuss the role of the following factors in maintaining homeostasis in the coagulation pathways:

a. Protein S   d. Platelet granules

b. Protein C   e. Endothelial cell

c. Platelets   f. Antithrombin III

31. Describe the use of adjunctive measures in the management of patients with vascular disease such as:

a. Antibiotics   c. Thrombolytic agents

b. Anticoagulants   d. Antiplatelet agents

32. Review the costs associated with providing surgical care to patients with vascular disorders.

33. Atherosclerosis:

a. Pathology of atherosclerosis (atherothrombosis) and complications.

b. Recognize risk factors for arterial disease

c. Natural history of lower limb arterial disease

34. Critical limb ischemia

a. Chronic Lower Limb Ischemia - Assessment

b.   Anatomy of arteries supplying the lower limb.

c.   Role of ultrasound and angiography and other imaging (e.g. MRA)

d.   Role of angioplasty

35.   Chronic lower limb ischemia - Surgery:

     a.   Indications for intervention

     b.   Surgical approaches to infra-inguinal vessels

     c.   Types of anesthesia

36.   Potential complications of vascular surgery

     Technical components of vascular anastomosis and commonly occurring problems

37.   Chronic lower limb ischemia - Conservative Management:

38.   Basic principles of management of hypertension and hyperlipidaemia and diabetes

     a.   Epidemiology of tobacco smoking

     b.   Role of antiplatelet drugs

39.   Amputation:

     a.   Types of amputation and advantages of each

     b.   Potential complications of amputation

40.   Diagnosis Intestinal ischemia

     a.   Patients at risk

     b.   Clinical features

     c.   Role and timing of investigation

     d.   nitial Management

     e.   Hypovolemia relevant to the condition

     f.   Understands importance of immediate intervention

     g.   Operation

     h.   Anatomy of the abdomen and major vessels

     i.   Basic physiology of aortic clamping

     j.   Coagulopathy

k.   Postoperative Care

l.   Nutrition

m.   Fluid Balance

n.   Respiratory and renal physiology

o.   Cardiac function

p.   Complications

q.   Early and late complications

r.   Indications for investigation such as CT scan

41.   Indications for surgery for varicose veins

a.   Anatomy of the venous system

b.   Complications of varicose veins

42.   Acute limb ischemia

a.   Pathophysiology of acute limb ischemia

b.   Anatomy of the arterial system

c.   Risk factors for acute limb ischemia

d.   Knowledge of causes of acute limb ischemia

e.   Indications for emergency intervention

f.   Indications for embolectomy, thrombolysis, primary amputation

g.   Subsequent management and investigation of patient with acute limb ischemia

h.   Complications of acute limb ischemia

i.   Ischemia reperfusion injury and systemic effects

j.   Ways of attenuating effects of reperfusion

k.   Thrombolysis

l.   Knowledge of methods and agents used for Thrombolysis

m.   Describe indications for Thrombolysis

n.   Describe complications of Thrombolysis

Senior Level:

1. Identify and describe vascular anatomy and regional anatomy related to vascular disease.

2. Discuss the broad range of vascular illnesses, including congenital vascular disease and diseases of the venous and lymphatic systems.

3. Explain the physiologic and organic manifestations of vascular disease, such as renovascular hypertension, portal hypertension, and renal failure.

4. Differentiate between the different operative approaches to the vascular system to include:

    a. Incisions and exposure

    b. Handling of vascular tissues

    c. Principles of vascular bypass grafting

    d. Emergency vascular surgery

    e. Reoperative vascular surgery

    f. Principles of endarterectomy

    g. Endovascular techniques

5. Illustrate the operative exposure of the major vessels, including:

    a. Aortic arch   e. Suprarenal aorta

    b. Proximal subclavian   f. Infrarenal aorta

    c. Carotid artery   g. Femoral artery

    d. Descending thoracic aorta   h. Popliteal artery

6. Outline the indications for operations for claudication, abdominal aortic aneurysm, carotid stenosis, and amputation.

7. Describe the indications for balloon angioplasty and vascular stent placement with its risks and complications.

8. Describe the pathogenesis and complications of aneurysmal disease.

9. Summarize the etiology, microbiology, and treatment of diabetic foot infection.

10. Categorize the prevention and management of operative and postoperative complications, including graft infections, ischemic bowel, graft thrombosis, and extremity ischemia.

11. Outline the manifestation of failing peripheral vascular grafts, contrasting angioplasty with reconstruction and amputation.

12. Discuss the principles of reoperative vascular surgery.

13. Outline procedures for managing vascular surgical emergencies such as acute tissue ischemia or major hemorrhage (traumatic or ruptured aneurysm).

14. Summarize the characteristics of congenital arterial, venous, and lymphatic diseases.

15. Analyze the options for treatment of patients with chronic venous insufficiency and venous ulceration.

16. Demonstrate a basic knowledge of the various types of graft and suture material available.

17. Analyze alternative measures for the diagnosis and management of renovascular hypertension.

18. Discuss alternative operative procedures for the management of portal hypertension.

19. Summarize the surgical techniques available for managing the following vascular disorders:

   a. Abdominal aortic bypass or aneurysmectomy

   b. Carotid stenosis

   c. Femoral-popliteal occlusion

   d. Tibial artery occlusion

20. Analyze the management of complex vascular problems considering the following factors:

   a. Morbidity and mortality

   b. Advanced surgical techniques

      (1) Endoscopy

      (2) Microvascular techniques

21. Review critical factors for decision making in vascular surgery:

   a. Risk: reward ratio

   b. Morbidity and mortality probability

   c. Preoperative and postoperative assessment

   d. Non-invasive laboratories, duplex scanning

e.　　Role of advanced radiologic techniques: Angioplasty, CT scanning, MRI/MRA imaging

22.　Apply the decision making process in analyzing complex vascular diseases, including the following:

a.　　Cerebrovascular problems

b.　　Mesenteric vascular disease

c.　　Renovascular disease

d.　　Aneurysmal disease

e.　　Lower extremity arterial occlusion

f.　　Venous disease

23.　Outline the management of prosthetic graft infections, including:

a.　　Diagnosis

b.　　Use of alternate routes for revascularization

c.　　Use of alternative graft materials

24.　Summarize complications of common major vascular procedures such as:

a.　　Carotid endarterectomy

b.　　Aortic reconstruction

c.　　Lower extremity vascular reconstruction

Patient Care that is compassionate, appropriate, and effective for the treatment of health problems and the promotion of health.

Junior Level:

1.　Evaluate patients for vascular disease.

2.　Demonstrate skill in basic surgical techniques, including:

a.　　Knot tying

b.　　Exposure and retraction

  c. Knowledge of instrumentation

  d. Incisions

  e. Closure of incisions

  f. Handling of graft material

3. Participate in surgery for varicose vein disease, including:

  a. Ligation and stripping

  b. Management of venous stasis ulcers

  c. Management of venous thrombosis

4. Participate in amputations with specific attention to:

  a. Demarcation levels

  b. Control of toxicity

5. Demonstrate proficiency in venous access procedures.

6. Demonstrate the ability to perform arterial access or arterio-venous access, including:

  a. Incisions

  b. Closure of incision

7. Obtain vascular control of diseased or traumatically occluded blood vessels using:

  a. Vascular clamp

  b. Vessel loop

  c. Balloon occlusion

8. Participate in thromboendarterectomy and thrombectomy.

9. Demonstrate appropriate vascular suture techniques.

10. Evaluate and manage sympathectomy procedures.

11. Perform the preoperative assessment and postoperative care of patients undergoing major vascular surgical procedures.

  a. Ability to take a relevant history and examine vascular system

  b. Use of ankle pressure measurements

    c.   Duplex ultrasound

    d.   Interpretation of angiograms

    e.   Selection for surgery and angioplasty

12.   Chronic lower limb ischemia Surgery:

    a.   Expose femoral vessels

    b.   Vascular anastomosis

    c.   Chronic lower limb ischemia - Conservative Management

13.   Management of graft surveillance program/clinic

         Ability to run risk factor clinic

14.   Technical Skills and Procedures

    a.   Chronic Lower Limb Ischemia - Assessment:

    b.   Percutaneous angiography

    c.   Chronic lower limb ischemia - Surgery:

    d.   Occlusive-Aorto-femoral bypass

    e.   Occlusive-Axillo-femoral bypass

    f.   Lower limb-femoro-femoral cross-over graft

    g.   Amputation:

    h.   amputation-digit(s)

    i.   Amputation-BK

    j.   Amputation-AK

16.   Aortic Surgery

    a.   Diagnosis

    b.   History and examination

    c.   Initial Management

    d.   Patient Selection

    e.   Operation Assist at operation

    f.   Recognizes signs of coagulopathy

    g.   Able to initiate basic treatment of coagulopathy

h. Postoperative care

i. Understands need for nutritional support

j. Fluid requirements

k. Complications

l. Clinical recognition of complications

m. Recognize need for early and late re-intervention

n. Carry out appropriate surgery with other disciplines as necessary

o. Technical Skills and Procedures

p. Operation

(1) AAA-bifurcated graft-complete operation

(2) AAA-tube graft-complete operation

17. Examination of the venous system of the lower limbs

a. Select patients who require preoperative investigations such as Duplex scanning

b. Select patients who require surgery

c. Non-operative management

d. Technical Skills and Procedures

e. Varicose veins - primary varicose veins

(1) 4 Vvs-long saphenous-SFJ lign and strip+/-avulsions

(2) 4 Vvs-SPJ ligation+/-strip+/-avulsions

(3) 4 Vvs-multiple stab avulsions

18. Acute Limb ischemia

a. History and examination to detect acute limb ischemia

b. Arrange appropriate urgent investigations: duplex, angiogram

c. Can recognize when intervention is not appropriate

d. Complications of acute limb ischemia

e. Manage patient when embolectomy fails

f. Manage patient with rhabdomyolosis

g. Peri-operative thrombolysis

h. Emergency bypass

i. Thrombolysis

j. Manage patient undergoing Thrombolysis

k. Management of complications of Thrombolysis

19. Technical Skills and Procedures

a. Thrombo-embolectomy-arterial-femoral

b. Peri-operative angiogram

c. Complications of acute limb ischemia

d. Fasciotomy

Senior Level:

1. Demonstrate the appropriate incisions and exposure of:

a. Abdominal aorta and its major branches

b. Portal venous system

c. Peripheral arterial system

d. Carotid arterial system

e. Arteriovenous fistula

2. Obtain vascular control of major vessels

a. Aorta　　　b. Vena cava

3. Participate in endarterectomy and bypass grafting.

4. Demonstrate ability to manage graft and suture materials.

5. Perform selected operative procedures or selected parts of the following operative procedures under supervision:

a. Aortic aneurysm repair

b. Carotid endarterectomy

c. Aorto-iliac occlusive disease

d. Femoral popliteal occlusive disease

e. Correction of portal hypertension

f.	Peripheral vascular trauma

6.	Discuss and demonstrate the role of adjunctive measures in operative procedures including angioscopy, and thrombolytic therapy.

7.	Select and use proper advanced techniques in managing patients with a variety of vascular disorders such as:

a.	Ruptured aortic aneurysm

b.	Central vascular trauma

c.	Supra-renal aortic aneurysm

d.	Renovascular hypertension

e.	Femoral tibial bypasses

8.	Perform alternative methods of bypass grafting such as:

a.	Extra-anatomic bypass, principles and techniques

b.	Indirect revascularization

c.	In situ techniques

d.	Sequential and composite techniques

9.	Manage prosthetic graft infections to include:

a.	Diagnosis

b.	Selection of alternate routes for revascularization

c.	Selection of appropriate graft materials

d.	Timing

10.	Manage complications of common major vascular procedures such as:

a.	Carotid endarterectomy

b.	Aortic reconstruction

c.	Lower extremity vascular reconstruction

Practice-Based Learning and Improvement that involves investigation and evaluation of their own patient care, appraisal and assimilation of scientific evidence, and improvements in patient care.

INFORMATION TECHNOLOGY AND POPULATION COMPARISONS
REFERENCES

Cameron JL (ed). Vascular system. Current Surgical Therapy (7th ed). St. Louis: Mosby, 2001; 790-1031.

Ernst CB, Stanley JC. Current Therapy in Vascular Surgery (3rd ed). St. Louis: Mosby, 1995.

Greenfield LJ, Mulholland M, Oldham KT, Zelenock GB, Lillemoe KD (eds). Arterial system. Surgery: Scientific Principles and Practice (2nd ed). Philadelphia: Lippincott-Raven, 1997;1585-1971.

Miller TA (ed). The peripheral vascular system. Modern Surgical Care: Physiologic Foundations and Clinical Applications (2nd ed). St. Louis: Quality Medical Publishing, Inc., 1998;1007-1088.

Moore WS. Vascular Surgery: A Comprehensive Review (5th ed). Philadelphia: WB Saunders Co., 1998;1-903.

Moore WS, Ahn SS (eds). Endovascular Surgery (3rd ed). Philadelphia: WB Saunders Company, 2001.

Ouriel K, Rutherford RB. Atlas of Vascular Surgery: Operative Procedures. Philadelphia: WB Saunders Co., 1998;1-285.

Rutherford RB. Vascular Surgery (4th ed). Philadelphia: WB Saunders Co., 1995.

http://www.svmb.org

http://www.vascsurg.org

11.11A   VASCULAR DISEASE IN THE ELDERLY PATIENT

The Vascular Disease in the Elderly unit was written by Jamal J. Hoballah, MD.

UNIT OBJECTIVES:

Demonstrate an understanding of the pathophysiology of vascular diseases in the elderly patient.

Demonstrate an understanding of the potential variations in the management of vascular diseases between the various age groups of the elderly and the younger population.

Demonstrate the ability to prepare elderly patients for definitive operative and non-operative interventions, rehabilitation, and discharge planning.

Medical Knowledge about established and evolving biomedical, clinical, and cognate (e.g. epidemiological and social-behavioral) sciences and the application of this knowledge to patient care.

Junior Level:

1. Demonstrate knowledge of the pathophysiology of abdominal aortic aneurysm (AAA) in the elderly patient with respect to:
   a. Incidence in patients 65-85 years old
   b. Annual growth rate and natural history of untreated AAA
   c. Incidence of rupture and risk factors associated with increased incidence of rupture

2. Mortality rate of elective AAA replacement in selected elderly patients in comparison with the younger population
3. Mortality rate of emergent AAA replacement in elderly patients in comparison with the younger population
4. Concept of chronological age vs. physiological age and the medical risk factors that increase the risk of AAA replacement such as cardiac disease, pulmonary insufficiency and chronic renal failure

5.   Perioperative cardiac screening and optimization of medical condition

6.   Preservation of the quality of life following AAA replacement in elderly patients

7.   Screening and diagnostic tests for AAA and the association between AAA and iliac, popliteal, and femoral aneurysms

8.   Approaches to AAA replacement

9.   Concept of endovascular aortic aneurysm replacement and its investigational status

Knowledge of the manifestation and management of lower extremity occlusive disease in the elderly patient with respect to:

1.   Ability to differentiate the symptoms of arterial claudication from neurogenic or venous claudication

2.   Natural history of intermittent claudication; the effects of smoking, diabetes, hypertension, and degree of ischemia upon presentation on the future risk of amputation

3.   Role of exercise, risk factor modification, and drug therapy in the management of claudication; their mechanism of action and their limitations

4.   Definition of rest pain and the risk of amputation if untreated

5.   Different presentation of the elderly patient with single and multilevel arterial disease

6.   Interpretation of noninvasive tests used for evaluating lower extremity ischemia:

    a.   Arm brachial index (ABI)

    b.   Segmental pressures

    c.   Toe pressures

    d.   Transcutaneous oxygen tension.

7.   ABI changes in patients with claudication, rest pain, tissue loss

8.   Limitations of the ABI in diabetic patients and the value of toe pressure measurements

9.   Predicting healing of an amputation based on noninvasive testing

10.   Morbidity, mortality, and ambulation rates after a major amputation in elderly patients

11.   Accepted indications for primary amputation in elderly patients

12. Morbidity, mortality and patency rates of the revascularization options for aortoiliac occlusive disease:

    a.   Aorto bifemoral bypass   d.   Balloon angioplasty

    b.   Axillo femoral bypass   e.   Primary stenting

    c.   Femoro femoral bypass

13. The patency rate and limb salvage rate following infrainguinal revascularization using autogenous veins and prosthetic conduits for:

    a.   Femoro-above knee popliteal bypass

    b.   Femoro-below knee popliteal bypass

    c.   Femoro-tibial bypass

14. Limitations and patency rates of balloon angioplasty in infrainguinal occlusive disease

15. Mortality and morbidity of distal revascularization in octogenarians

Demonstrate knowledge of the manifestation and management of carotid disease in the elderly patient with respect to:

1. Significance of stroke as cause of mortality and disability in elderly patients

2. Risk factors for stroke development

3. Changes in stroke incidence with every decade of life

4. Contribution of carotid disease to the incidence of stroke

5. Significance of carotid bruit in elderly patients

6. Proven measures for stroke prevention

7. Advantages and disadvantages of diagnostic methods (duplex ultrasonography, angiography, MRA, intracranial doppler and CT scan)

8. Role of duplex ultrasonography in assessing the degree of carotid disease

9. Measurements of the degree of carotid stenosis based on angiography

10. Natural history of asymptomatic vs. symptomatic carotid disease

11. Benefits of Carotid endarterectomy in symptomatic patients

12. Benefits of Carotid endarterectomy in asymptomatic patients.

13. Risk of stroke or death following CEA in asymptomatic patients, patients with TIA, and patients with prior stroke

14. Mortality and morbidity of CEA in octogenarians

15. Limitations of the prospective randomized CEA trials with respect to the octogenarians

Medical Knowledge about established and evolving biomedical, clinical, and cognate (e.g. epidemiological and social-behavioral) sciences and the application of this knowledge to patient care.

Senior Level:

Demonstrate the ability to provide competent care to elderly patients with AAA with respect to:

1. Management of concomitant intra-abdominal pathology such as cholelithiasis, colonic cancer, renal tumors, and prostatic disease

2. Ability to recognize and treat possible postoperative complications, such as myocardial infarction, distal embolization, and ischemic colitis

3. Importance of preserving pelvic circulation through reperfusion of at least one hypogastric artery, the significance of previous colectomy, and the indications for reimplantation of the inferior mesenteric artery

4. Management of concomitant renovascular occlusive disease, mesenteric occlusive disease, or suprarenal extension of the aneurysmal pathology

Demonstrate knowledge of the management of carotid disease in elderly patients with respect to:

1. Effect of ulceration, degree of stenosis, and presenting symptoms on the risk of stroke in patients with symptomatic carotid disease managed medically without CEA

2. Effect of life expectancy and female gender on the benefits of CEA in asymptomatic patients

3. Causes of stroke during CEA

4. Understanding the etiology of recurrent carotid disease and the indications for intervention

5. Causes and management of stroke during and after CEA

6.   Investigational role of carotid angioplasty and stenting in the management of carotid disease

Practice-Based Learning and Improvement that involves investigation and evaluation of their own patient care, appraisal and assimilation of scientific evidence, and improvements in patient care.

INFORMATION TECHNOLOGY
REFERENCES

Aronow WS, Stemmer EA, Wilson SE (eds). Vascular Disease in the Elderly. Armonk, NY: Futura Publishing Company, 1997;1-574.

Bernstein EF, Chan EL. Abdominal aortic aneurysm in high risk patients: outcome of selective management based on size and expansion rate. Ann Surg 1984;200:255-263.

Coyle KA, Smith RB III, Salam AA, et al. Carotid endarterectomy in the octogenarian. Ann Vasc Surg 1994;8:417-420.

Currie IC, Robson AK, Scott DJA, et al. Quality of life of octogenarians after aneurysm surgery. Ann R Coll Surg 1992;74:269-273.

Dean RH, Woody JD, Enarson CE, et al. Operative treatment of abdominal aortic aneurysms in octogenarians: when is it too much too late? Ann Surg 1993;217:721-728.

Friedman SG, Kerner BA, Friedman MS, et al. Limb salvage in elderly patients: is aggressive surgical therapy warranted? J Cardiovasc Surg 1989;30:848-851.

Hoballah JJ, Martinasevic M, Chalmers RTA, et al. Management of infrarenal abdominal aortic aneurysms in the elderly: "the geriatric abdominal aortic aneurysm." Internat J Angiol 1996;5:222-225.

Hoballah JJ, Nazzal MM, Jacobovicz C, et al. Entering the ninth decade is not a contraindication for carotid endarterectomy. Angiology. (In press).

O'Hara PJ, Hertzer NR, Krajewski LP, et al. Ten-year experience with abdominal aortic aneurysm repair in octogenarians: early results and late outcome. J Vasc Surg 1995;21:830-838.

O'Mara CS, Kilgore TL, Jr, McMullan MH, et al. Distal bypass for limb salvage in very elderly patients. Am Surgeon 1987;53(2):66-70.

Plecha FR, Bertin VJ, Plecha EJ, et al. The early results of vascular surgery in patients 75 years of age and older: an analysis of 3,259 cases. J Vasc Surg 1985;2:769-774.

Scher LA, Veith FJ, Ascer E, et al. Limb salvage in octogenarians and nonagenarians. Surgery 1986;90(2):160-165.

SECTION 11.13   SURGICAL ENDOSCOPY

UNIT OBJECTIVE:

Demonstrate knowledge of and the ability to use a variety of endoscopic instruments in the screening, diagnosis, and treatment of various diseases.

Medical Knowledge about established and evolving biomedical, clinical, and cognate (e.g. epidemiological and social-behavioral) sciences and the application of this knowledge to patient care.

<u>Junior Level:</u>

1. Review normal anatomy and physiology of the gastrointestinal tract, airway, mediastinum, and thorax.

2. Demonstrate a working knowledge of the anatomical landmarks in the following organs. Describe and contrast the normal and pathological appearance of the:

   a. Esophagus   e. Colon

   b. Stomach   f. Airways

   c. Duodenum   g. Mediastinum

   d. Small bowel   h. Thorax

3. Identify the indications for endoscopy and common pathological conditions outlined below:

   a. Esophagus

      (1) Classes of esophagitis   (5) Ulcers

      (2) Esophageal varices   (6) Strictures

      (3) Barrett's Esophagus   (7) Infections

      (4) Neoplasms (benign/malignant)

   b. Stomach

      (1) Ulcers: benign/malignant

      (2) Gastric varices

      (3) Gastric polyps: benign/malignant

      (4) Erosive gastritis

(5)   Gastric outlet obstruction

(6)   Gastric Bezoar

(7)   Marginal ulcer

(8)   The postoperative stomach

c.   Duodenum

(1)   Ulcers

(2)   Polyps: benign/malignant

(3)   Inflammatory conditions (Duodenal Crohn's)

(4)   Tumors of the duodenum and ampulla of Vater

d.   Small bowel

(1)   Indications for enteroclysis

(2)   Ileal Crohn's

(3)   Angiodysplasia

(4)   Leiomyoma

e.   Large bowel

(1)   Polyps: benign and malignant; sessile and polypoid

(2)   Diverticulosis/Diverticulitis

(3)   Inflammatory conditions

(a)   Ulcerative colitis

(b)   Crohn's Colitis

(c)   Pseudomembranous colitis

(4)   Intestinal ischemia

(5)   Tumors: benign and malignant

(6)   Melanosis Coli

4.   Identify the various anatomical landmarks during endoscopy:

a.   Esophagus

       GE junction/Z-line

b.   Stomach

(1)   Cardia   (4)   Incisura angularis

(2)   Fundus   (5)   Antrum

| | | (3) | Body | (6) | Pylorus |
| c. | Duodenum |

        (1)   Duodenal bulb   (3)   Papilla of Vater

        (2)   Duodenal mucosa

  d.   Colon

        (1)   Rectum

        (2)   Sigmoid

        (3)   Descending

        (4)   Splenic flexure

        (5)   Transverse

        (6)   Hepatic flexure

        (7)   Ascending colon

        (8)   Ileocecal valve

        (9)   Cecum, confluence of tinea coli, and appendiceal orifice

5. Describe the fundamental mechanics and physics of endoscopic equipment and accessories (e.g., rigid and flexible scopes, multichannel scopes, types of snares, and biopsy forceps).

6. Be familiar with the routine operation of endoscopes and their support systems, including:

  a.   Ability to troubleshoot minor malfunctions

  b.   Knowledge of established procedures for cleaning, sterilization, and routine handling

7. Summarize methodological issues in endoscopy to include:

a.	Patient preparation	d.	Cytology techniques
b.	Intubation	e.	Specimen handling
c.	Biopsy techniques	f.	Polypectomies

8. Review surgical journals (e.g., SAGES publications) and other medical and surgical sources of information regarding screening, diagnostic, and therapeutic uses of various endoscopic procedures.

9. Understand the various access techniques for laparoscopic surgery, including:

   a. Veress needle   d. Optical trocars

   b. Closed   e. Combination techniques

   c. Open

10. Describe factors that account for the principal physiologic effects and benefits of laparoscopy, including:

    a. Reduced tissue trauma

    b. Carbon dioxide pneumoperitoneum

    c. Use of Helium, Argon, or Nitrous oxide

    d. Gasless laparoscopy

11. Outline the indications for performing diagnostic and therapeutic:

    a. Laryngoscopy   g. Proctosigmoidoscopy

    b. Bronchoscopy   h. Thoracoscopy

    c. Colonoscopy   i. Mediastinoscopy

    d. Laparoscopy

    e. Choledochoscopy

    f. Esophagogastroduodenoscopy (EGD)

12. Summarize the use of sedatives (conscious sedation) and analgesics during endoscopic procedures, including:

    a. Mode of onset   d. Reversing agents

    b. Principles of monitoring   e. monetary considerations

    c. Side effects

13. Describe potential advantages of thoracoscopy over an open procedure, discussing:

    a. Pain

b.   Length of hospital stay

c.   Tissue trauma

d.   Costs (hospital, disability, additional procedures)

e.   Cosmesis

14.   Analyze the purpose of established guidelines for the management of various gastrointestinal disease states as developed by:

a.   Society for Surgery of the Alimentary Tract (SSAT)

b.   Society of American Gastrointestinal Endoscopic Surgeons (SAGES)

c.   American Society for Gastrointestinal Endoscopy (ASGE)

Senior Level:

1.   Explain the pathophysiology of disease entities in which proctosigmoidoscopy, rigid or flexible, is indicated, including:

a.   Ulcerative colitis   e.   Ischemic colitis

b.   Crohn's Disease   f.   Rectal ulcers

c.   Rectal polyps and tumors   g.   Anorectal tumors

d.   Pseudomembranous colitis   h.   Sigmoid volvulus

2.   Differentiate between the following therapeutic maneuvers utilizing the endoscope:

a.   Dilatation

b.   Laser ablation

c.   Endomucosal resection

d.   Sclerotherapy

e.   Electrocautery (bipolar, monopolar, heater probe)

f.   Polyp excision

3.   Analyze the use of endoscopes in the diagnosis and treatment of upper and lower gastrointestinal hemorrhage.

4.   Assess the complications that may result from flexible endoscopic procedures, including:

a.   Hemorrhage

b.   Perforation and the various causes

5.   Determine and categorize the essential features of a wide variety of diseases as seen through the endoscopes listed in #8 above.

6.   Evaluate the uses of laparoscopy in surgical procedures to include:

   a.   Indications and contraindications

   b.   Technical and procedural considerations.

   c.   Post-procedure care

   d.   Comparison of open and laparoscopic procedures in regards to morbidity and mortality

   e.   Complications

7.   Understand the significance of laparoscopy and endoscopy in elderly patients:

   a.   Elective, corrective action

   b.   Sedation

   c.   Continuous monitoring

   d. CO_2 effects

   e.   Length of stay

8.   Assess the significance of physiologic effects of Carbon dioxide pneumoperitoneum, including:

   a.   Heart rate   e.   Decrease in venous return

   b.   Mean arterial blood pressure   f.   Cardiac output

   c.   Systemic vascular resistance   g.   Cardiac index

   d.   Central venous pressure

9.   Identify potential complications of thoracoscopic pulmonary resection, describing the significance of:

   a.   Pneumothorax   d.   Lung injury

   b.   Air leak   e.   Infection

   c.   Air embolism   f.   Equipment malfunction

10.   Summarize the legal and ethical issues associated with the use of endoscopic procedures.

Patient Care that is compassionate, appropriate, and effective for the treatment of health

problems and the promotion of health

Junior Level:

1.   Observe flexible and rigid endoscopic procedures.

2.   Under supervision, manipulate the endoscope for routine endoscopic procedures.

3.   Discuss pathological findings and their significance as they relate to the patient's clinical

history or condition.

4.   Observe and monitor appropriate anesthetic techniques used to sedate the patient.

5.   Prepare patients for various routine and elective endoscopic procedures.

6.   Under supervision, demonstrate proper cleansing and sterilization of endoscopic

instruments.

7.   Participate in hands-on experience in rigid sigmoidoscopy in the operating room and in

the endoscopic suite or clinic.

8.   Distinguish between the indications for use and the preparation methods of the following:

   a.   Biopsy   c.   Culture

   b.   Smears (cytologic)   d.   Cytology

9.   Use the flexible sigmoidoscope under direct supervision, beginning with elective cases.

10.   Use models to improve eye-hand coordination and experience with endoscopic

instruments, including:

   a.   Computer simulators

   b.   Trainer boxes

   c.   Inanimate models

   d.   Animal models

11.   Assist in the performance of diagnostic and therapeutic:

a. Esophagoscopy (rigid and flexible):

b. Esophagogastroduodenoscopy (EGD)

c. Colonoscopy

d. Laparoscopy

e. Bronchoscopy

f. Thoracoscopy

g. Mediastinoscopy

h. Endoscopic retrograde cholangiopancreatography

i. Operative choledochoscopy

Senior Level:

1. Demonstrate, under proper senior supervision, the performance of a rigid proctosigmoidoscopy.

2. Observe, recognize, and interpret normal and abnormal findings by the use of the endoscopic procedures listed in #11 immediately above.

3. Perform flexible sigmoidoscopy under supervision.

4. Perform uncomplicated therapeutic endoscopic maneuvers under direct supervision such as:

a. Excision of pedunculated colonic polyps

b. Performance of percutaneous endoscopic gastrostomy (PEG)

5. Perform all portions of esophagoscopy, esophagogastro-duodenoscopy, and colonoscopy under supervision.

6. Perform the following uncomplicated endoscopic procedures independently with supervision available if needed:

a. Rigid and flexible sigmoidoscopy

b. Anoproctoscopy

7. Initiate and correlate the management of surgical patients who require various endoscopic procedures.

8.   Demonstrate knowledge of the indications and contraindications for various medications used at your institution in the preparation and performance of endoscopic procedures.

9.   Describe and demonstrate knowledge of the anatomy of the biliary tree as it relates to the use and limitations of the choledochoscope.

10. Assist in therapeutic endoscopic procedures such as:

   a.   Sclerotherapy of esophageal varices

   b.   Electrocoagulation of upper and lower bleeding lesions

   c.   Removal of foreign bodies

   d.   Endoscopic polypectomy

   e.   Percutaneous gastrostomy

11. Observe and assist in more complicated therapeutic procedures such as:

   a.   Coagulation of mucosal ulcers

   b.   Palliative treatment of intestinal malignancies

   c.   Palliative stent placement

12. Describe the indications for and employ the best use of rigid and flexible bronchoscopy in patients, including:

   a.   Evacuation of mucous plugs

   b.   Brush biopsy techniques

   c.   Collection of bronchoscopic washings for culture and cytology

   d.   Removal of foreign bodies from the respiratory tract

   e.   Biopsy of endobronchial masses

Practice-Based Learning and Improvement that involves investigation and evaluation of their own patient care, appraisal and assimilation of scientific evidence, and improvements in patient care.

INFORMATION TECHNOLOGY AND POPULATION COMPARISONS

REFERENCES

Adkins RB, Jr., Avant GR, Eller R, Ladipo JK. Endoscopy and laparoscopic surgery. In: Adkins RB, Jr., Scott HW, Jr. (eds), Surgical Care for the Elderly (2nd ed). Philadelphia: Lippincott-Raven Publishers, 1998;89-102.

Eubanks S. Endosurgical principles. In: Greenfield LJ, Mulholland M, Oldham KT, Zelenock GB, Lillemoe KD (eds), Surgery: Scientific Principles and Practice (2nd ed). Philadelphia: Lippincott-Raven, 1997;735-743.

Eubanks WS, Swanstrom LL, Soper, NJ. Mastery of Endoscopic and Laparoscopic Surgery. Philadelphia: Lippincott Williams and Wilkins, 1999.

Fink AS. Endoscopy. In: Zinner MJ, Schwartz SI, Ellis H (eds), Maingot's AbdominalOperations (10th ed). CT: Appleton & Lange 1997;189-238.

Green FL, Ponsky JL. Endoscopic Surgery. Philadelphia: WB Saunders, 1994.

McFadyen BV, Ponsky JL. Operative Laparoscopy and Thoracoscopy. Philadelphia: Lippincott-Raven, 1996.

Ponsky JL. Atlas of Surgical Endoscopy. St. Louis: Mosby Year Book, 1992. SAGES. Curriculum Guide for Resident Education in Surgical Endoscopy. Santa Monica, CA: Society American Gastrointestinal Endoscopic Surgeons, 1998:1-25.

Toouli J, Gossot D, Hunter JG. Endoscopy. New York: Churchill Livingstone, 1996.

http://www.asge.org

http://www.sages.org

SECTION 11.14   PEDIATRIC SURGERY

NEONATAL SURGERY

UNIT OBJECTIVES:

Understand the unique anatomic, pathophysiologic, and genetic conditions that affect the fetus and neonate.

Learn the principles of stabilization, appropriate preoperative diagnosis, and preparation of the sick neonate.

Understand the anatomic and physiologic principles which guide successful operative repair of neonatal diseases.

Learn principles of routine postoperative care and postoperative critical care management.

Understand how new techniques, such as fetal surgery, may offer alternatives for treatment of certain neonatal diseases.

Medical Knowledge about established and evolving biomedical, clinical, and cognate (e.g. epidemiological and social-behavioral) sciences and the application of this knowledge to patient care.

Junior Level:

Learn the embryology, anatomy and physiology of common neonatal surgical diseases:

1.   Describe the cardiac, pulmonary, blood volume, and gastrointestinal changes of postpartum transitional physiology.

2.   Describe relevant mechanisms (conductive, convective, evaporative, and radiant) of neonatal thermoregulation.

3.   Describe how neonatal renal function (decreased concentrating ability) affects the pharmacokinetics of commonly used drugs and antibiotics.

4.   Describe factors influencing neonatal immunologic immaturity and how this increases susceptibility to common neonatal pathogens.

5.   Describe appropriate fluid and electrolyte management of the full-term neonate.

6. Describe the nutritional requirements of the full-term neonate, and calculate appropriate enteral and parenteral nutritional support.

7. Describe the embryology of neonatal organ systems and their common congenital anomalies, including:

   a. Craniocervical: dermoid cysts, branchial cleft cysts, and fistulas

   b. Foregut: esophageal atresia/tracheoesophageal fistula, duodenal atresia

   c. Respiratory: cystic adenomatoid malformation, congenital diaphragmatic hernia

   d. Cardiac: common cyanotic and acyanotic cardiac malformations

   e. Midgut: intestinal atresia, malrotation, meconium ileus

   f. Hindgut: Hirschsprung's disease, imperforate anus, meconium plug syndrome, small left colon syndrome

   g. Body wall defects: gastroschisis, omphalocele, umbilical and inguinal hernias

   h. Renal: ureteral obstruction, vesicoureteral reflux

   i. Lower GU tract: urethral valves, hypospadias

8. Explain the pathophysiology of necrotizing enterocolitis.

9. Describe the arterial and venous anatomy of the neonate.

Diagnose common neonatal problems and describe surgical procedures for their correction:

1. Describe the diagnosis, preoperative evaluation, and management of the common congenital anomalies listed above.

2. Outline the technical principles involved in the following procedures:

   a. Gastrostomy

   b. Colostomy

   c. Inguinal and umbilical herniorrhaphy

   d. Circumcision

   e. Central venous access

3. Explain the perioperative care of neonates, including:

   a. Basic ventilator management

   b. Fluid, electrolyte, and nutritional management

c. Correction of coagulopathies

d. Indications for transfusion

e. Diagnosis of sepsis and antibiotic use

Senior Level:

The senior-level resident should function as an effective consultant to the nursery, and be able to provide expertise in the evaluation and definitive treatment of elective surgical conditions as well as be able to perform emergent surgical procedures (including but not limited to vascular access, orotracheal intubation, tube thoracostomy, exploratory laparotomy, and exploratory thoracotomy) with little or no immediate supervision. The senior-level resident should be prepared to direct the management of the pediatric surgical service, including the education of junior residents and medical students on surgical clerkships.

Learn the embryology, anatomy, and physiology of basic and advanced neonatal surgical diseases. The resident is responsible for all conditions listed above in junior-level objectives, plus:

1. Describe the pathophysiology and evaluation of:

   a. Respiratory distress
   b. Cyanosis
   c. Gastroesophageal reflux
   d. Jaundice
   e. Bilious emesis
   f. Abdominal distention
   g. Bloody diarrhea
   h. Body wall defects

2. Describe the complications and appropriate treatment of necrotizing enterocolitis.

3. Describe appropriate fluid and electrolyte management of the premature neonate.

4. Describe the nutritional requirements of premature neonates, and calculate appropriate enteral and parenteral nutritional support.

5. Describe the embryology of basic anomalies (listed above) and more complex congenital anomalies, including:

   a. Craniocervical: choanal atresia, cleft lip and palate
   b. Foregut: laryngotracheal cleft, duodenal web and duplication,

annular pancreas, preduodenal portal vein, biliary atresia

    c.   Respiratory: congenital lobar emphysema and sequestrations

    d.   Cardiac: complex cyanotic and acyanotic cardiac malformation

    e.   Midgut: intestinal duplication, volvulus, meconium peritonitis

    f.   Hindgut: neuronal intestinal dysplasia, total colonic and ultrashort Hirschsprung's disease, cloacal exstrophy

    g.   Body wall defects: pentalogy of Cantrell, Jeune's thoracic dystrophy

    h.   Renal: renal agenesis, fusion and ectopia; bladder exstrophy, prune-belly syndrome

    i.   Lower GU tract: ambiguous genitalia, urogenital sinus abnormalities

Diagnose common neonatal problems and describe surgical procedures for their correction:

1.   Describe the diagnosis, preoperative evaluation, operative management, and postoperative care of the congenital anomalies listed above.

2.   Describe the immediate care, operative correction, and postoperative management of life-threatening anomalies:

    a.   Congenital diaphragmatic hernia

    b.   Midgut volvulus

    c.   Necrotizing enterocolitis

    d.   Gastroschisis

    e.   Prune-belly syndrome

3.   Describe respiratory support of the neonate, including high frequency ventilation and extracorporeal membrane oxygenation.

4.   Describe neonatal nutritional assessment and supervision of long-term nutritional support for neonates with short-gut syndrome.

5.   Describe indications for and technical aspects of endoscopic evaluation of the neonate.

6.   Describe indications for and technical aspects of intubation, tube thoracostomy, and percutaneous central venous access in the neonate.

Patient Care that is compassionate, appropriate, and effective for the treatment of health problems and the promotion of health.

Junior Level:

1. Perform a comprehensive evaluation of a neonate with suspected surgically correctable conditions.

2. Establish percutaneous venous and arterial access in neonates over 2 kg.

3. Assist or perform under supervision:

    a. Peripheral venous and arterial cutdown access

    b. Placement of umbilical catheters

    c. Placement of central venous access

    d. Tube thoracostomy

    e. Incision and drainage of cysts and abscesses

    f. Hernia reduction

4. Participate in the perioperative care of the neonate by recording appropriate assessments and treatment plans in daily progress notes, including:

    a. Ventilator management

    b. Fluid, electrolyte, and nutritional management

    c. Antibiotic use

5. Complete oral or written examination of topics listed in junior level knowledge objectives.

6. Assist or perform surgical repairs of congenital diseases listed in junior-level knowledge objectives.

Senior Level:

1. Describe the capabilities and limitations of various diagnostic modalities used in neonatal care.

2. Formulate a care plan for neonates with problems such as:

a.	Respiratory distress	e.	Bilious emesis
b.	Cyanosis	f.	Abdominal distention
c.	Gastroesophageal reflux	g.	Bloody diarrhea
d.	Jaundice	h.	Body wall defects

3. Perform or assist in all major surgical procedures performed on the pediatric surgical service.

4. Personally conduct comprehensive preoperative evaluation and postoperative management for all critically ill neonates, and direct junior residents in the management of routine surgical problems.

5. Complete oral or written examination of topics listed in senior-level knowledge objectives.

Practice-Based Learning and Improvement that involves investigation and evaluation of their own patient care, appraisal and assimilation of scientific evidence, and improvements in patient care.

INFORMATION TECHNOLOGY AND POPULATION COMPARISONS REFERENCES

Avery GB, Fletcher MA, MacDonald MG (eds). Neonatology: Pathophysiology and Management of the Newborn (4th ed). Philadelphia: JB Lippincott Company, 1994.

Avery ME, First LR (eds). Pediatric Medicine (2nd ed). Baltimore: Williams & Wilkins, 1994.
Carlson BM. Human Embryology and Developmental Biology. Baltimore: Mosby-Year Book, Inc., 1994.

Fuhrman BP, Zimmerman JJ (eds). Pediatric Critical Care (2nd ed). Baltimore: Mosby-Year Book, Inc., 1998.

O'Neill JA, Rowe MI, Grosfeld JL, Fonkalsrud EW, Coran AG (eds). Pediatric Surgery (5th ed).
St. Louis: Mosby-Year Book, Inc., 1998.

Stringer MD, Oldham KT, Mouriquand PDE, Howard ER (eds). Pediatric Surgery and Urology:
Long Term Outcomes. Philadelphia: WB Saunders Company, Ltd., 1998.

PEDIATRIC SURGERY

UNIT OBJECTIVES:

Understand the unique anatomic, pathophysiologic, and genetic conditions that affect children.
Learn the principles of stabilization, appropriate preoperative diagnosis, and preparation of the
sick child.
Understand the anatomic and physiologic principles which guide successful operative repair of
pediatric diseases.
Learn principles of routine postoperative care and postoperative critical care management.

Medical Knowledge about established and evolving biomedical, clinical, and cognate (e.g.
epidemiological and social-behavioral) sciences and the application of this knowledge to
patient care.

<u>Junior Level:</u>

1. Describe the development of children in terms of the following criteria:
   a. Weight, length, and head size
   b. Nutritional requirements
   c. Renal function
   d. Hormonal influences on development
   e. Response to stress and infection

2. Classify congenital malformations of the newborn by type, origin, and the need for
   surgical intervention:
   a. Head and neck: thyroglossal duct cyst, lymphadenopathy, cystic hygroma

b.   Gastrointestinal: pyloric stenosis, appendicitis

c.   Respiratory: tracheal lesions

d.   Abdominal wall defects: omphalomesenteric and urachal malformations

e.   Genitourinary: polycystic kidneys, undescended testis, torsion of the testis

f.   Inborn and genetic errors: trisomy 13, trisomy 18, Down's syndrome

g.   Orthopedic anomalies which commonly occur with other malformations

3.   Summarize the basic approach to the diagnosis and management of more common surgical problems of infancy and childhood, such as:

a.   Pyloric stenosis

b.   Perforated appendicitis

c.   Intussusception

4.   Identify the technical aspects of the following procedures:

a.   Excision of skin and subcutaneous lesions

b.   Incision and drainage of abscesses

c.   Lymph node biopsy

d.   Chest tube placement

e.   Oral intubation

f.   Herniorrhaphy in older children

5.   Describe the fundamental considerations in the pre- and post- operative care of infants and children in the cases listed above.

6.   Explain the principles of diagnosis and treatment for common causes of gastrointestinal hemorrhage in the neonate, infant, child, and adolescent.

<u>Senior Level:</u>

The senior-level resident should function as an effective consultant to the nursery, and be able to provide expertise in the evaluation and definitive treatment of elective surgical conditions as well as be able to perform emergent surgical procedures (including but not limited to vascular access, orotracheal intubation, tube thoracostomy, exploratory laparotomy, and exploratory thoracotomy) with little or no immediate supervision. The senior level resident should be prepared to direct the management of the pediatric surgical service, including the education of junior residents and medical students on surgical clerkships.

Learn the embryology, anatomy, and physiology of basic and advanced neonatal surgical diseases. The resident is responsible for all conditions listed above in junior-level objectives, plus:

1. Explain the approach to surgical management, (i.e., diagnosis, perioperative care, surgical therapy, and postoperative follow-up) of more complex surgical procedures for infants and children such as:

  a. Large skin grafts and musculocutaneous flaps

  b. Thoracotomy for pulmonary resection and vascular cardiac repair

  c. Flexible endoscopy

  d. Antireflux procedure

  e. Bowel resection

  f. Repair of hepatic, biliary, and pancreatic injury

  g. Splenectomy and splenorrhaphy

  h. Management of the seriously injured patient

2. Analyze the pathophysiology, diagnosis, and management options in the treatment of short-gut syndrome.

3. Demonstrate an understanding of the special psychological, social, and education issues confronting selected pediatric trauma/ postoperative patients.

Patient Care that is compassionate, appropriate, and effective for the treatment of health problems and the promotion of health.

Junior Level:

1. Evaluate surgical conditions in the pediatric population through a comprehensive history, physical examination, and appropriate diagnostic studies.

2. Participate in the management of simple surgical problems in the pediatric population, including:

    a.   Integument

        (1)   Excision of skin and subcutaneous lesions

        (2)   Incision and drainage of abscesses

    b.   Head and Neck

        (1)   Excision of dermoid cysts and small skin lesions

        (2)   Lymph node biopsy

    c.   Thoracic

        (1)   Chest tube placement

    d.   Cardiovascular

        (1)   Central venous catheter placement

        (2)   Venous cutdown

        (3)   Arterial line placement

    e.   Gastrointestinal

        (1)   Pyloromyotomy

        (2)   Appendectomy

        (3)   Herniorrhaphy (umbilical; inguinal in patients 2 years and up)

    f.   Genitourinary

        (1)   Circumcision

        (2)   Orchiopexy

    g.   Gynecology

        (1)   Oophorectomy, simple

        (2)   Vaginoscopy for foreign body or biopsy

    h.   Musculoskeletal

        (1)   Ganglion cyst excision

        (2)   Excision of supernumerary digit

        (3)   Muscle biopsy

3. Develop a working relationship with members of the pediatric intensive care unit in managing postoperative pediatric patients.

1. Evaluate pediatric patients for problems requiring more complex surgical intervention.

2. Participate in preoperative, operative, and postoperative care of more complex problems in pediatric surgery such as:

    a. Integument

        (1)   Pedicle graft

        (2)   Large skin grafts for burns

        (3)   Subcutaneous mastectomy

    b. Craniocervical

        (1)   Branchial cleft and thyroglossal duct cysts

        (2)   Cystic hygroma

    c. Thoracic

        (1)   Laryngoscopy, bronchoscopy, esophagoscopy

        (2)   Tracheostomy

        (3)   Thoracotomy for biopsy, lung resection

        (4)   Diaphragm repair

    d. Cardiovascular

        (1)   Resection of small vascular cutaneous lesions such as (A-V) malformation, hemangioma, or lymphangioma

        (2)   Repair of patent ductus arteriosus

        (3)   Repair of aortic anomaly/injury

        (4)   Support of a child with extracorporeal membrane oxygenation (ECMO)

    e. Gastrointestinal

        (1)   Flexible endoscopy

        (2)   Antireflux procedure

        (3)   Bowel resection for inflammatory bowel disease, intussusception, intestinal duplications

        (4)   Hodgkin's staging

        (5)   Biopsy of tumor (open, laparoscopic or endoscopic)

        (6)   Laparotomy for trauma

        (7)   Splenectomy (laparoscopic or open), splenorrhaphy

        (8)   Repair of hepatic injury, renal and/or bladder injury

        (9)   Cholecystectomy (open or laparoscopic)

        (10)   Omphalomesenteric duct and urachal anomalies

    f.   Oncologic

        (1)   Neuroblastoma

        (2)   Wilms' tumor

        (3)   Rhabdomyosarcoma

        (4)   Teratomas

        (5)   Germ cell tumors

        (6)   Hepatoblastoma

        (7)   Sarcomas

        (8)   Hodgkin's and non-Hodgkin's lymphomas

        (9)   ALL

    g.   Genitourinary

        (1)   Polycystic kidney

        (2)   Ambiguous genitalia

    h.   Musculoskeletal

        (1)   Torticollis

Practice-Based Learning and Improvement that involves investigation and evaluation of their own patient care, appraisal and assimilation of scientific evidence, and improvements in patient care.

INFORMATION TECHNOLOGY AND POPULATION COMPARISONS REFERENCES

Avery ME, First LR (eds). Pediatric Medicine (2nd ed). Baltimore: Williams & Wilkins, 1994.

Carlson BM. Human Embryology and Developmental Biology. Baltimore: Mosby-Year Book, Inc., 1994.

Cox CC, Marvin RG, Lally KP, et al. Physiologic problems in the pediatric surgical patient. In: Miller TA (ed), Modern Surgical Care: Physiologic Foundations and Clinical Applications (2nd ed). St. Louis: Quality Medical Publishing, Inc., 1998;1337-1361.

Fuhrman BP, Zimmerman JJ (eds). Pediatric Critical Care (2nd ed). Baltimore: Mosby-Year Book, Inc., 1998.

O'Neill JA, Rowe MI, Grosfeld JL, Fonkalsrud EW, Coran AG (eds). Pediatric Surgery (5th ed). St. Louis: Mosby-Year Book, Inc., 1998.

Stringer MD, Oldham KT, Mouriquand PDE, Howard ER (eds). Pediatric Surgery and Urology: Long Term Outcomes. Philadelphia: WB Saunders Company, Ltd., 1998.

http://www.eapsa.org

SECTION 11.15   OTOLARYNGOLOGY AND HEAD AND NECK SURGERY
PART A: OTOLARYNGOLOGY

UNIT OBJECTIVES:

Demonstrate knowledge of the anatomy, physiology, and pathophysiology of the ear, nose, and throat pertinent to the practice of general surgery.

Demonstrate the ability to manage ear, nose, and throat problems associated with the practice of general surgery.

Medical Knowledge about established and evolving biomedical, clinical, and cognate (e.g. epidemiological and social-behavioral) sciences and the application of this knowledge to patient care.

1.   Identify the anatomy and explain the physiology of the ear, nose, oral cavity, and throat.

2.   Summarize the essential components of a focused history and physical examination for common otolaryngologic problems.

3.   Discuss the significance of the cornerstones of the physical examination, including:

   a.   Visual inspection c. Palpation

   b.   Auscultation d. Percussion

4.   Analyze the clinical management of ear, nose, and throat (ENT) patients in the intensive care unit (ICU), including:

   a.   Respiratory infection management

   b.   Airway management

   c.   Wound care

5.   Describe and compare the pathophysiology of the following common ENT diseases:

   a.   Sinusitis   c.   Neck abscess

   b.   Sialadenitis   d.   Epiglottitis

6. Describe and explain the pathophysiology of presbycusis as it can be:

   a. Conductive

   b. Metabolic and toxic

   c. Neural

   d. Cochlear

   e. Tumor-related

   f. Age-dependent

7. Explain how physical examination differs for delineation of conductive versus neurosensory hearing loss.

8. Explain the principal causes of simple epistaxis and describe its management.

9. Evaluate patients with facial trauma and develop a treatment plan for the management of:

   a. Fractures   c. Hemotympanum

   b. Lacerations   d. Epistaxis

10. Describe the indications for tracheostomy in adults and children.

11. Discuss the indications for biopsy of lesions of the skin of the face, neck, and oral cavity.

12. Compare the use of the following procedures in evaluating ENT problems:

    a. Radiography

    b. Contrast studies

    c. Ultrasound

13. Describe the indications for simple endoscopy and its diagnostic contributions such as:

    a. Nasopharyngoscopy   c. Esophagoscopy

    b. Direct laryngoscopy

14. Summarize the characteristics of the common neoplasms of the ear, nose, and throat, and describe appropriate surgical intervention.

15. Outline the diagnostic approaches to otolaryngologic neoplasia, including:

    a. Direct visualization   c. Use of radiography

    b. Indirect visualization   d. Fine-needle biopsy

16. Describe diagnostic and therapeutic procedures utilized in treating the following:

    a. Abscess   c. Oral ulcer

    b. Neck mass   d. Salivary gland mass

17. Describe and demonstrate methods for removing foreign bodies from the trachea, bronchus, and esophagus.

18. Compare surgical approaches using surgical flaps for repair of ENT defects and trauma of the lip, alar rim, and helix.

19. Outline the diagnosis and repair of facial fractures of the mandible, nose, and frontal sinus.

20. Summarize diagnostic and therapeutic considerations in the management of caustic injury to the mouth, nasopharynx, trachea, and esophagus.

21. Discuss the management of airway in patients with terminal carcinoma of the thyroid and trachea.

22. Describe the signs and symptoms and discuss the health care significance to elderly patients from the pathophysiology of:

    a. Tinnitus   c. Cerumen impaction

    b. Vertigo   d. Basilar artery stenosis

Patient Care that is compassionate, appropriate, and effective for the treatment of health problems and the promotion of health.

1. Perform and record a focused ENT history and physical examination.

2. Manage the emergent/elective airway; using visual inspection, radiographic evaluation, indirect invasive and non-invasive visualization techniques (direct speculum and indirect mirror evaluations, direct fiberoptic and rigid evaluations); with consideration for:

    a. Nose, nasal passages   d. Larynx

    b. Nasopharynx   e. Trachea

    c. Oropharynx

3. Be prepared to manage airway obstruction as the result of:

    a. Edema   d. Anaphylaxis

    b. Secretion   e. Foreign body

    c. Benign and malignant tumors (including, vascular malformations and infectious processes)

4. Evaluate patients with facial trauma, including fractures, lacerations, hemotympanum, and epistaxis.

5. Perform tracheostomy on adults under direct supervision.

6. Perform biopsies of lesions of skin of face, neck, and oral cavity.

7. Perform evaluation of a neck mass, and provide appropriate treatment.

8. Correctly differentiate between the indications for and management of cricothyroidotomy and tracheostomy, demonstrating varying techniques and choice of instrumentation for emergent airway management and ventilation in each.

9. Interpret radiologic examinations of sinuses.

10. Perform simple endoscopy including:

    a. Nasopharyngoscopy   c. Esophagoscopy

    b. Direct laryngoscopy

11. Evaluate head and neck tumor patients, and be prepared to perform a tumor biopsy.

12. Perform tracheostomy on children with supervision.

13. Evaluate radiologic studies of the head and neck, including computed axial tomography (CAT) scanning.

14. Evaluate and treat head and neck abscesses and other masses.

15. Remove esophageal foreign bodies endoscopically.

16. Perform diagnostic bronchoscopy.

17. Reconstruct facial and neck defects with transposition and myocutaneous flaps.

18. Manage facial fractures with appropriate consultation.

19. Evaluate and treat caustic injury.

20. Manage airway in patients with terminal thyroid or tracheal carcinoma.

PART B: HEAD AND NECK SURGERY
UNIT OBJECTIVES:

Demonstrate understanding of the anatomy, physiology, and pathophysiology of the head and neck amenable to surgical intervention.

Demonstrate the ability to manage surgical problems of the head and neck in a variety of settings.

Medical Knowledge about established and evolving biomedical, clinical, and cognate (e.g. epidemiological and social-behavioral) sciences and the application of this knowledge to patient care.

1. Define and discuss the three-dimensional anatomy of the head and neck region with regard to:
   a. Interrelationships of anatomy
   b. Fascial planes
   c. Path and course of cranial nerves
   d. Major arterioles and venous structures
   e. Musculature of face and neck
   f. Anatomy of larynx and cervical trachea
   g. Location of cricothyroid membrane
   h. Cervical anatomy of nasopharynx, pharynx, esophagus (special emphasis on sinuses, eustachian tubes, middle and external ear structures)

2. Describe laryngeal function as it relates to voice production.
3. Describe the interrelationship of pharyngeal and laryngeal function.
4. Identify the bones of the skull, face, and cervical spine. Explain their relationship to major neurologic and neurovascular structures of the head and neck.
5. Analyze predisposing factors for head and neck cancer.
6. Differentiate between neoplastic and non-neoplastic neck masses.

7. Explain the tumor, nodes, and metastases (TNM) classification system for tumors of the head and neck.

8. Prepare a protocol for evaluating intraoral cancer.

9. Outline the principles associated with the repair of avulsion of ear and nose.

10. Indicate how to examine a patient with severe facial laceration to rule out damage to the following:

    a. Lacrimal drainage systems

    b. Parotid gland and duct

    c. Facial nerve

11. Identify and delineate

    a. Pathophysiology of cranial nerve dysfunctions and injuries

    b. Brachial plexus injuries

    c. Anatomy/location of parotid and submandibular ductal drainage systems

12. Define and describe the Le Fort maxillary fracture classification system.

13. Define and demonstrate knowledge of Angle's classification of dental occlusion.

14. Identify and delineate Zones I, II, and III of penetrating injuries to the neck and their associated management.

15. Describe the roles of the following diagnostic modalities in the evaluation of head and neck lesions and facial fracture:

    a. Plain x-rays   e. Isotope scans

    b. CT scanning   f. Ultrasound

    c. Sialography

    d. Magnetic resonance imaging (MRI)

16. Describe the anatomy of the fascial spaces of the neck and their importance in neck abscesses and infections.

17. Discuss indications for radical and modified radical neck dissection.

18. Distinguish between the following kinds of grafts in the management of head and neck problems:

a. Split-thickness grafts

b. Full-thickness skin grafts

c. Rotational flaps

d. Free flaps

19. Describe the anatomy and the advantages and disadvantages of regional flaps available for head and neck reconstruction.

20. Compare and contrast the use of the following local flaps:

a. Advancement e. Z-plasty

b. Rotational f. W-plasty

c. Pedicle g. V-Y advancement

d. Rhomboid (Limberg)

21. Outline the advantages and disadvantages of irradiation, chemotherapy, and resection of neoplastic lesions of the:

a. Tongue   d. Retromolar trigone

b. Floor of mouth   e. Alveolar ridge

c. Buccal mucosa   f. Palate

22. Discuss the frequency of benign and malignant head and neck tumors in the pediatric population.

23. Outline the microbiology and treatment of deep neck abscesses.

24. Explain the techniques of scar revision, including:

a. Primary excision   d. Geometric broken line closure

b. Z-plasty   e. Use of cosmetics

c. Serial excision

Patient Care that is compassionate, appropriate, and effective for the treatment of health problems and the promotion of health.

1. Perform head and neck examinations, including nasopharyngoscopy and fiberoptic direct laryngoscopy.

2. Administer postoperative care (ICU, wards, discharge planning, follow-up appointments, patient/family counseling, home health care) for head and neck patients.

3. Provide emergency airway management, including performance of:

   a. Intubation

   b. Emergency cricothyrotomy

   c. Emergency tracheostomy

4. Administer treatment for sialadenitis.

5. Diagnose and evaluate infectious illness (viral, bacterial, fungal), acute and chronic, affecting:

   a. CNS

   b. Sinuses

   c. Bones

   d. Soft tissues of face

6. Demonstrate a clear understanding of the pathophysiology of:

   a. Ludwig's angina

   b. Necrotizing fasciitis of the neck

   c. Mucormycosis of sinus

   d. Epiglottitis

   e. Gustatory sweating (Frye's syndrome)

7. Perform biopsy of all intraoral lesions.

8. Care for contaminated wounds, including animal bites of face and neck.

9. Assist with incisions for head and neck surgery, including:

   a. Radical neck dissection

   b. Salivary gland surgery

   c. Tracheostomy

   d. Laryngeal/tracheal trauma

   e. Considerations for incisions of previously irradiated tissues

10. Formulate a plan for the management of an unknown primary tumor of the head and neck.

11. Perform fine-needle biopsies.

12. Perform simple operative incisions with supervision (tracheostomy, intubation, simple lesions of head and neck).

13. Assist with repair of avulsion of ear and nose.

14. Perform simple operative incisions without direct supervision.

15. Perform radical neck dissection under direct supervision.

16. Manage postoperative complications, including nerve paralysis and cutaneous fistulas from the aerodigestive tract.

17. Manage trauma to the upper airway.

Practice-Based Learning and Improvement that involves investigation and evaluation of their own patient care, appraisal and assimilation of scientific evidence, and improvements in patient care.

INFORMATION TECHNOLOGY AND POPULATION COMPARISONS
REFERENCES

Britt LD, Riblet JL. Penetrating neck trauma. In: Cameron JL (ed), Current Surgical Therapy (6th ed). St. Louis: Mosby, 1998;1000-1004.

Castle JM, Rees R. Head and neck cancer. In: Adkins RB, Jr., Scott HW, Jr. (eds), Surgical Care for the Elderly (2nd ed). Philadelphia: Lippincott-Raven Publishers, 1998;457-466.

Cobbs EL, Duthie EH, Jr, Murphy JB (eds). Hearing impairment. Oral diseases and disorders. Hearing handicap inventory. Geriatrics Review Syllabus: A Core Curriculum in Geriatric Medicine (4th ed). Dubuque IA: Kendall/Hunt Publishing Company, 1999.

Cummings CW, Krause CJ, Schuller DE, et al. (eds). Otolaryngology: Head and Neck Surgery (3rd ed). St. Louis: Mosby Year Book, 1998.

Fortune DS, Netterville JL. Rhinolaryngologic problems. In: Adkins RB, Jr., Scott HW, Jr. (eds), Surgical Care for the Elderly (2nd ed). Philadelphia: Lippincott-Raven Publishers, 1998;175-192.

Manson PN. Facial injuries. In: Cameron JL (ed), Current Surgical Therapy (6th ed). St. Louis: Mosby, 1998;990-1000.

Mulrow CD, Lichtenstein MJ. Screening for hearing impairment in the elderly. J Gen Intern Med 1991;6:249-258.

Neifeld JP. Head and neck. In: Greenfield LJ, Mulholland M, Oldham KT, Zelenock GB, Lillemoe KD (eds), Surgery: Scientific Principles and Practice (2nd ed). Philadelphia: Lippincott-Raven, 1997;635-651.

Paparella MM. Otolaryngology. Philadelphia: WB Saunders Co., 1991.

http://www.entnet.org

SECTION 11.16 NEUROSURGERY

UNIT OBJECTIVES:

Demonstrate the ability to recognize neurological or neurosurgical disease or injury so that appropriate consultation/referral can be obtained.

Demonstrate the ability to manage neurological or neurosurgical problems which require attention prior to, or in conjunction with, consultation or referral.

Medical Knowledge about established and evolving biomedical, clinical, and cognate (e.g. epidemiological and social-behavioral) sciences and the application of this knowledge to patient care.

1.   Demonstrate knowledge of and skills in neurological examination of patients with neurological or neurosurgical disease or injury so that:

   a.   An accurate history can be taken

   b.   A sufficient physical examination can be performed

   c.   Logical conclusions can be drawn regarding location and nature of neuropathology

2.   Apply basic knowledge of the following neuroradiological methods in terms of deciding, after conducting the neurological history and examination, which diagnostic tests or interventions would provide the least risk and most useful information for subsequent interpretation:

   a.   Plain skull and spine radiographs

   b.   Computed axial tomography of the head and spine

   c.   Magnetic resonance imaging (MRI)

3.   Demonstrate an understanding of the management of head injuries to include:

   a.   Selection, prioritizing, and performance of resuscitation efforts

   b.   Analyzing components and results of baseline neurological examination to determine and evaluate changes in patient neurological status

c. Treatment of a scalp wound

d. Initial treatment of compound depressed skull fractures

e. Management of increased intracranial pressure

f. Recognition of cerebral herniation syndromes

g. Initiation, management, and interpretation of intracranial pressure monitoring

h. Recognition and initial management of post-traumatic intracranial hemorrhage

4. Apply knowledge of cervical and thoracolumbar spine injuries, including:

a. Means of stabilization of spine (sandbags, tongs, halo)

b. Recognition of level of injury by neurological deficit found on physical examination

c. Pathophysiological responses in quadriplegic or paraplegic patient

5. Demonstrate the ability to assess and manage diseases of the cervical and lumbar discs according to:

a. Anatomical structures involved: disc (cartilage), annulus (ligament), joint capsule, pedicle, nerve root, foramen

b. Conservative management: traction, rest, physical therapy, and analgesic medications

c. Selection and usefulness of radiological modalities: plain spine films, CT, MRI, myelography

d. Indications for surgical management: intractable radicular pain, neurological deficit

6. Demonstrate the ability to describe and diagnose intracranial and intraspinal mass lesions (neoplasm, abscess, hematoma) utilizing:

a. Signs and symptoms of intracranial and intraspinal mass lesions

b. Classification of intracranial and intraspinal tumors

c. Pathophysiology of intracranial and intraspinal abscess

d. Pathophysiology of cerebral aneurysms and vascular lesions

e. Pathophysiology of spontaneous intracranial and intraspinal hemorrhage

f. Pathophysiology of hydrocephalus

7. Summarize several factors to consider when making critical decisions about treatment options for the elderly neurosurgical patient, to include:

    a. Patient views

    b. Quality of life issues

    c. Acceptable risks

8. Demonstrate an understanding of important non-surgical problems and postoperative complications relating to neurosurgery, including:

    a. Closed head injury: problems related to coma, brain swelling, increased intracranial pressure (ICP), ICP monitoring

    b. Spinal cord injury: problems related to paralysis, sensory deficit, roto bed, tongs, halo

    c. Airway and respiratory problems secondary to coma or high cord injury: arterial blood gases, respirator, endotracheal tube, tracheostomy

    d. Vascular problems: hypo- and hyper- tension, cerebral circulation, cerebral ischemia

    e. Bladder problems: secondary to brain, cord, or cauda pathology

    f. Metabolic problems: hypopituitary, hypoadrenal, hyponatremia, water intoxication

9. Clarify and explain the challenge of making an accurate diagnosis for the elderly patient who exhibits signs of the following disorders. Suggest diagnostic tools for making a differential diagnosis.

    a. Alterations of consciousness

    b. Personality changes

    c. Focal neurologic deficits to cerebrovascular disease

    d. Senile dementia

10. Discuss ethical and socioeconomic issues relating to neurosurgery (e.g., brain death, mental incompetence, dysphasia, compensation neuroses, and intractable or chronic pain).

11. Demonstrate an understanding of the importance of early referral of head and spinal cord injury patients to rehabilitation services; recognize the potential impact of these services for long-term prognosis.

Patient Care that is compassionate, appropriate, and effective for the treatment of health problems and the promotion of health.

1. Perform neurological history and examination of patients at various levels of consciousness; obtain appropriate radiologic studies, and plan operative and medical management with appropriate supervision.

2. Assist during neurosurgical procedures, gaining exposure to and hands-on experience with:
   a. Craniotomy, laminectomy
   b. Hemostasis
   c. Protection of neural tissues
   d. Removal of specific lesions: tumor, abscess, hematoma, disc
   e. Vascular repair: carotid endarterectomy, clipping of aneurysm
   f. Problems related to cerebrospinal fluid circulation: hydrocephalus
   g. Repair/replacement of dura and bone

3. Perform limited neurosurgical procedures under direction such as:
   a. Diagnostic lumbar puncture
   b. Insertion of ICP monitor
   c. Repair of scalp lacerations
   d. Burr hole for sub-dural hematoma
   e. Elevation of simple depressed skull fracture
   f. Application and management of skeletal traction by tongs or halo

4. Manage patients with closed head injuries.

5. Formulate appropriate postoperative care, including:
   a. Address potential complications

b.   Provide information/instructions to patient and family

c.   Prepare a discharge plan

d.   Plan adequate post hospital care

Practice-Based Learning and Improvement that involves investigation and evaluation of their own patient care, appraisal and assimilation of scientific evidence, and improvements in patient care.

INFORMATION TECHNOLOGY AND POPULATION COMPARISONS REFERENCES

Cameron JL (ed). Current Surgical Therapy (7th ed). St. Louis: Mosby, 2001.

Gerszten PC, Marion DW. Spine and spinal cord injuries. In: Cameron JL (ed). Current Surgical Therapy (7th ed). St. Louis: Mosby, 2001;1151-1160.

Hoff JT, Boland MF. Central nervous system. In: Greenfield LJ, Mulholland M, Oldham KT, Zelenock GB, Lillemoe KD (eds), Surgery: Scientific Principles and Practice (2nd ed). Philadelphia: Lippincott-Raven, 1997;2165-2197.

Margolin RA, Kwentus JA. Neuropsychiatric aspects of surgery. In:
Adkins RB, Jr., Scott HW, Jr. (eds), Surgical Care for the Elderly (2nd ed). Philadelphia: Lippincott-Raven Publishers, 1998;131-150.

Miller TA (ed). The central and peripheral nervous systems. Modern Surgical Care: Physiologic Foundations and Clinical Applications (2nd ed). St. Louis: Quality Medical Publishing, Inc., 1998;935-1006.

Smith RD, Tiel R, Johnson RJ. Basic neuroscience. In: O'Leary JP (ed), The Physiologic Basis of Surgery (2nd ed). Baltimore: Williams and Wilkins, 1996;522-560.
Young B, Meacham WF. Neurosurgical diseases. In: Adkins RB, Jr., Scott HW, Jr. (eds), Surgical Care for the Elderly (2nd ed). Philadelphia: Lippincott-Raven Publishers, 1998;403-410.

SECTION 11.17   ORTHOPEDIC SURGERY

UNIT OBJECTIVES:

Demonstrate knowledge of the anatomy, physiology, and pathophysiology of the musculoskeletal system.

Demonstrate the ability to manage preoperative, operative, and postoperative care of surgical patients with orthopedic disorders in a variety of settings.

Medical Knowledge about established and evolving biomedical, clinical, and cognate (e.g. epidemiological and social-behavioral) sciences and the application of this knowledge to patient care.

1.   Describe the gross anatomical structures of the skeletal system.
2.   Explain the physiology and biochemistry of bone growth and maturation.
3.   Describe the function of the specific bones of the body.
4.   Analyze the orthopedic role in evaluation of the following:
   a.   Musculoskeletal trauma
   b.   Inflammatory, infectious, and metabolic disorders (rheumatoid arthritis, systemic lupus erythematosus, pyogenic arthritis, osteomyelitis, osteomalacia, hypothyroidism)
   c.   Musculoskeletal tumors
   d.   Degenerative conditions (osteoarthritis, traumatic arthritis, osteoporosis)

5.   Outline a protocol for the assessment of the skeletal system using appropriate skills of history taking and physical examination.
6.   Discuss the use of radiographic imaging such as magnetic resonance imaging (MRI), computed axial tomography (CAT) scan, radionucleotide, arteriography, and plain films in the evaluation and management of the following orthopedic pathology:
   a.   Musculoskeletal tumors   d.   Pelvic trauma
   b.   Isolated extremity injury   e.   Vascular injury

c. Spinal injury or fracture f. Urologic injury

7. Identify considerations for basic care of patients with acute trauma to the musculoskeletal system, including accurate assessment and documentation of the neurovascular status of all extremities.

8. Discuss specific areas of concern when considering total hip replacement for the elderly patient, including:

  a. Comorbid conditions d. Bleeding dyscrasias

  b. Thromboembolic disease e. Occult infections

  c. Urinary retention

9. Explain the fundamental principles of management of orthopedic trauma, including:

  a. Compartment pressure problems and use of fasciotomy

  b. Indications and limitations of closed reduction and casting

  c. Indications for open reduction and internal fixation of fractures

  d. Indications and methods for application of skeletal traction

  e. Principles of early mobilization and rehabilitation

  f. Diagnosis and management of fat embolism

10. Explain the management of open fractures, including:

  a. Timing d. Early fixation

  b. Stabilization priorities e. Mobilization

  c. Irrigation and debridement

11. Discuss the role of arthroscopy in the evaluation and therapy of orthopedic pathology (specifically for the knee).

12. Determine the management of selected congenital and developmental musculoskeletal defects and fractures in children to include:

  a. Epiphyseal fractures: Salter-Harris Classification

  b. Supracondylar elbow fractures in children

    (1) Risk of Volkmann's ischemic contracture

(2)   Role of the vascular surgeon in evaluation and treatment

c.   Supracondylar femur fracture (adjacent role of the vascular surgeon)

d.   Cervical spine congenital deformity versus pseudosubluxation in a young child

e.   Developmental hip dislocation

f.   Talipes equinovarus (club foot)

13.   Discuss common causes of deterioration in elderly patients that most frequently lead to the need for total knee replacement. Include:

a.   Frequency of occurrence

b.   Associated medications,

c.   Pain and degeneration

d.   Quality of life decisions for:

(1)   Osteoarthritis   (3)   Post-traumatic arthritis

(2)   Rheumatoid arthritis   (4)   Osteonecrosis of femoral condyles

14.   Describe contraindications to knee replacement in the elderly patient with advanced arthritis of the knee.

15.   Explain the management of the following kinds of diseases affecting the musculoskeletal system:

a.   Inflammatory diseases (rheumatoid arthritis, systemic lupus erythematosus [SLE], psoriatic arthritis, Reiter's syndrome)

b.   Infectious diseases (septic arthritis, osteomyelitis)

c.   Metabolic diseases (osteomalacia, hyperparathyroidism, hyperthyroidism)

16.   Describe the following fracture classifications:

a.   Malgaigne

b.   Complex extremity and soft tissue

c.   Pelvic

17. Diagram gross and roentgen graphic characteristics of histological and pathological conditions of the musculoskeletal system, including:

   a. Osteoporosis
   c. Primary tumors
   b. Metastatic disease of the skeleton
   d. Trauma

18. Outline the management of musculoskeletal tumors, including:

   a. Evaluation and staging: Enneking Classification

   b. Selection and performance of appropriate biopsy such as:

      (1) Open- versus fine- needle aspiration

      (2) Frozen section versus permanent section

   c. Adjuvant therapy options

      (1) Chemotherapy

      (2) Radiation

19. Explain the management of nerve injury associated with musculoskeletal trauma and other pathology, including:

   a. Response of nervous tissue to injury

   b. Evaluation of nerve injury

   c. Transmission of impulses at various points in the peripheral nervous system

   d. Operative repair options

20. Analyze the principal concepts of pain causation and perception.

21. Demonstrate the evaluation of back and leg pain using a standard algorithm.

22. Fractures in the elderly population typically occur as the result of low-energy impacts. Discuss the significance of frequency and outcome of the following disease entities/abnormalities:

   a. Osteoporosis (include gender)

   b. Paget's disease

   c. Infection

   d. Malignancy

   e. Marrow dysplasias

f. Osteomalacia

g. Metabolic derangements (hyperthyroidism, hyperparathyroidism)

h. Elder abuse and neglect

23. Compare the indications and contraindications for joint aspiration.

24. Analyze the indications for and surgical approaches to amputation in the following situations:

a. Trauma   d. Tumors

b. Ischemia   e. Prostheses

c. Infection

25. Summarize the role of joint replacement in the management of orthopedic pathology.

26. Summarize the characteristics of infection/sepsis secondary to prosthetic implants or orthopedic hardware; discuss treatment strategies.

27. Explain the importance and timing of physical therapy in the care of postoperative orthopedic repairs.

28. Describe the surgical technique utilizing a "clean air" environment, covering these broad aspects of control:

a. Needs assessment regarding procedure

b. Consideration of laminar flow systems

c. Use of ultraviolet light

d. Operating room traffic

e. Soft tissue handling

f. Use of prophylactic antibiotics

Patient Care that is compassionate, appropriate, and effective for the treatment of health problems and the promotion of health.

1. Perform and record a focused history and physical examination of orthopedic disorders, including:

a.	Trauma	d.	Inflammatory processes
b.	Congenital malformations	e.	Neoplasia
c.	Degenerative diseases		

2. Request and interpret appropriate diagnostic imaging and laboratory studies of orthopedic pathology:

   a. Preoperative laboratory evaluation as needed for safe surgical intervention

   b. Plain film analysis (specifically cervical spine and major skeleton films)

   c. CT scan for spinal fracture, pelvis, and extremity injury

   d. MRI spine and knee

3. Perform immobilization of cervical spine.

4. Triage patients with musculoskeletal injuries in a mass casualty situation.

5. Participate in the management of orthopedic trauma to extremities, including such procedures as:

   a. Splinting closed fractures

   b. Closed reduction of fractures

   c. Reducing dislocations

   d. Applying traction

   e. Applying casts

   f. Debriding and irrigating open extremity fractures

   g. Open reduction and internal fixation of extremity fractures

6. Monitor compartment pressure in orthopedic trauma and begin appropriate therapy, including the performance of fasciotomy, if indicated.

7. Monitor trauma patients for indications of fat embolism syndrome and begin appropriate therapy.

8. Perform joint aspirations in appropriate situations.

9. Participate in diagnostic and therapeutic arthroscopy procedures such as:

   a. Partial meniscectomy (knee)

   b. Arthroscopy of shoulder (diagnostic)

10.   Participate in the management of amputations:

      a.   Determine amputation level

      b.   Perform lower extremity amputation in appropriate cases

      c.   Direct rehabilitation of an amputee in appropriate cases

11.   Participate in the management of musculoskeletal tumors, including:

      a.   Planning and performing an incisional biopsy of a soft tissue tumor

      b.   Performing preoperative evaluation and staging of soft tissue tumors

      c.   Assisting in the planning and resection of soft tissue tumors and considerations for limb salvage

12.   Assist in prosthetic joint replacement.

13.   Participate in the management of congenital, developmental, and other musculoskeletal deficiencies in children such as:

      a.   Cerebral palsy

      b.   Myelomeningocele

      c.   Muscular dystrophy

      d.   Developmental hip/dislocation

      e.   Talipes equinovarus

Practice-Based Learning and Improvement that involves investigation and evaluation of their own patient care, appraisal and assimilation of scientific evidence, and improvements in patient care.

INFORMATION TECHNOLOGY AND POPULATION COMPARISONS
REFERENCES

Browner BD. Skeletal Trauma: Fractures, Dislocations, Ligamentous Injuries. Philadelphia: WB Saunders Co., 1992.

Donato KC. The musculoskeletal system. In: O'Leary JP (ed), The Physiologic Basis of Surgery (2nd ed). Baltimore: Williams and Wilkins, 1996;507-521.

Green NE, Swionkowski MF. Skeletal Trauma in Children. Philadelphia: WB Saunders Co., 1993.

Healey MA, Winchell RJ. Orthopedic and spinal injuries. In: Greenfield LJ, Mulholland M, Oldham KT, Zelenock GB, Lillemoe KD (eds), Surgery: Scientific Principles and Practice (2nd ed). Philadelphia: Lippincott-Raven, 1997;373-377.

Hoppenfeld S, DeBoer P, Hutton R. Surgical Exposures in Orthopaedics: The Anatomic Approach (2nd ed). Philadelphia: JB Lippincott Co., 1994.

Ling SM, Bathon JM. Osteoarthritis in older adults. Amer J Geriatr Soc 1998;46(2):216-225.

Loeser RF, Jr. Musculoskeletal and connective tissue disorders. Clinics in Geriatr Med 1998; August.

Matthews LS, Goldstein SA. Orthopedic surgery. In: Greenfield LJ, Mulholland M, Oldham KT, Zelenock GB, Lillemoe KD (eds), Surgery: Scientific Principles and Practice (2nd ed). Philadelphia: Lippincott-Raven, 1997;2141-2152.

Rosen C, Glowacki J, Bilezikian (eds). The Aging Skeleton. San Diego: Academic Press, 1999;1-632.

Rosenthal RE. Musculoskeletal diseases. In: Adkins RB, Jr., Scott HW, Jr. (eds), Surgical Care for the Elderly (2nd ed). Philadelphia: Lippincott-Raven Publishers, 1998;383-402.

Sanders AB (ed). Trauma and falls. Abuse and neglect. Emergency Care of the Elder Person. St. Louis: Beverly Cracom Publications, 1996;153-170; 171-196.

Zuckerman JD, Spivak JM. Orthopaedic surgery in the elderly. In: Katlic MR (ed), Geriatric Surgery: Comprehensive Care of the Elderly Patient. Baltimore: Urban & Schwarzenberg, 1990;597-674.

SECTION11.18   OPHTHALMOLOGY

UNIT OBJECTIVES:

Demonstrate an understanding of the anatomy and function of the eye.

Demonstrate working knowledge of the pathophysiology of common eye problems relevant to the practice of general surgery.

Demonstrate the ability to initiate management and arrange appropriate care of eye problems associated with the practice of general surgery.

Medical Knowledge about established and evolving biomedical, clinical, and cognate (e.g. epidemiological and social-behavioral) sciences and the application of this knowledge to patient care.

1.   Describe the anatomy of the eye and its surrounding structures, including:

    a.   Adnexa (lids, tarsal plates, gray line, levator muscles, orbital septum, innervation, vascular supply, nasolacrimal system, orbital bones, lacrimal gland)

    b.   Extraocular muscles and innervation

    c.   Anterior Segment (conjunctiva, cornea, anterior chamber, iris, lens)

    d.   Posterior Segment (ciliary body, vitreous, optic nerve, retina, macula, fovea, choroid)

    e.   Retrobulbar Structures (optic nerve, optic canal, chiasm, sella turcica)

2.   Diagram and summarize the principles of vision, including:

    a.   Refraction caused by lenses (tear film, cornea, lens, vitreous)

    b.   Encoding of image (retina, including fovea and macula)

    c.   Transmission of image (nerve fiber layer, optic disc, optic nerve, chiasm, optic radiations, occipital lobe)

    d.   Muscle control centers (cranial nerves III, IV, VI)

    e.   Pupillary control (cranial nerve III and parasympathetic nerves)

3.   Explain fundamental ocular physiology by considering the following questions:

    a.   How do the adnexal structures ensure that the eye is lubricated and shielded from trauma?

    b.   What would a paresis of any of the innervating cranial nerves do to the movement of the eye?

    c.   When the cornea is damaged, what effect is there upon comfort or vision? Knowing the innervation of the iris, what information might an anisocoria indicate? What is a Marcus Gunn, afferent pupillary defect, or a Horner's pupil?

    d.   What purpose do the ciliary body and the vitreous serve? What do the macula, the fovea, and the optic nerve do?

    e.   What difference would it make in the examination of the eye (vision, visual field, and appearance of the nerve) if damage occurred at the site of the optic nerve, optic canal, optic chiasm, or in a retrochiasmal location?

4.   Outline common eye pathology, including:

    a.   Trauma to eye, orbit, and supporting structure

        (1)   Diagnosing a perforated globe

        (2)   Indications for referral and repair of a blowout fracture

        (3)   Diagnosing a corneal epithelial defect

        (4)   Identifying a hyphema

        (5)   Treatments for severe loss of vision with optic nerve trauma

    b.   Infections of the eye (blepharitis, hordeola, chalazia, corneal ulcers, endophthalmitis, conjunctivitis, keratoconjunctivitis, iritis, uveitis)

    c.   Burns of the eye (different effects of a thermal, alkali, or acid burn of the cornea)

    d.   Anisocoria (Horner's syndrome, iatrogenic, belladonna induced, diabetic, third cranial nerve, Marcus Gunn, afferent pupillary defect)

    e.   Sudden loss of vision (from migraine, traumatic neuropathy, ischemic optic neuropathy, temporal arteritis, optic neuritis, central retinal vein or artery occlusion)

f.   Eye pain (different descriptions of pain from iritis vs. corneal abrasion vs. herpes simplex keratitis)

g.   Eye donation (methods of tissue removal: whole eye and anterior segment)

5.   Discuss the following important microbiologic considerations of the eye and its surrounding structures:

    a.   Indications for cultures:

        (1)   Hyperpurulent or unresponsive conjunctivitis

        (2)   Neonatal conjunctivitis

        (3)   Corneal ulcers

        (4)   Localized lid infections

        (5)   Suspected orbital cellulitis

        (6)   Penetrating trauma

    b.   Sampling technique

        (1)   Swab and transport media (acceptable for mild infections)

        (2)   Direct culture on agar plates (for more serious disease)

        (3)   Spatula scraping and direct agar plating (for corneal ulcers by ophthalmologist)

        (4)   Blood cultures for orbital cellulitis

    c.   Risks for patients who cannot blink fully (as in eyes drying in intensive care unit)

        (1)   Predisposes to severe infection

        (2)   Possible globe perforation by Pseudomonas or N. gonorrhea

6.   Outline the essential elements of a focused eye examination for each of the problems in #5 above to include significant aspects of the following:

    a.   History

    b.   Visual acuity and confrontational visual fields

    c.   External exam (appearance of adnexa)

    d.   Anterior segment (cornea, iris, anterior chamber)

    e.   Pupillary exam (direct, consensual, indirect, afferent)

    f.   Extraocular muscles (ductions, vergences, exotropia, esotropia, convergence)

g. Posterior segment (including red reflex, direct ophthalmoscopy)

7. Discuss the pros and cons of performing elective or emergency eye operations on elderly patients who also present with comorbidity.

8. What is the level of importance of these elderly patient situations to the outcome of eye surgery?

   a. Renal transplant recipient

   b. Bone marrow transplant recipient

   c. End-stage renal patient

   d. Insulin-dependent diabetes mellitus patient

9. Summarize the criteria for appropriate referral and follow-up for the management of common eye problems to include the following questions:

   a. Is there information that will help me assess the systemic condition of the patient? (vascular and neurologic information especially important)

   b. Is there a vision-threatening problem? (consultation with ophthalmologist is essential if patient is obtunded, does not blink, and there is a developing corneal ulcer)

   c. What is the source of the patient's ocular complaint or condition? Is it acute (inpatient consult) or chronic (outpatient consult)?

10. Explain the principles of management for common eye problems to include the following:

    a. Exposure keratopathy   d. Iritis

    b. Conjunctivitis   e. Blow out fracture

    c. Herpes simplex keratitis   f. Corneal abrasion

11. Describe the etiology (include appropriate racial differences), signs and symptoms of, and primary treatment or rehabilitative strategy for the following disorders as they affect the vision of the elderly population:

    a. Presbyopia   g. Retinal detachment

b.	Essential blepharospasm	h.	Macular degeneration
c.	Ptosis	i.	Diabetic retinopathy
d.	Glaucoma	j.	Herpes zoster
e.	Cataracts	k.	Pterygium
f.	Noncicatricial ectropion; entropion		

12. Determine appropriate surgical management of common eye problems utilizing precepts such as the following:

    a. Indications for repair of blow out fracture

        (1) Persistent findings after approximately seven days of symptomatic diplopia, or symptomatic enophthalmos; positive forced traction test

        (2) Possible hypesthesia

        (3) Presence of a fracture by itself is not necessarily an indication

    b. Current controversy and possible therapy for sudden, profound vision loss associated with traumatic optic neuropathy

13. Describe the pathophysiology of uncommon eye problems associated with surgical practice, including:

    a. Tumors of the eye

        (1) Retinoblastoma

        (2) Melanoma

        (3) Metastatic

    b. Congenital abnormalities of the eye

        (1) Glaucoma

        (2) Cataract

        (3) Exotropia/esotropia

14. Determine the emergency surgical management of eye and orbital injuries, including:

a.	Blow out fracture	d.	Corneal foreign bodies
b.	Rupture of the globe	e.	Hyphema
c.	Corneal laceration	f.	Vitreous hemorrhage

Patient Care that is compassionate, appropriate, and effective for the treatment of health problems and the promotion of health.

1. Complete a basic history and eye examination.

2. Apply eye dressings or appropriate eye medications for corneal abrasion and corneal perforation or globe rupture.

3. Apply local anesthetic, repair simple eyelid lacerations, and remove foreign bodies.

    a. Diagnose injuries

    b. Review special techniques for repair

    c. Call the ophthalmologist if the following situation(s) exists: laceration involving: margin of lid, levator muscle, canaliculus, or nasolacrimal system

4. Interpret imaging studies in the evaluation of common eye problems such as:

    a. Ocular prosthesis   c. Blow out fracture

    b. Ocular foreign body   d. Zygomatic fracture

5. Treat orbital injuries and assign priority in management in a multiple-injured patient.

6. Identify appropriate candidates and arrange for eye donation: Review criteria of the Eye Bank Association of America for donors

    a. Essentially no age limits on donation

    b. Tissue that is "too old" or "too young" for routine transplant may still be useful for emergency repairs or for research

    c. Contagious diseases are contraindications (syphilis, AIDS, Creutzfeldt-Jacob, rabies, death from unknown causes)

7. Participate in enucleation for corneal harvesting under supervision.

8. Participate in management of orbital injuries.

9. Manage the treatment of common and uncommon eye problems with appropriate consultation.

Practice-Based Learning and Improvement that involves investigation and evaluation of their own patient care, appraisal and assimilation of scientific evidence, and improvements in patient care.

INFORMATION TECHNOLOGY AND POPULATION COMPARISONS REFERENCES

Cobbs EL, Duthie EH, Jr, Murphy JB (eds). Vision impairment. Geriatrics Review Syllabus: A Core Curriculum in Geriatric Medicine (4th ed). Dubuque IA: Kendall/Hunt Publishing Company, 1999.

Elliott JH, Feman SS. Ophthalmic diseases. In: Adkins RB, Jr., Scott HW, Jr. (eds), Surgical Care for the Elderly (2nd ed). Philadelphia: Lippincott-Raven Publishers, 1998;201-210.

Friedberg MA, Rapuano CJ. Office and Emergency Room Diagnosis and Treatment of Eye Disease. Philadelphia: JB Lippincott Co., 1990.

Weinstock FJ. Ophthalmic surgery in the elderly. In: Katlic MR (ed), Geriatric Surgery: Comprehensive Care of the Elderly Patient. Baltimore: Urban & Schwarzenberg, 1990;703-719.

http://www.aao.org

SECTION 11.19   PLASTIC AND RECONSTRUCTIVE SURGERY
UNIT OBJECTIVES:

Demonstrate an understanding of the nature and principles of correction and reconstruction of congenital and acquired defects of the head, neck, trunk, and extremities.

Demonstrate the ability to manage the treatment of acute, chronic, and neoplastic defects not requiring complex reconstruction.

Recognize benign lesions of skin and subcutaneous tissue and treat when appropriate.

Diagnosis of benign lesions of skin and subcutaneous tissues: Recognize benign lesions of skin and subcutaneous tissue.

Treatment of benign lesions of skin and subcutaneous tissues: Appropriate management of benign lesions of skin and subcutaneous tissue.

Recognize and appropriately manage malignant skin lesions.

Basal cell carcinoma: Diagnose and treat appropriately small basal cell carcinomas.

Malignant melanoma: Diagnose malignant melanoma and refer appropriately.

Squamous cell carcinoma: Diagnose squamous cell carcinoma and refer appropriately if large.

Medical Knowledge about established and evolving biomedical, clinical, and cognate (e.g. epidemiological and social-behavioral) sciences and the application of this knowledge to patient care.

1.   Outline the components of a comprehensive focused history and physical examination pertinent to the evaluation and correction of congenital or acquired defects under the realm of plastic and reconstructive surgery.

2.   Discuss and compare skin and connective tissue according to:

   a.   Anatomy

   b.   Normal physiology and biochemistry

   c.   Pathophysiology of benign and malignant skin disorders

   d.   Unique pathophysiology of connective tissue disorders

3.	Explain the basic techniques for surgical repair of superficial incisions and lacerations of the head, neck, trunk, and extremities to include the following considerations:

	a.	Skin

	b.	Subcutaneous tissue

	c.	Superficial muscle and fascia

	d.	Dressings

	e.	Splints

	f.	Suturing and knot tying

4.	Describe the physiology of various techniques of skin and composite tissue transplantation with particular regard to component tissue circulation:

	a.	Skin grafts (split- vs. full- thickness)

	b.	Bone (cartilage grafts)

	c.	Composite grafts

	d.	Skin flaps

	e.	Muscle flaps

	f.	Myocutaneous flaps

	g.	Bone flaps

	h.	Osteocutaneous flaps

	i.	Myo-osseous flaps

	j.	Vascularized versus nonvascularized flaps

	k.	Neurocutaneous flaps

5.	Categorize the pathophysiology of thermal, chemical, and electrical burns, including consideration of:

	a.	Systemic pathophysiology	c.	Cardiac depression

	b.	Local pathophysiology	d.	Pulmonary compromise

6.	Describe the "classical" chemical agents causing burns; list their antidotes.

7.	Outline the components of a comprehensive examination of the naso-, oro-, and hyo-pharynx to include:

a. Normal anatomy

b. Common congenital anomalies

c. Evolution of neoplastic disease

8. Explain the assessment of facial skeletal trauma according to the following systems:

a. LeFort I, II, and III classification of maxillary fractures

b. Nasoethmoidal disruption classification

c. Zygomatic, orbit, and mandibular fractures

d. Disruption classification

9. Define the tumor, node, and metastases (TNM) classification system as used for neoplasms of skin, soft tissue, and head and neck.

10. Discuss epidemiology, risk factors, treatment, and prevention of cutaneous malignancies in the geriatric patient, including:

a. Skin cancer rates (basal cell carcinoma [BCC], squamous cell carcinoma [SCC])

b. Average age of onset for BCC/SCC

c. Etiology of BCC/SCC

d. Usual modes of treatment for BCC/SCC (Mohs Technique, radiation, chemotherapy)

e. Prevention using medications (isotretinoin, beta-carotene)

11. Explain the methods for performing incisional and excisional biopsies of skin and oral cavity.

12. Demonstrate the systematic examination of the hand to assess motor and sensory function, including:

a. Intrinsic tendon and muscle function

b. Extensive tendon and muscle function

c. Median nerve

d. Ulnar nerve

e. Radial nerve

f. Circulation

g.   Bones

13.   Describe the physiology of local and general anesthetics in these categories:

    a.   Narcotics

    b.   Sedatives

    c.   Analgesics

        (1)   Local anesthesia

        (2)   General anesthetics

14.   Outline appropriate diagnostic studies needed to supplement the physical examination when developing a treatment plan for:

    a.   Surgery of the hand

    b.   Facial fractures

    c.   Congenital structural anomalies of the head/neck and hand/trunk.

15.   Summarize the evaluation of patients with head and neck cancer, and develop a treatment plan according to the following criteria:

    a.   Location of lesion

    b.   Size of primary lesion

    c.   Presence of metastatic disease

16.   Demonstrate a working knowledge of the safe use of nasopharyngoscopy, laryngoscopy, esophagoscopy, and other endoscopic procedures utilized in the evaluation of patients with head and neck cancer.

17.   Discuss the use of the reconstructive ladder (including skin grafts, local flaps, and regional and free microvascular flaps) in the definitive management of traumatic or excised wounds.

18.   Explain considerations in a geriatric patient undergoing major reconstructive operation, to include the implications of:

    a.   Decreased functional physiologic reserve

    b.   Multiple medical problems

c. Slower wound healing (consider significance of: age, concomitant illnesses, medications)

d. Preoperative evaluation procedures

e. Invasive operative monitoring

f. Intensive postoperative monitoring

19. Discuss the surgical treatment of:

   a. Common hand injuries and tumors

   b. Surgical repair of facial trauma, soft tissue, and bony defects

   c. Resection and reconstruction of the simple, soft tissue defects following resection of neoplasms of the head and neck

   d. Resection of skin and soft tissue neoplasms requiring complex reconstruction

   e. Reconstruction of the breast for congenital and acquired defects

   f. Management of the burned hand and face

   g. Reconstruction of congenital craniofacial defects

20. Analyze treatment options for the comprehensive care of the burn patient, including:

   a. Excision of burn

   b. Homografting

   c. Xenografting

   d. Autografting

   e. Tissue engineering and prefabrication

21. Assess basic lines of research in plastic and reconstructive surgery to include:

   a. Current hypotheses dealing with:

      (1) Craniofacial growth and development

      (2) Perfusion of the skin and muscle

      (3) Wound healing

      (4) Skin, bone, and cartilage grafts

      (5) Tumor biology

      (6) Reconstructive hand surgery

(7)   Bone reconstruction

(8)   Bone distraction

(9)   Tissue transplantation

b.   Avenues for new investigation

22.   Summarize currently accepted surgical techniques for treating the following:

    a.   Correction of congenital lesions of the head/neck and hand/trunk

    b.   Craniofacial anomalies, including cleft lip and palate

    c.   Breast reconstruction after mastectomy

    d.   Reconstruction and ablative head and neck surgery

    e.   Aesthetic rejuvenation of the face and body

    f.   Pathology of common lesions, such as naevi, sebaceous cysts, vitiligo, Campbell de Morgan spots, basal cell papillomas

Patient Care that is compassionate, appropriate, and effective for the treatment of health problems and the promotion of health.

1.   Complete a comprehensive physical examination and clinical data history, including pertinent diagnostic laboratory and radiographic findings.

2.   Evaluate and treat simple and intermediate abrasions and burns of the face, trunk, and extremities.

3.   Perform simple incisional biopsies and excise small lesions on the skin and subcutaneous tissue of the trunk or extremities.

4.   Provide definitive treatment plans for superficial incised and lacerated wounds of the neck, trunk, and extremities.

5.   Participate in the perioperative evaluation and management of congenital or acquired defects (traumatic and surgical).

6.   Apply and remove dressings of the head, neck, hand, trunk, and extremities, including:

    a.   Occlusive   d.   Casts

    b.   Non-occlusive   e.   Alginate

    c.   Wet to dry   f.   Colloidal

7. Debride and suture major non-facial wounds and burns.

8. Participate in the acute resuscitation, evaluation, and initial treatment of a burned patient.

9. Harvest and apply split-thickness skin grafts.

10. Perform simple, localized skin flaps for wound coverage.

11. Participate in the evaluation and formulation of treatment plans for:

a.	Hand injuries	d.	Congenital anomalies
b.	Facial fractures	e.	Breast deformities
c.	Head and neck cancer	f.	Burn patients

12. Under the direction of a plastic surgeon, assist in the planning and performance of complex reconstructive operations.

13. Harvest and apply full-thickness skin grafts and local flaps.

14. Reconstruct defects with random flaps, composite flaps, and grafts.

15. Act as first assistant and attending-supervised surgeon for major resectional and reconstructive surgery of the head, neck, breast, trunk and extremities.

16. Raise muscle and skin-muscle flaps under direct supervision.

17. Perform major excision of burns, escharotomy, and skin grafting.

18. Assess and act as first assistant and attending-supervised surgeon for the following:

    a. Complex soft tissue injury

    b. Fractures requiring operative and non-operative reduction

    c. Nerve, tendon, and bone surgery of the hand

    d. Vascular injuries

19. Act as first assistant or attending supervised surgeon for:

    a. Reconstruction and reparative surgery of the hand

    b. Surgical repair of facial trauma

    c. Resection of neoplasms of the head and neck

    d. Resection of major skin and soft tissue neoplasms requiring complex reconstruction

    e. Surgical repair of craniomaxillofacial congenital defects

f.   Reconstruction of the breast

g.   Complex wound reconstruction using flap both local, regional, and free microvascular

20.   Basal cell carcinoma:

a.   Assess skin lesion

b.   Biopsy of large skin lesions to plan treatment

c.   Closure of large defects after excision by split skin grafts, full thickness grafts, flap closure

21.   Malignant melanoma:

a.   Assess skin lesion

b.   Indications for wider excision, lymph node biopsy, axillary or groin block dissection based on staging

22.   Squamous cell carcinoma:

a.   Assess skin lesion including incisional biopsy

b.   Technical Skills and Procedures

23.   Basal cell carcinoma

24.   Malignant skin lesion-excision biopsy

a.   Malignant melanoma:

b.   Malignant skin lesion-excision biopsy

Practice-Based Learning and Improvement that involves investigation and evaluation of their own patient care, appraisal and assimilation of scientific evidence, and improvements in patient care.

INFORMATION TECHNOLOGY AND POPULATION COMPARISONS
REFERENCES

Bentz ML. Pediatric Plastic Surge. CT: Appleton and Lange, 1998;1-1099.

Georgiade NG. Textbook of Plastic, Maxillofacial, and Reconstructive Surgery (3rd ed). Baltimore: Williams & Wilkins, 1996.

Goldberg JA, Alpert BS, Lineaweaver WC, et al. Microvascular reconstruction of the lower extremity in the elderly. Clinics of Plastic Surg 1991;18(3):459-465.

Grabb WC, Smith JW, Aston SJ. Grabb and Smith's Plastic Surgery (5th ed). Boston: Little, Brown and Co., 1997.

Greenfield LJ, Mulholland M, Oldham KT, Zelenock GB, Lillemoe KD (eds). Skin and soft tissue. Surgery: Scientific Principles and Practice (2nd ed). Philadelphia: Lippincott-Raven, 1997;2231-2289.

Kaldor J, Shugg D, Young B, et al. Nonmelanoma skin cancer: ten years of cancer registry-based surveillance. Int J Cancer 1993;53:886-891.

Levin LS. Reconstructive plastic surgery. In: Greenfield LJ, Mulholland M, Oldham KT, Zelenock GB, Lillemoe KD (eds), Surgery: Scientific Principles and Practice (2nd ed). Philadelphia: Lippincott-Raven, 1997;2280-2289.

Malata CM, Cooter RD, Batchelor R, et al. Microvascular free-tissue transfers in elderly patients: the Leeds Experience. J Plastic and Reconstr Surg 1996;98(7):1234-1241.

Reece GP, Schusterman MA, Miller MJ, et al. Morbidity associated with free-tissue transfer after radiotherapy and chemotherapy in elderly cancer patients. J Reconstr Microsurg 1994;10(6):375-382.

Sennett BJ, Savoie FH. Surgery of the hand. In: Greenfield LJ, Mulholland M, Oldham KT, Zelenock GB, Lillemoe KD (eds), Surgery: Scientific Principles and Practice (2nd ed). Philadelphia: Lippincott-Raven, 1997;2153-2163.

Strom SS, Yamamura Y. Epidemiology of nonmelanoma skin cancer. Clinics of Plastic Surg 1997;24(4):627-636.

Wood RJ, Jurkiewicz MJ. Plastic and reconstructive surgery. In: Schwartz SI (ed), Principles of Surgery (6th ed). New York: McGraw-Hill, Inc., 1994;2025-2074.

SECTION 11.20   UROLOGY

UNIT OBJECTIVES:

Demonstrate an understanding of the anatomy, physiology, and pathophysiology of the genitourinary system.

Demonstrate the ability to manage routine and emergency genitourinary problems in a variety of settings.

Medical Knowledge about established and evolving biomedical, clinical, and cognate (e.g. epidemiological and social-behavioral) sciences and the application of this knowledge to patient care.

1.   Describe the normal anatomy and physiology of the genitourinary system to include the following structures:

    a.   Kidneys

    b.   Ureters

    c.   Bladder

    d.   Prostate seminal vesicles and vas deferens

    e.   Urethra (male and female)

2.   Summarize the basic science of genitourinary disease to include the following:

    a.   Anatomy, physiology, biology, biochemistry, microbiology, immunology, and embryology of the genitourinary system

    b.   Pathophysiology of urinary tract disease

    c.   Endocrine function of kidney

3.   Discuss the components of a focused genitourinary history and physical examination to include:

    a.   History

        (1)   Pain (location)

        (2)   Hematuria

414

                    (a)   Painful, painless

                    (b)   Initial, terminal, total

                    (c)   Presence of clots

           (3)   Lower urinary

                    (a)   Irritative

                    (b)   Obstructive

           (4)   Incontinence (stress, urge)

           (5)   Sexual dysfunction

    b.   Physical Examination

           (1)   Kidneys

                    (a)   Flank masses

                    (b)   Peritoneal signs

                    (c)   Signs of nerve root irritability

           (2)   Bladder

           (3)   Penis

           (4)   Scrotum and contents

           (5)   Rectal examination (to include prostate)

           (6)   Pelvic examination in female

4.   Explain the following clinical science study factors/variables as they relate to genitourinary disease:

    a.   Anatomy

    b.   Embryology of genitourinary tract

    c.   Renal physiology

    d.   Bacteriology and antibiotic management

    e.   Renal calculus disease

    f.   Urologic oncology

    g.   Female urology

    h.   Urologic trauma

5.   Describe the pathologic anatomy and pathophysiology of non-complex genitourinary diseases such as:

    a.   Tumors (renal, ureteral, bladder, testicular, prostate)

    b.   Calculi (renal, ureteral, bladder)

    c.   Trauma (testis, upper and lower urinary tract)

    d.   Renal infections

    e.   Benign prostatic hyperplasia and bladder outlet obstruction

    f.   Vesicoureteral reflux and pyelonephritis

    g.   Varicocele

    h.   Incontinence (stress, overflow, neurogenic, urgency)

    i.   Impotence and Peyronie's disease

    j.   Urethral stricture disease

    k.   Priapism

6.   Explain the tumor, nodes, and metastases (TNM) classification of tumors of the kidney, bladder, prostate, and testis.

7.   Summarize the indications for routine diagnostic procedures in urology such as:

    a.   Cystoscopy (ureteral catheterization)

    b.   Bladder catheterization

    c.   Intravenous pyelogram

    d.   Cystogram (retrograde ureteropyelogram)

    e.   Computed tomography and ultrasound of the GU tract

    f.   Urography in trauma

    g.   Indications for using MRI

    h.   Retrograde urethrogram

    i.   Transrectal ultrasound

    j.   Renal arteriography

    k.   Renography and renal perfusion scanning (I 131)

    l.   Urinalysis, biochemical and radioimmunoassay

8.   Discuss the nature and indication for routine therapeutic procedures in genitourinary disease such as:

   a.   Bladder catheterization

   b.   Passage of Coudé tips and filiform catheters

   c.   Meatotomy if necessary for catheterization

   d.   Suprapubic punch cystostomy

   e.   Dorsal slit for phimosis

9.   Analyze the etiology of urinary incontinence in elderly patients. Consider the following:

   a.   Factors that may be associated with aging

      (1)   Bladder capacity

      (2)   Amount of residual urine

      (3)   Frequency of involuntary bladder contractions

      (4)   Incidence of impaired mobility

      (5)   CNS disorder

      (6)   Congestive heart failure

      (7)   Medications

   b.   Female elderly patients

      (1)   Decline in bladder outlet

      (2)   Decline in urethral resistance pressure

         (a)   Influence of estrogen

         (b)   Pelvic structures associated with childbirth

         (c)   Surgeries

   c.   Male elderly patients : Prostatic enlargement

      (1)   Obstructed urethra (overflow incontinence)

      (2)   Detrusor motor instability (urge incontinence)

10.   Describe the rationale for transurethral prostate resection and other endoscopic urologic procedures.

11.   Describe cancer of the prostate, citing disease rates that make it the:

   a.   Most commonly diagnosed malignancy in men

b.   Second leading cause of cancer death in men

12.   Describe the embryology of the GU tract to include a discussion of the following:
        Congenital abnormalities

        a.   Ureteropelvic junction (UPJ) with hydronephrosis

        b.   Reflux

        c.   Polycystic kidney

        d.   Urethral valves with hydronephrosis

13.   Describe the types of incisions and exposure required for genitourinary surgery, including
        those for:

        a.   Nephrectomy

        b.   Radical nephrectomy

        c.   Ureterolithotomy

        d.   Radical cystectomy

        e.   Radical retropubic prostatectomy

        f.   Perineal prostatectomy

        g.   Orchiectomy

        h.   Radical orchiectomy

        i.   Laparoscopic urologic surgery (nephrectomy, partial nephrectomy,
                prostatectomy)

14.   Discuss treatment options in the management of ureteral injuries to include:

        a.   Primary repair e. Percutaneous drainage

        b.   Ureteroureterostomy f. Emergent nephrectomy

        c.   Neoureterocystostomy g. Ureteral stenting

        d.   Psoas hitch

15.   Outline recommended screening guidelines for prostate cancer.

16.   Summarize considerations for appropriate treatment of incidentally detected carcinoma of
        the prostate, found on simple prostatectomy, when these conditions exist:

a.   Low-grade lesion with combined Gleason score <5

b.   Transurethral resection (TUR) shows lesion occupies 5% or less of tissue resected

c.   Lesion is considered clinical stage A-1

Patient Care that is compassionate, appropriate, and effective for the treatment of health problems and the promotion of health.

1.   Complete and record a focused urological history and physical examination.

2.   Work up a prostatic mass on a routine rectal examination, including processing necessary radiologic and laboratory studies.

3.   Plan and initiate appropriate therapy for urological disorders such as:

     a.   Hematuria work up

     b.   Obstructive uropathy work-up

     c.   Simple infections

     d.   Resistant infections

     e.   Initiate therapy for: calculus disease, renal neoplasm, transitional cell neoplasm

     f.   Maintain a working knowledge of carcinoma of the prostate

4.   Perform a bladder catheterization (including passage of Coudé tips).

5.   Perform a <u>urologic evaluation</u> (history and physical exam), <u>diagnostic studies</u> (retrograde urethrogram, cystogram, CT, angiography), and <u>treatment</u> (cystostomy, cystorrhaphy, ureteral repair, ureteral reconstruction, renal artery and vein repair, nephrectomy) in a trauma setting.

6.   Interpret Computed Tomography scans and ultrasound results in genitourinary diseases.

7.   Perform cystoscopy and urethral catheterization.

8.   Request intravenous pyelography (IVP), CT, and ultrasound genitourinary procedures in appropriate cases.

9.   Perform nephrectomies for disease.

10.   Perform suprapubic prostatectomy.

11.   Manage urologic emergencies such as torsion of testicle, scrotal masses, and urinary retention.

12.   Manage complex intra-abdominal and pelvic general surgery that involves the genitourinary system.

Practice-Based Learning and Improvement that involves investigation and evaluation of their own patient care, appraisal and assimilation of scientific evidence, and improvements in patient care.

INFORMATION TECHNOLOGY AND POPULATION COMPARISONS REFERENCES

Beck LH (ed). Genitourinary problems. Clinics in Geriatr Med 1998; May.

Campbell MF, Walsh PC (eds). Campbell's Urology (7th ed). Philadelphia: WB Saunders Co., 1998.

Grossman HB, Belville WD, Faerbea GJ. Male anatomy and physiology. In: Greenfield LJ, Mulholland M, Oldham KT, Zelenock GB, Lillemoe KD (eds), Surgery: Scientific Principles and Practice (2nd ed). Philadelphia: Lippincott-Raven, 1997;2199-2216.

Hurt WG, Soper DE. Female genital system. In: Greenfield LJ, Mulholland M, Oldham KT, Zelenock GB, Lillemoe KD (eds), Surgery: Scientific Principles and Practice (2nd ed). Philadelphia: Lippincott-Raven, 1997;2216-2229.

Jordan GH, Whelan TV, Horstman WG, et al. Urology/urinary system. In: O'Leary JP (ed), The Physiologic Basis of Surgery (2nd ed). Baltimore: Williams and Wilkins, 1996;581-601.

Miller TA (ed). The urinary system. Modern Surgical Care: Physiologic Foundations and Clinical Applications (2nd ed). St. Louis: Quality Medical Publishing, Inc., 1998;851-934.

O'Donnell P. Geriatric urology. In: Adkins RB, Jr., Scott HW, Jr. (eds), Surgical Care for the Elderly (2nd ed). Philadelphia: Lippincott-Raven Publishers, 1998;363-370.

Webster GG, Goldwasser B (eds). Urinary Diversion. Oxford: Isis Medical Media 1995;1-351.

http://www.auanet.org

SECTION 11.21   GYNECOLOGY AND OBSTETRICS
PART A: GYNECOLOGY

UNIT OBJECTIVES:

Demonstrate the ability to identify basic gynecologic pathologic conditions, and differentiate between gynecological and abdominal pathology requiring surgical intervention.

Demonstrate the ability to manage gynecologic problems, including emergency procedures and pathology/trauma involving pelvic and abdominal organs.

Recognize that gynecological disease may present to the general surgeon.

Pelvic inflammatory disease/Endometriosis/salpingitis: Diagnosis and initial management of pelvic sepsis.

Obstruction secondary to Ovarian Carcinoma: Recognition that bowel obstruction may be due to ovarian carcinoma.

Intra-abdominal hemorrhage due to ruptured Ovarian cyst or Ectopic Pregnancy: Recognize the possibility of ectopic pregnancy and refer to the appropriate team.

Iatrogenic injury: Recognize that an iatrogenic injury may be the cause of the patient's symptoms and consult with senior.

Medical Knowledge about established and evolving biomedical, clinical, and cognate (e.g. epidemiological and social-behavioral) sciences and the application of this knowledge to patient care.

1. Describe the components of a complete gynecological assessment, including an accurate history and physical examination. Note how the examination and findings would likely differ for a postmenopausal woman without estrogen replacement therapy.

2. Outline the anatomical relationships of the pelvic organs and the lower intra-abdominal organs.

3. Explain the physiology and endocrinology relating to endometrial function (e.g., hypothalamic pituitary ovarian axis and menstrual function).

4. Discuss the physiology and pathophysiology of gynecologic conditions and disease, including:

a.   Intrauterine pregnancy

b.   Benign diseases of the ovaries (e.g., cysts and the risks of torsion, hemorrhagic corpus luteum)

c.   Ectopic pregnancy

d.   Carcinoma of the ovary, uterus, cervix uteri, vagina, and vulva

e.   Advanced uterine prolapse in a postmenopausal woman

f.   Uterine leiomyoma in a postmenopausal woman

g.   Urinary and rectal incontinence

5.   Outline the differential diagnoses for pelvic pathology such as:

a.   Salpingitis versus appendicitis

b.   Mittelschmerz versus bleeding ovarian cyst

c.   Fibroid uterus versus other intra-abdominal masses

6.   Discuss the differential diagnosis of a pelvic mass to include considering:

a.   Cysts

         (1)   Benign ovarian cysts (functional, neoplastic)

         (2)   Malignant ovarian cysts

b.   Tumors

         (1)   Benign solid tumors (uterus, tubes, ovaries)

         (2)   Malignant solid tumors (primary or metastatic)

c.   Infectious processes (tubo-ovarian abscess)

d.   Gastrointestinal processes (diverticular disease)

7.   Summarize the categories of information provided by the following types of studies:

a.   Imaging (ultrasound—including Doppler flow, computed axial tomography, magnetic resonance imaging)

b.   Cytology of ascitic fluid

c.   Intravenous pyelography and cystoscopy

d.   Gastrointestinal contrast studies and sigmoidoscopy

8.	Explain the basis of preferred treatment for the following conditions:

  a.	Uterine bleeding

  b.	Ectopic pregnancy (ruptured versus unruptured)

  c.	Ovarian cysts with bleeding, enlargement

  d.	Adnexal torsion (role of detorsion, color flow Doppler)

  e.	Endometriosis

  f.	Carcinoma of the ovary, uterus, vagina, and vulva

  g.	Fibroids; fibroids in a 70-year-old woman

  h.	Normal pregnancy and its complications requiring Caesarean section

9.	Discuss the significance of postmenopausal vaginal bleeding, including:

  a.	Etiology	d.	Alleviation of symptoms

  b.	Evaluation	e.	Treatment alternatives

  c.	Diagnostic studies (including endometrial stripe assessment, saline-infusion sonohysterography)

10.	Identify and discuss pelvic support defects in the elderly woman, including:

  a.	Restoration of normal genital tract anatomy

    (1)	Bladder neck	(4)	Vaginal length

    (2)	Anterior vaginal wall	(5)	Posterior vaginal wall

    (3)	Apex of vagina	(6)	Perineal body

  b.	Options to surgery

  c.	Associated risks and benefits

    (1)	Quality of life decisions

    (2)	Healthy life-style

11.	Describe the indications for hysterectomy.

12.	Explain the appropriate surgical approach to radical groin dissection and vulvectomy for carcinoma.

13.	Describe the surgical and pathological staging of ovarian and uterine neoplasia.

14.	Summarize the principles of the following surgical procedures:

a. Hysterectomy   d. Laparoscopy

b. Salpingectomy   e. Vulvectomy

c. Oophorectomy   f. Radical groin dissection

15. Explain the principle of uterine artery embolization procedures.

16. Describe the relation of the ureters to the pelvic anatomy and the most common locations for ureteral compromise.

17. Explain the principles of chemotherapy and radiotherapy in the management of gynecologic malignancies.

18. Discuss the management of an ovarian mass unsuspected at laparotomy by considering:

   a. Biopsy versus oophorectomy

   b. Surgical staging (peritoneal washings, contralateral ovarian biopsy, omentectomy)

   c. Consultation (family, gynecologist)

   d. Morphology (size, septations, surface texture)

19. Adenocarcinoma of the endometrium is the most common invasive gynecologic malignancy in the U.S. Describe:

   a. Mean age at diagnosis

   b. Most common presenting complaint (90% of cases)

   c. High-risk factors (including Tamoxifen use and familial predisposition)

20. Pelvic inflammatory disease/Endometriosis/salpingitis:

   a. Anatomy and physiology of Pelvic organs

   b. Infective intra abdominal conditions

   c. Appropriate management of likely conditions /Antibiotic treatment /referral pathway

21. Obstruction secondary to Ovarian Carcinoma:

   a. Anatomy and physiology of Pelvic organs

   b. Understand investigation of the obstructed colon

   c. Understand modern management of Ovarian carcinoma

22. Intra-abdominal hemorrhage due to ruptured Ovarian cyst or Ectopic Pregnancy:

    a.   Anatomy and physiology of pelvic organs

    b.   Management of abnormality discovered

23. Iatrogenic injury:

    a.   Anatomy and physiology of abdominal organs

Patient Care that is compassionate, appropriate, and effective for the treatment of health problems and the promotion of health.

1. Perform pelvic examinations, only initially under direct supervision:

    a.   Part of every woman's general physical examination (includingrectovaginal exam)

    b.   Significant for patient to be evaluated for abdominal or pelvic symptoms

    c.   Critical for patients who must undergo abdominal or pelvic surgery

    d.   Evaluation of traumatically injured female

2. Participate as part of the surgical team in performing multiple gynecological surgery procedures:

    a.   Perform as surgical assistant during earliest training stages

    b.   Perform surgical procedures when experienced and under supervision:

        (1)   Pelvic laparoscopy   (3)   Salpingectomy

        (2)   Oophorectomy   (4)   Hysterectomy

3. Formulate differential diagnoses of pelvic infection and masses to consider:

    a.   Common infections (endometritis, salpingitis, tubo-ovarian abscess, bacterial vaginosis)

    b.   Common organisms (gonococcus, chlamydia, anaerobic bacteria)

    c.   Differentiating findings on pelvic and abdominal examination (mass, tenderness, signs of peritoneal irritation, ultrasound imaging, fever, leucocytosis)

4. Identify all normal pelvic structures visually and through palpation during laparotomy.

5. Manage general surgical problems of the pregnant patient (appendicitis, cholecystitis, breast mass, intestinal obstruction, ovarian torsion).

6. Diagnose ectopic pregnancy (role of quantitative B-HCG and transvaginal ultrasound, discriminatory zone)

7. Perform a salpingostomy under direct supervision. (evaluate contralateral Fallopian tube and consider salpingectomy)

8. Perform an emergency hysterectomy (beware the ureters).

9. Perform a radical groin dissection and assist in the performance of related gynecological surgery for carcinoma such as:

   a. Pelvic and inguinal lymph node dissection

   b. Bowel resection

   c. Cystectomy

   d. Pelvic exenteration with urinary and/or bowel diversion

10. Organise pelvic ultrasound /Pregnancy test /CT/tumor markers:
    Give Prognosis and discuss future therapy

PART B: OBSTETRICS
UNIT OBJECTIVES:

Demonstrate an understanding of the process of pregnancy.

Demonstrate the ability to manage common surgical problems that occur during pregnancy.

Medical Knowledge about established and evolving biomedical, clinical, and cognate (e.g. epidemiological and social-behavioral) sciences and the application of this knowledge to patient care.

1. Describe the physiologic changes in pregnancy, including:

   a. Cardiovascular d. Genital

   b. Respiratory

   c. Breasts

    d.   Gastrointestinal

2.   Describe normal intrauterine growth and development with consideration for the following:

    a.   Basic science principles of placental and fetal development

    b.   Fetal developmental physiology

3.   Explain the stages of fetal development, including

    a.   Characteristics of each trimester of pregnancy

    b.   Assessment of the fetus

    c.   Risk of surgery in each trimester.

4.   Outline major issues involved in managing surgical conditions in the pregnant patient, including:

    a.   Appendicitis (difficult to diagnose; necessity for different surgical approach)

    b.   Cholecystitis (medical management before resorting to surgery)

    c.   Intestinal obstruction (confusing symptoms; operative approach; postoperative nutritional support)

    d.   Breast mass (confusion with physiologic changes in breast; special considerations at surgery; postoperative complications with lactation)

    e.   Trauma (management of mother and fetus; special diagnostic measures)

    f.   Ovarian torsion (diagnosis and treatment options, risk of oophorectomy in the first trimester)

5.   Specify possible physiologic effects to the pregnant woman and/or the developing child exposed to the following agents:

    a.   Anesthesia

        (1)   Effects of common anesthetic agents, inhalation, and conduction

        (2)   Catastrophic events: failed endotracheal intubation, pulmonary aspiration, total spinal block

    (3) Anesthetic management in obstetric complications: amniotic fluid embolism, hemorrhage, hypertension

    (4) Position on operating room table and relevance to hemodynamics

  b. Medication

    (1) Understanding risk factors and categories assigned to all drugs

    (2) Fetal effects of drugs which cross the placenta

  c. Radiation

    (1) Effect on fertility

    (2) Effect on fetus (trimester specific, Rad/Gray levels considered safe)

6. Discuss the differential diagnosis of ectopic pregnancy, including:

  a. Signs and symptoms

  b. Qualitative human chorionic gonadotrophin (hCG)

  c. Quantitative hCG

  d. Abdominal and vaginal ultrasonography: correlation with hCG for presence of intrauterine fetal sac or adnexal mass (discriminatory zone)

7. Outline the indications and contraindications for laparoscopy in the pregnant patient, discussing:

  a. Diagnosis and treatment of ectopic pregnancy

  b. Contraindications: including multiple previous laparotomies, Class IV cardiac disease, peritonitis or obstruction with bowel distension

Patient Care that is compassionate, appropriate, and effective for the treatment of health problems and the promotion of health.

1. Diagnose pregnancy, utilizing:

  a. History: include menstrual history and symptoms of early pregnancy

  b. Physical examination: expected changes in the uterine cervix and corpus

  c. Laboratory tests for pregnancy

2.   Diagnose common gynecological problems that affect pregnant women, including:

    a.   Sexually transmitted diseases

    b.   Acquired Immunodeficiency Syndrome

    c.   Human papillomavirus infections (especially condylomata)

    d.   Leiomyomata uteri

3.   Deliver a baby during an uncomplicated delivery.

4.   Perform a Cesarian section in an emergency situation.

5.   Manage a pregnant surgical patient during acute trauma (mother comes first!).

6.   Perform laparoscopy under direct supervision for a pregnant patient (usually ectopic pregnancy).

Practice-Based Learning and Improvement that involves investigation and evaluation of their own patient care, appraisal and assimilation of scientific evidence, and improvements in patient care.

INFORMATION TECHNOLOGY AND POPULATION COMPARISONS REFERENCES

Cobbs EL, Duthie EH, Jr, Murphy JB (eds). Osteoporosis. Urinary incontinence. Gynecologic diseases and disorders. Disorders of sexual function. Geriatrics Review Syllabus: A Core Curriculum in Geriatric Medicine (4th ed). Dubuque IA: Kendall/Hunt Publishing Company, 1999.

Gabbe SG, Niebyl JR, Simpson JL. Obstetrics: Normal and Problem Pregnancies (3rd ed_. New York: Churchill Livingstone, 1996.

Hansen KA, Nolan TE. Female reproductive biology. In: O'Leary JP (ed). The Physiologic Basis of Surgery (2nd ed). Baltimore: Williams and Wilkins, 1996;269-284.

Hurt WG (ed). Urogynecologic Surgery. Gaithersburg, MD: Aspen Publishers, Inc., 1992.

Hurt WG, Soper DE. Female genital system. In: Greenfield LJ, Mulholland M, Oldham KT, Zelenock GB, Lillemoe KD (eds), Surgery: Scientific Principles and Practice (2nd ed). Philadelphia: Lippincott-Raven, 1997;2216-2229.

Johnson SR. The gynecologic history. The gynecologic examination. In: Sciarra JJ (ed), Gynecology and Obstetrics. Philadelphia: JB Lippincott, Co., 1994; Chapt. 6-7.

Jones HW, III, Burnett LS. Gynecologic diseases. In: Adkins RB, Jr., Scott HW, Jr. (eds), Surgical Care for the Elderly (2nd ed). Philadelphia: Lippincott-Raven Publishers, 1998;371-382.

Miller TA (ed). The urinary system. Modern Surgical Care: Physiologic Foundations and Clinical Applications (2nd ed). St. Louis: Quality Medical Publishing, Inc., 1998;851-934.

Mishell DR, Stenchever MA, Droegemueller W, Herbst A. Comprehensive Gynecology (3rd ed). St.Louis: Mosby, 1997.

Nelson ME, Fisher EC, Dilmanian FA, et al. A 1-year walking program and increased dietary calcium in postmenopausal women: effects on bone. Am J Clin Nutr 1991;53:1304-1311.

Prince RL, Smith M, Dick IM, et al. Prevention of postmenopausal osteoporosis; a comparative study of exercise, calcium supplementation, and hormone-replacement therapy. N Engl J Med 1991;325:1189-1195.

http://www.acog.com

SECTION 11.22   CARDIOTHORACIC SURGERY

UNIT OBJECTIVES:

Demonstrate an understanding of the anatomy, physiology, and pathophysiology of thoracic conditions pertinent to general surgery, exhibiting knowledge of how these change with age and how those changes alter one's considerations.

Effectively apply this understanding to the diagnosis, evaluation, and treatment of patients with thoracic problems who are to be managed by general surgery.

_Medical Knowledge about established and evolving biomedical, clinical, and cognate (e.g. epidemiological and social-behavioral) sciences and the application of this knowledge to patient care.

Junior Level:

1.   Describe thoracic anatomy and physiology, including anatomic and functional relationships:

    a.   Chest wall (including spine)

    b.   Accessory muscles of respiration

    c.   Diaphragm (including subjacent abdominal organs)

    d.   Mediastinum

    e.   Trachea, segmental and subsegmental bronchi

    f.   Lungs

    g.   Esophagus

    h.   Heart and pericardium

    i.   Great vessels and their immediate branches

    j.   Peripheral nerves (vagus, sympathetics, intercostals, phrenic, recurrent laryngeal)

    k.   Thoracic duct

    l.   Azygous and Hemiazygous veins

2.   Summarize and discuss the embryological development of:

    a.   Upper airway

b.   Lower airway

c.   Lungs

d.   Esophagus

e.   Heart and great vessels

f.   Mediastinal contents

g.   Lymphatic drainage of esophagus and lungs

3.   Review and analyze the basic principles and critical factors involved in:

a.   Ventilation

b.   Perfusion

c.   Control of respiration

d.   Lung function tests

e.   Respiratory failure

f.   Oxygen therapy

g.   Function of the diseased lung (obstructive, restrictive, and vascular)

4.   Summarize the modalities listed below, stating their indications and limitations in thoracic surgical procedures:

a.   Endoscopy/thoracoscopy

b.   Standard and positional roentgenograms

c.   Arteriography

d.   Ultrasonography

e.   Computed axial tomography (CAT), magnetic resonance imaging (MRI), and positron emission tomograph (PET)

f.   Nuclear medicine

g.   Ventilatory methods

h.   Tracheostomy

i.   Intubation and vent support

j.   Central venous catheters

k.   Pacemakers/defibrillators

l.   Thoracostomy tubes

m.　Stents (coronary, esophageal, tracheal, and bronchial)

5.　Discuss the following conditions, then choose and justify the appropriate diagnostic and therapeutic modalities:

a.　Pneumothorax

b.　Hydrothorax and hemothorax

c.　Combinations of a and b

d.　Chylothorax

e.　Pulmonary infiltrates or masses

f.　Abnormal cardiac silhouettes

g.　Congenital anomalies

h.　Pleural effusions

i.　Fractures (clavicles, sternum, ribs, scapulae, and spine)

j.　Mediastinal masses

k.　Infectious processes (parenchymal and pleural)

l.　Neoplastic processes (esophageal, pulmonary, extrapulmonary)

m.　Reactive processes (esophageal)

6.　Explain the various types of anesthetic agents and equipment used in thoracic surgery.

7.　Discuss and justify the indications for the following procedures:

a.	Needle aspiration	g.	Thoracotomy
b.	Chest tube placement	h.	Bilateral thoracotomy
c.	Mediastinoscopy	i.	Heller myotomy
d.	Thoracoscopy	j.	Thal patch
e.	Median sternotomy	k.	Stent use
f.	Mediastinotomy	l.	Bronchoscopy

8.　Evaluate a patient as a candidate for thoracic surgery and discuss:

a.　Operative risks

b.　Diagnostic tests important in assessing probable outcome

c.　Potential complications

d. Operation choices

e. Informed consent

f. Advanced directives

g. Living wills

h. Power of attorney

9. Explain the mechanics and applications of pulmonary function studies in evaluating patients for thoracic surgery.

10. Recommend when to use such diagnostic and therapeutic procedures as:

a. Bronchoscopy and esophagoscopy (flexible and rigid)

b. Thoracoscopy/Video Assisted Thoracoscopic Surgery (VATS)

c. Emergency room thoracotomy

d. Aortic cross clamping

e. Standard thoracotomy and median sternotomy (Chamberlain and book procedures)

f. Pericardial window/pericardiocentesis

g. Lung biopsy/fine-needle aspiration (FNA)

h. Pulmonary resection

i. Lung volume reduction operations

j. Mediastinoscopy

k. Dilatation

l. Manometry (esophageal)

m. 24-hour pH monitoring

11. Demonstrate an understanding of the mechanics of ventilatory support and the clinical application of mechanical ventilation by completing the following activities:

a. Contrast types of ventilators

b. Specify indications for ventilators

c. Demonstrate management of ventilators

d. Differentiate modes of ventilation

e. Explain weaning

f. Evaluate weaning parameters

g. Analyze complex ventilation problems

h. Discuss indications for tracheostomy

12. Identify indications for the following therapeutic modalities; and then justify/critique their use:

 a. Extra corporeal membrane oxygenation

 b. Ventricular assist devices (LVAD, RVAD, BVAD)

 c. Intra-aortic balloon pump (IABP)

 d. High frequency jet ventilation

 e. Laser (used endoscopically)

 f. Endoscopic thoracic procedures

 g. Alveolar (pulmonary) lavage

 h. Autotransfusion

 i. Cell saver

 j. Pulmonary artery catheterization

13. Analyze changes in thoracic anatomy and physiology resulting from the following:

 a. Abdominal operations g. Spine operations

 b. Mediastinoscopy h. Neck operations

 c. Thoracotomies i. General anesthesia

 d. Sternotomies j. Epidural anesthesia

 e. Thoracoscopy

 f. Thoracoplasties

14. Illustrate the various types of incisions used in thoracic surgery for:

 a. Apical resections

 b. Pneumonectomy

 c. Esophagectomy

 d. Mediastinal procedures

 e. Tracheal/bronchial procedures

f.   Esophageal stenosis and diverticula

g.   Thoracoplasty

h.   Diaphragmatic operations

Senior Level:

1.   Discuss the general diagnostic and operative approaches to treating blunt and penetrating trauma to the thorax and its contents.

2.   Describe specific surgical management of trauma to the thorax and its contents:

a.   Neck

b.   Esophagus

c.   Nerves

d.   Mediastinum

e.   Bony thorax

f.   Diaphragm

g.   Vessels

h.   Trachea/lungs

i.   Heart

3.   Integrate the pathophysiology and surgical management of the following:

a.   Aortic aneurysms

b.   Aortic dissections

c.   Trauma to heart and great vessels

d.   Occlusive disease

4.   Evaluate infiltrates, infectious processes, and neoplastic processes in the thorax, and recommend appropriate management.

5.   Discuss and list thoracic tumor types, staging for each, including descriptions of nodal drainage sites and levels.

6.   Summarize the causes and appropriate management of cardiac arrhythmias, including:

a.   Pharmacotherapeutics   c.   Pacemakers

b.   Cardioversion   d.   Defibrillators

7. Describe the diagnosis and discuss therapy of such surgical complications as:

   a. Fistulas: bronchopleural, pleurocutaneous, tracheoesophageal (TE), arteriovenous (AV) and thoracic duct

   b. Esophageal leak/stenosis/obstruction

   c. Loculated hemothorax

   d. Postoperative bleeding

   e. Empyema

   f. Air leaks

   g. Bronchial obstructions

   h. Endstage COPD/pulmonary fibrosis

8. Identify indications for and be prepared to interpret results of the following diagnostic modalities:

   a. Plain and positional chest x-rays

   b. Gastrointestinal contrast studies

   c. CAT, MRI, and PET scans

   d. Bronchograms

   e. Pulmonary function studies

   f. Ventilation-perfusion studies

   g. Nuclear medicine studies

   h. Ultrasound

   i. Split pulmonary functions

9. Specify and justify the diagnostic or therapeutic indications for the use of the following modalities:

   a. Rigid and flexible bronchoscopy

   b. Esophagoscopy (rigid and flexible)

   c. Mediastinoscopy (cervical and parasternal)

   d. Thoracoscopy/VATS

   e. Laser

   f. Stents

g.   Lung transplant

10.   Assess and recommend the surgical procedures involved in:

    a.   Tracheal, bronchial, and esophageal obstructing lesions

    b.   Thoracoplasty

    c.   Esophageal resection/reconstruction

    d.   Anti-reflux procedures

    e.   Sleeve resection of the trachea/bronchus for tumor

    f.   Chest wall reconstruction using myocutaneous flaps and/or synthetic materials

11.   Select and specify diagnostic and therapeutic maneuvers to manage problem areas following thoracic surgery:

    a.   Cardiovascular and pulmonary medical complications

    b.   Renal failure

    c.   Liver failure

    d.   Diabetes mellitus

    e.   Malnutrition

    f.   Metabolic dysfunction

    g.   Immune system suppression

12.   Discuss quality assurance, cost-cutting measures, and patient-care pathways as they relate to thoracic surgery.

Patient Care that is compassionate, appropriate, and effective for the treatment of health problems and the promotion of health.

<u>Junior Level</u>:

1.   Evaluate thoracic pathophysiology; order and interpret appropriate tests.

2.   Diagnose and provide initial management of fractures of ribs, clavicle, sternum, scapulae, and spine.

3. Evaluate patients for thoracic surgery with regard to risk factors, candidacy for surgical resection, pulmonary function studies, and possible postoperative disability.

4. Manage general thoracic perioperative procedures.

5. Use, set, and regulate mechanical ventilators.

6. Observe and then:

    a. Insert chest tubes

    b. Perform thoracentesis

    c. Insert central venous access lines

    d. Execute simple endoscopic procedures

    e. Perform tracheostomies

    f. Institute naso-oropharyngeal/tracheal anesthesia for endoscopic procedures

7. Use data obtained from diagnostic and therapeutic procedures to assess and plan treatment for thoracic pathology.

8. Perform bronchoscopy, esophagoscopy, nasotracheal, and orotracheal intubation, including double lumen tubes.

9. Manage empyemas surgically.

10. Insert Swan-Ganz catheter and perform cardiovascular monitoring calculations for:

    a. Pressures

    b. Cardiac output

    c. Systemic vascular resistance

11. Supervise ventilator regulation.

<u>Senior Level</u>:

1. Perform and/or supervise all thoracic diagnostic and therapeutic endoscopic procedures.

2. Resect ribs, treat empyema cavities, perform pleural and lung biopsies.

3. Manage thoracic trauma.

4. Manage thoracic aortic aneurysms and dissections.

5. Direct complex ventilator-dependent patient management.

6. Perform lung resections, rib resections, mediastinoscopies, and mediastinotomies.

7. Provide surgical management of neoplasms of the thorax and its contents.

8. Provide medical and surgical management of infectious processes in the thorax.

9. Manage cardiac arrhythmias.

10. Perform and/or supervise pacemaker/defibrillator selection and placement.

11. Manage all pharmacotherapeutics associated with thoracic surgery.

12. Treat medical conditions associated with thoracic surgical procedures.

13. Place esophageal and bronchial stents.

Practice-Based Learning and Improvement that involves investigation and evaluation of their own patient care, appraisal and assimilation of scientific evidence, and improvements in patient care.

INFORMATION TECHNOLOGY AND POPULATION COMPARISONS REFERENCES

Cameron JL (ed). Current Surgical Therapy (7th ed). St. Louis: Mosby, 2001.

Crim C. Physiology of respiration. In: Miller TA (ed), Modern Surgical Care: Physiologic Foundations and Clinical Applications (2nd ed). St. Louis: Quality Medical Publishing, Inc., 1998;729-737.

Hood RM, Arnold HS, Calhoon JH. Techniques in General Thoracic Surgery (2nd ed). Philadelphia: Lea & Febiger, 1993.

Iannettoni MD, Orringer MB. Chest wall, pleura, mediastinum, and nonneoplastic lung disease. In: Greenfield LJ, Mulholland M, Oldham KT, Zelenock GB, Lillemoe KD (eds), Surgery: Scientific Principles and Practice (2nd ed). Philadelphia: Lippincott-Raven, 1997;1440-1482.

Mack MJ, Scrubbs GR, Kelly KM, et al. Video-assisted thoracic surgery: has technology found its place? Ann Thoracic Surg 1997;64:211-215.

McKenna RJ, Jr. Thoracoscopy. In: Cameron JL (ed), Current Surgical Therapy (6th ed). St. Louis: Mosby, 1998;1240-1244.

Moulton AL, Greenburg AG. The pulmonary system. In: O'Leary JP (ed), The Physiologic Basis of Surgery (2nd ed). Baltimore: Williams and Wilkins, 1996;376-405.

Mountain CF. Revisions in the international system for staging lung cancer. Chest 1997;111:1710-1717.

Mountain CF, Dresler CM. Regional lymph nodes classification for lung cancer staging. Chest 1997;111:1718-1723.

Peters RM, Mark JBD. Pulmonary disease and mediastinal surgery. In: Adkins RB, Jr., Scott HW, Jr. (eds), Surgical Care for the Elderly (2nd ed). Philadelphia: Lippincott-Raven Publishers, 1998;251-268.

Richardson JD. Common pulmonary derangements, respiratory failure, and adult respiratory distress syndrome. In: Miller TA (ed), Modern Surgical Care: Physiologic Foundations and Clinical Applications (2nd ed). St. Louis: Quality Medical Publishing, Inc., 1998;738-764.

Rusch VW. Lung neoplasms. In: Greenfield LJ, Mulholland M, Oldham KT, Zelenock GB, Lillemoe KD (eds), Surgery: Scientific Principles and Practice (2nd ed). Philadelphia: Lippincott-Raven, 1997;1417-1440.
Sabiston DC, Spender FC (eds). Surgery of the Chest (6th ed). Philadelphia: WB Saunders Co., 1995.

Shields TW. General Thoracic Surgery (4th ed). Baltimore: Williams & Wilkins, 1994.

http://www.sts.org

SECTION 11:22B **CARDIAC AND GREAT VESSELS SURGERY**
UNIT OBJECTIVES:

Demonstrate knowledge of the anatomy, physiology, and pathophysiologic conditions of the heart and great vessels which are amenable to surgical correction.

Demonstrate the ability to clinically manage patients with pathologic conditions of the heart and great vessels.

Medical Knowledge about established and evolving biomedical, clinical, and cognate (e.g. epidemiological and social-behavioral) sciences and the application of this knowledge to patient care.

<u>Junior Level:</u>

1. Describe and demonstrate a working knowledge of the heart and great vessels, including:

    a.   Cardiac chambers (atria and ventricles)

    b.   Cardiac valves (mitral, aortic, tricuspid, pulmonic)

    c.   Coronary arteries

    d.   Intrinsic neural conduction system

    e.   Extrinsic neural innervation (sympathetic and parasympathetic)

    f.   Great vessels (cavae, aorta, innominate artery, carotid arteries, and subclavian arteries)

2. Describe and demonstrate working knowledge of cardiac physiology, including:

    a.   Electrophysiology (action potential, depolarization, repolarization, mechanisms of rhythm control)

    b.   Determinants of cardiac output (heart rate and stroke volume)

    c.   Interactions and control mechanisms (preload, afterload, contractility, Frank-Starling Law, peripheral resistance)

    d.   Determinants of myocardial oxygen consumption

    e.   Normal pressures, waveforms, and oxygen saturation in cardiac chambers

443

3.   Identify the control mechanisms and normal physiology of peripheral vessels. Relate each of these to a clinical example:

   a.   Arterial autoregulation

   b.   Venous flow regulation

   c.   Interrelationship of cardiac output, peripheral blood flow, and autoregulation

4.   Discuss the information obtained from the history and physical examination pertinent to cardiac and peripheral vascular pathophysiology. Determine the interactions of those details and their implications on planned surgical procedures and outcomes. Consider the following for risk assessment and perioperative management:

   a.   Patient age

   b.   Risk factors for cardiovascular disease (family history, smoking, hypertension, diabetes mellitus, hyperlipidemia, and obesity)

   c.   Symptoms/signs associated with coronary artery disease, ventricular dysfunction, and valvular dysfunction

   d.   Pulmonary dysfunction (pulmonary hypertension, chronic obstructive pulmonary disease [COPD], previous pulmonary resection)

   e.   Neurologic abnormalities

   f.   Renal dysfunction

   g.   Hematologic abnormalities

   h.   Hepatic dysfunction

   i.   Cerebrovascular, peripheral vascular or aneurysmal disease

   j.   Gastrointestinal considerations

   k.   Metabolic, nutritional, genetic, immune, and oncologic abnormalities

   l.   Psychiatric conditions, psychological and social interactions

   m.   Re-operative chest surgery

   n.   Miscellaneous considerations (prior operations including vascular or valvular prostheses, substance abuse, dental status, interactions of medications)

5.   Discuss the use and interpretation of cardiovascular diagnostic tests in identification of cardiovascular pathology, including:

a. Electrocardiography

b. Echocardiography (transthoracic and transesophageal)

c. Traditional roentgenography

d. Cardiac catheterization and arteriography

e. Peripheral vascular arteriography

f. Vascular ultrasonography

g. Computer and magnetic resonance imaging

h. Radionuclide scintigraphy (multi-gated acquisition [MUGA], stress, and Persantine thallium)

6. Demonstrate the use and principles associated with various cardiac monitoring methods, including:

a. Intra-arterial and central venous pressure transducers

b. Pulmonary artery catheters

c. Left atrial catheters

d. Temporary percutaneous and intracardiac pacing wires

7. Discuss techniques, mechanisms of action, and potential complications for mechanical and pharmacologic support of the circulation, including:

a. Inotropic agents (dopamine, dobutamine, epinephrine, norepinephrine, amrinone, isoproterenol)

b. Pre- /after- load agents (Nipride, nitroglycerine, Neo-synephrine)

c. Intra-aortic balloon pump

d. Ventricular assist devices

e. Cardiac pacing

8. Describe and assess the operative indications, risk, and expected outcomes associated with several cardiac surgical procedures, including:

a. Coronary artery bypass and minimally invasive direct coronary artery bypass surgery

b. Valvular replacement/repair (aortic, mitral, tricuspid)

c.   Operations of the ascending aorta, aortic arch and descending thoracic aorta

d.   Permanent pacemaker/automatic defibrillator insertion

e.   Pericardial drainage procedure

9.   Discuss the complications of cardiac surgery and methods used to reduce their incidence. Complications: death, myocardial infarction, stroke, bleeding, arrhythmias, low cardiac output syndrome, cardiac tamponade, pneumothorax, sternal and extremity wound infections, respiratory and renal failure

10.   Review the management of postoperative cardiac surgery patients in the intensive care unit.

<u>Senior Level</u>:

1.   Discuss the pathophysiology of congenital cardiac disease, including:

a.   Coarctation of the aorta

b.   Patent ductus arteriosus

c.   Atrial septal defects

d.   Ventricular septal defects

e.   Complex cyanotic cardiac disease

(1)   Transportation of great vessels

(2)   Tetralogy of Fallot

(3)   Pulmonary atresia

(4)   Total anomalous venous return

2.   Discuss the pathophysiology of acquired cardiac disease including:

a.   Myocardial ischemia

b.   Valvular heart disease (stenotic and regurgitant)

c.   Endocarditis

d.   Ventricular aneurysms

e.   Thoracic aneurysms

f.   Trauma to the heart and great vessels

3. Summarize the management of the following post-cardiac surgery variances, including the monitoring, prevention, and the therapeutic intervention of:

    a. Arrhythmias (ventricular and atrial)

    b. Bleeding (correction of coagulopathy, indications for re-exploration)

    c. Infection (methods of prophylaxis, empiric and culture-specific therapy)

    d. Low cardiac output and hypotension

    e. Postoperative hypertension

4. Demonstrate working knowledge and use of the following postoperative support systems:

    a. Cardiac drugs (inotropic, chronotropic, afterload-reducing, anti-platelet, beta blockade, ACE inhibition, diuretics)

    b. Mediastinal and pleural drainage

    c. Mechanical ventilation, airway management systems

    d. Temporary and permanent pacemakers

    e. Intra-aortic balloon pumps and other ventricular assist devices

    f. Dialysis and ultrafiltration

    g. Cardiopulmonary bypass and extracorporeal membrane oxygenation

5. Summarize the diagnostic evaluation and indications for each of the following surgical procedures:

    a. Adult valvular repair and replacement procedures (mechanical vs. bioprosthetic)

    c. Resection of ventricular aneurysms

    d. Resection and grafting of thoracic aneurysms

    e. Combination operations of valve replacement and coronary artery bypass grafting

    f. Surgical treatment of idiopathic hypertrophic subaortic stenosis

6. Discuss the evaluation and therapeutic options available for surgical management of cardiac trauma such as:

    a. Traumatic transection of the aorta and other great vessels

    b. Blunt and penetrating cardiac and great vessel injury

7. Outline the post-hospitalization follow-up and management of cardiac surgery patients to include:

   a. Instructions to the patient

   b. Follow-up clinic visit (including physical examination, electrocardiogram [ECG], Chest x-ray)

   c. Long-term follow-up for coronary and valve patients (including anticoagulation adjustment where indicated)

Patient Care that is compassionate, appropriate, and effective for the treatment of health problems and the promotion of health.

<u>Junior Level:</u>

1. Perform preoperative evaluation, history, and physical examination of cardiac surgery patients.

2. Obtain and interpret indicated diagnostic studies.

3. Discuss diagnostic and therapeutic approaches to specific acquired and congenital cardiac diseases with the attending physicians.

4. Assist with selected cardiac and general surgery cases, such as:

   a. Pacemaker and defibrillator insertions

   b. Saphenous vein harvest and wound closure for coronary bypass operations

   c. Valve and coronary operations

   d. Pericardial drainage operations

   e. Tracheostomy

   f. Minor vascular repairs

5. Provide postoperative cardiac surgery follow-up care for the following cases:

   a. Coronary surgery

   b. Valve surgery

   c. Thoracic aortic surgery

   d. Pacemaker and defibrillator placement

6.   Perform percutaneous insertion of chest tubes and intravenous, intra-arterial, and pulmonary artery catheters with supervision.

                                Senior Level:

1.   Serve as first assistant on selected major cardiothoracic cases, including:

        a.   Coronary artery bypass surgery, minimally invasive direct coronary artery bypass

        b.   Valvular replacements and repairs, including minimally invasive procedures

        c.   Thoracic aortic surgery

        d.   Congenital cardiac surgery

        e.   Complex defibrillators

        f.   Emergency thoracotomies

2.   Perform cardiac procedures, under supervision, including the following:

        a.   Insert intra-aortic balloon pump

        b.   Pacemaker implantation

        c.   Median sternotomy incision

        d.   Aortic cannulation for cardiopulmonary bypass

        e.   Saphenous vein and internal thoracic artery harvest

        f.   Perform proximal coronary anastomoses

        g.   Repair of vascular trauma

        h.   Graft replacement of aorta in selected cases

3.   Coordinate the work-up of emergency cardiac surgery cases with:

        a.   Emergency room or trauma team

        b.   Cardiac catheterization laboratory

        c.   Diagnostic imaging services

        d.   Laboratory (including blood bank)

        e.   Anesthesia

        f.   Operating room

        g.   Perfusion services

449

4.   Assist with emergency cardiac surgery, including trauma cases.

5.   Recognize and prescribe treatment for complications of cardiac surgery such as:

    a.   Gastrointestinal bleeding

    b.   Cerebrovascular accident

    c.   Endocrine abnormalities

    d.   Pulmonary complications

    e.   Renal dysfunction

    f.   Coagulopathy

    g.   Dysrhythmias

    h.   Low cardiac output status

Practice-Based Learning and Improvement that involves investigation and evaluation of their own patient care, appraisal and assimilation of scientific evidence, and improvements in patient care.

INFORMATION TECHNOLOGY AND POPULATION COMPARISONS REFERENCES

Baumgartner WA, Owens SG, Cameron DE, Reitz BA (eds). Johns Hopkins Manual of Cardiac Surgical Care. St. Louis: Mosby Year Book, 1994.

Clary BM, Milano CA (eds). The Handbook of Surgical Intensive Care: Practices of the Surgical Residents at Duke University Medical Center (5th ed). St.Louis: Mosby, 2000.

Eagle KA, Brundage BH, Chaitman BR, et al. Guidelines for perioperative cardiovascular evaluation for noncardiac surgery. Circulation 1996;93:12780-1317.

Foster ED, Davis KB, Carpentier JA, et al. Risk of noncardiac operation in patients with defined coronary disease: the coronary artery surgery study (CASS) registry experience. Ann Thor Surg 1986;41(1):42-50.

Goldman L, Caldera DI, Nussbaum SR, et al. Multifactorial index of cardiac risk in noncardiac surgical procedures. N Engl J Med 1977;297:845-850.

Higgins TL, Estafanous FG, Loop FD, et al. Stratification of morbidity and mortality outcome by preoperative risk factors in coronary artery bypass patients: a clinical severity score. JAMA 1992;267:2344-2348.

Kirklin JW, Barratt-Boyes BG. Cardiac Surgery: Morphology, Diagnostic Criteria, Natural History, Techniques, Results, and Indications (2nd ed). New York: Churchill Livingstone, Inc., 1993.

Mangano DT, Goldman L. Preoperative assessment of patients with known or suspected coronary disease. N Engl J Med 1995;333:1750-1756.

Rosengart TA, deBois W, Francalancia NA. Adult heart disease. In: Norton JA, Bollinger RR, Chang AE, et al. (eds). Surgery: Basic Science and Clinical Evidence. New York: Springer-Verlag, 2000.

Sabiston DC, Spencer FC (eds). Surgery of the Chest (6th ed). Philadelphia: WB Saunders Co., 1995.

Vlahakes GJ (ed). Handbook of Patient Care in Cardiac Surgery (5th ed). Boston: Little, Brown and Co., 1994.

SECTION 11.22C: CARDIOTHORACIC SURGERY IN ELDERLY PATIENTS

Medical Knowledge about established and evolving biomedical, clinical, and cognate (e.g. epidemiological and social-behavioral) sciences and the application of this knowledge to patient care.

1.   Discuss the epidemiological impact of cardiovascular disease in the elderly.
2.   Identify the cardiovascular risk factors associated with surgical morbidity and mortality.
3.   Discuss the cardiac surgical procedures performed most often in the elderly.
4.   Discuss the indications for valvular heart surgery in the elderly.
5.   Discuss the pathophysiologic changes in the cardiovascular system that accompanies aging.
6.   Discuss the case management of elderly patients with coronary artery disease with respect to surgical risk.

Practice-Based Learning and Improvement that involves investigation and evaluation of their own patient care, appraisal and assimilation of scientific evidence, and improvements in patient care.

INFORMATION TECHNOLOGY AND POPULATION COMPARISONS
REFERENCES

Akins CW, Daggett WM, Vlahakes GJ, et al. Cardiac operations in patients 80 years old and older. Ann Thor Surg 1997;64:606-615.

Alexander KP, Anstrom KJ, Muhlbaier LH, et al. Outcomes of cardiac surgery in patients [3] 80 years: results from the National Cardiovascular Network. J Am Coll Cardiol 2000;35(3):731-738.

Boucher JM, Dupras A, Jutras N, et al. Long-term survival and functional status in the elderly after cardiac surgery. Can J Cardiol 1997;13:646-652.

Chesler E (ed). Clinical Cardiology in the Elderly (2nd ed). Armonk NY: Futura Publishing Company, Inc., 1999;1-840.

Davis EA, Gardner TJ, Gillinov AM, et al. Valvular disease in the elderly: influence on surgical results. Ann Thor Surg 1993;55:333-338.

Detsky AS, Abrams HB, Forbath N, et al. Cardiac assessment for patients undergoing noncardiac surgery: a multifactorial clinical risk index. Arch Intern Med 1986;146:2131-2134.

Duncan AK, Vittone J, Fleming KC, Smith HC. Cardiovascular disease in elderly patients. Mayo Clin Proc 1996;71:184-196.

Eagle KA, Brundage BH, Chaitman BR, et al. Guidelines for perioperative cardiovascular evaluation for noncardiac surgery. Circulation 1996;93:12780-1317.

Fernandez J, Chen C, Anolik G, et al. Perioperative risk factors affecting hospital stay and hospital costs in open heart surgery for patients 3 65 years old. Eur J Cardiothorac Surg 1997;11(6):1133-1140.

Foster ED, Davis KB, Carpentier JA, et al. Risk of noncardiac operation in patients with defined coronary disease: the coronary artery surgery study (CASS) registry experience. Ann Thor Surg 1986;41(1):42-50.

Fried GM, Clas D, Meakins JL. Minimally invasive surgery in the elderly patient. In: Zenilman ME, Roslyn JJ (eds), Surgery in the elderly patient, Surg Cl of N Amer 1994;74(2):375-387.

Fried LP, Kronmal RA, Newman AB, et al. Risk factors for 5-year mortality in older adults. The Cardiovascular Health Study. JAMA 1998;279:585-592.

Goldman L, Caldera DI, Nussbaum SR, et al. Multifactorial index of cardiac risk in noncardiac surgical procedures. N Engl J Med 1977;297:845-850.

Higgins TL, Estafanous FG, Loop FD, et al. Stratification of morbidity and mortality outcome by preoperative risk factors in coronary artery bypass patients: a clinical severity score. JAMA 1992;267:2344-2348.

Ivanov J, Weisel RD, David TE, Naylor CD. Fifteen-year trends in risk severity and operative mortality in elderly patients undergoing coronary artery bypass graft surgery. Circulation 1998;97:673-680.

Josephson R, Fannin S. Cardiovascular disease. In: McLeskey CH (ed). Geriatric Anesthesiology. Baltimore: Williams & Wilkins, 1997;43-55.

Lee EM, Porter JN, Shapiro LM, Wells FC. Mitral valve surgery in the elderly. J Heart Valve Dis 1997;6(1):22-31.

Mangano DT, Goldman L. Preoperative assessment of patients with known or suspected coronary disease. N Engl J Med 1995;333:1750-1756.

Merrill WH. Cardiac surgery. In: Adkins RB, Jr., Scott HW, Jr. (eds), Surgical Care for the Elderly (2nd ed). Philadelphia: Lippincott-Raven Publishers, 1998;233-240.

Mullany CJ, Mock MB, Brooks MM, et al. Effect of age in the Bypass Angioplasty Revascularization Investigation (BARI) randomized trial. Ann Thorac Surg 1999;67(2):3960403.

Paul SD, O'Gara PT, Mahjoub ZA, et al. Geriatric patients with acute myocardial infarction: cardiac risk factor profiles, presentation, thrombolysis, coronary interventions, and prognosis. Am Heart J 1996;131(4):710-715.

Rao V, Christakis GT, Weisel RD, et al. Changing pattern of valve surgery. Circulation 1996;94(9 Suppl):II113-120.

Shapira OM, Kelleher RM, Zelingher J, et al. Prognosis and quality of life after valve surgery in patients older than 75 years. Chest 1997;112(4):885-894.

Chapter 12

ASSOCIATED SPECIALTIES

SECTION 12.1   EMERGENCY MEDICINE

UNIT OBJECTIVES:

Manage a variety of surgical conditions in an emergency setting.

Demonstrate knowledge of patient stabilization, transport, and physician-to-physician communication in an emergency situation.

Demonstrate the ability to evaluate and effectively manage all acute or life-threatening conditions, including major trauma in an emergency setting.

Demonstrate knowledge of disaster management, including the role of triage; and display the ability to apply this knowledge to the emergency setting.

Medical Knowledge about established and evolving biomedical, clinical, and cognate (e.g. epidemiological and social-behavioral) sciences and the application of this knowledge to patient care.

<u>Junior Level</u>:

1.   Complete the coursework and testing to obtain Basic and Advanced Cardiac Life Support (BLS and ACLS), Advanced and Trauma Life Support (ATLS), and Fundamental Critical Care Support (FCCS) certification.

2.   Describe the initial management of the injured patient(s) in the following stages of care:

    a.   Care in pre-hospital setting including BLS

    b.   Triage in emergency department

    c.   Serve as team leader and member during ATLS

    d.   Coordinate patient transport to tertiary facility

3.   Outline the basic principles of triage in the emergency department, including:

    a.   Immediate treatment

    b.   Ambulatory treatment

    c.   Delayed treatment

    d.   Expectant treatment

    e.   Psychiatric considerations

4.   Explain priorities for the diagnosis and/or assessment of illness/injury for patients presenting to the emergency department, keeping the following issues in mind:

    a.   Discuss requests for diagnostic studies comparing the urgency of the need to know with:

        (1)   The time required to obtain results

        (2)   Potential danger to unstable patient

        (3)   Quality of information obtained if a stat procedure compromises preparation of the patient

    b.   Compare the need for provision of expedient, cost effective work-ups against the appropriateness of using the emergency setting for extensive work-ups at the risk of over utilizing limited resources.

5.   Explain the ATLS protocol for the emergency resuscitation and stabilization of a seriously ill or injured patient:

    a.   Cite working knowledge of the ABC's of resuscitation

    b.   Define the essentials of AMPLE history (Allergy, Medications, Past illnesses, Last meal, Events of illness/injury)

    c.   Define the essentials of the Primary and Secondary Surveys

6.   Describe the considerations for establishing an airway appropriate to the patient's condition, including:

    a.   Nasal trumpets/nasopharyngeal airway

    b.   Bag-mask assistance

    c.   Endotracheal tube

    d.   Surgically Created Airways (cricothyrotomy-needle or tube)

7.   Describe the typical case scenarios for the following life-threatening problems requiring appropriate urgent/emergent action:

    a.   Multiple system trauma

    b.   Shock (cardiogenic, neurogenic, septic, and hypovolemic)

      c.   Traumatic neurological injuries

           (1)   Head injury without altered consciousness

           (2)   Head injury with altered consciousness, including deteriorating mental status

           (3)   Subarachnoid/subdural hemorrhage

           (4)   Penetrating head trauma

      d.   Chest injuries (penetrating and blunt)

      e.   Abdominal and pelvic injuries (penetrating and blunt)

      f.   Vascular injuries (penetrating and blunt)

      g.   Myocardial infarction

           (1)   Complicated (with congestive heart failure [CHF], hypotension, dysrhythmia)

           (2)   Uncomplicated

      h.   Pulmonary embolus

      i.   Diabetic ketoacidosis and other metabolic derangements

           (1)   Hyper- and hypo- kalemia

           (2)   Hyper- and hypo- natremia

           (3)   Hyper- and hypo- calcemia

      j.   Gastrointestinal bleeding

      k.   Pancreatitis

      l.   Ectopic pregnancy

      m.   Phlebitis

      n.   Burns, including inhalation injury

      o.   Poisoning

      p.   Hypothermia

8.   Describe the principles of evaluation and management for the following less-serious problems:

      a.   Drug abuse and suicide attempts

      b.   Seizures/coma

      c.   Facial injuries

        (1)   Lacerations of face and scalp

        (2)   Fractures of facial bones and jaw

        (3)   Epistaxis

  d.   Pneumonia

  e.   Cardiac versus other chest pain

  f.   Acute abdominal pain

  g.   Hand injuries

  h.   Long bone fractures

9.   Discuss the principles of evaluation and management for the following common minor problems:

  a.   Laceration evaluation

  b.   Tetanus prophylaxis

  c.   Wound treatment

  d.   Surgical repair of wounds

  e.   Appropriate dressings

  f.   Soft tissue infections

  g.   Headache

  h.   Eye, ear, nose, and throat infections

  i.   Bronchitis

  j.   Gastroenteritis

  k.   Hemorrhoids

  l.   Wildlife injuries (animal bites, insect and marine envenomations)

  m.   Follow-up instructions

10.   Explain the indications and appropriate methods for:

  a.   Peritoneal lavage

  b.   Insertion of chest tubes

  c.   Pericardiocentesis

  d.   Suprapubic catheter insertion

  e.   Central line insertion

f.   External/transvenous pacemaker placement

g.   Cricothyrotomy

h.   Rapid rewarming BAIR Hugger, CAVR (Continuous arterial venous rewarming)

11.   Recommend ways in which the ED physical environment can be adapted to better meet the special needs of elderly patients. Discuss these problems:

      a.   Little privacy or confidentiality

      b.   Poor lighting

      c.   High ambient noise level

      d.   Lack of adequate communication and/or reassuring dialogue

12.   Analyze the medicolegal responsibilities of the physician in the field as an accepting physician coordinating transport.

13.   Define the requirements for informed consent in the emergency setting:

      a.   Life-threatening conditions

      b.   Minor surgery

      c.   Patients who are minors

      d.   Patients unable to provide informed consent (non compis mentis)

            (1)   Amnesia for event

            (2)   Drug or alcohol use

            (3)   Dementia

14.   Summarize significant steps in the examination for and treatment of dental/oral emergencies with which a general surgeon should be familiar:

      a.   Toothache

      b.   Gingival bleeding (gingivitis, periodontitis, HIV-related hemorrhagic conditions)

      c.   Buccolingually displaced tooth or teeth

      d.   Dental or periodontal abscess or fistulous tract

      e.   Cellulitis, including Ludwig's Angina

      f.   Peritonsillar abscess (Quinsy)

1. Outline the essential elements of a team approach to the management of life threatening illness or injury. Review responsibilities of the team leader and right- and left- side team members.

2. Describe the indications for emergency thoracotomy and the appropriate operative approach.

3. Analyze the decision process in evaluating the need for emergency operative intervention in trauma or disease.

4. Review, analyze, and design a hospital disaster plan that includes:
   a. Multiple victims
   b. Burns
   c. Radiation injury
   d. Chemical exposure
   e. Environmental injury
      (1) Immersion
      (2) Lightening strike
      (3) Hypothermia
      (4) Infections of epidemic proportions

5. Discuss the principles of advanced trauma care, including:
   a. Public education and outreach
   b. Emergency medical services management
   c. Public training in basic cardiopulmonary resuscitation (CPR)

6. Evaluate the functions of the leader of a multi-specialty team in emergency medicine.

7. Design a geriatric emergency care model that will foster optimal ED management and disposition.

Patient Care that is compassionate, appropriate, and effective for the treatment of health problems and the promotion of health.

<u>Junior Level:</u>

Under the guidance and supervision of more senior residents, attending surgeons, or emergencydepartment attendings:

1.   Perform triage of emergency trauma patients.

2.   Establish emergency stabilization of the traumatized patient via the following precautions:

   a.   Fracture management/stabilization

   b.   Cervical spine protection

   c.   Prevention of hypothermia

3.   Assess patients presenting emergency conditions using the appropriate diagnostic protocol.

4.   Prioritize requests for diagnostic studies based on need to know and the time required to obtain results.

5.   Establish the following airways:

   a.   Perform bag-mask ventilation

   b.   Insert nasopharyngeal or oropharyngeal airways

   c.   Perform endotracheal intubation (oro- and naso- pharyngeal)

   d.   Perform a cricothyrotomy

6.   Establish access to the central venous system.

7.   Assist with acute resuscitation procedures as indicated.

8.   Discuss patient's condition and future care with family.

9.   Provide appropriate treatment for non-emergency problems presenting to the emergency department.

10.   Function as a surgical consultant, assessing and developing differential diagnoses and discussing recommendations with senior resident or attending.

11.   Ascertain the severity of injury and identify patients requiring operative intervention.

12.   Perform emergency diagnostic and therapeutic procedures such as:

a. Peritoneal lavage

b. Insertion of chest tubes

c. Pericardiocentesis

d. Suprapubic catheter insertion

e. Central line insertion

f. External/ transvenous pacemaker

g. Insertion of intracranial pressure monitoring device

13. Perform minor surgical procedures such as:

a.	Drainage of abscesses	d.	Wound debridement
b.	Wound closure	e.	Bladder catheterization
c.	Removal of foreign bodies		

14. Perform emergent dental procedures prior to referral to a dentist, oral surgeon, or maxillofacial prosthodontist, including:

a. Examination and recommendation of palliative treatment for toothache

b. Reinsertion of avulsed tooth

c. Recognition and stabilization of fractured tooth/teeth

d. Alleviation and/or prescription preparation for abscess or fistula

e. Diagnosing and immediately managing cellulitis, especially extending to the neck

15. Explain patient's condition and proposed therapy to his/her family and obtain appropriate informed consent.

16. Discuss management options with the patient and his/her family.

17. Recommend further diagnostic and/or radiographic studies to clarify diagnosis and focus patient management.

18. Communicate the importance of injury prevention to patients, patient families, and staff in the quest for control of trauma as a disease of modern society.

Senior Level:

Under the guidance and supervision of more senior residents, attending surgeons, or emergency department attendings:

1. Perform triage of several sets of multiply-traumatized patients (single victims) requiring in-hospital resuscitation or operative intervention.

2. Perform triage of several sets of multiply-traumatized patients (multiple victims) in the emergency care center.

3. Perform resuscitative thoracotomies as necessary.

4. Treat traumatized patients and perform needed operative repair.

5. Demonstrate the ability to perform as senior trauma leader in coordinating the patient's care, delegating duties to junior team members, and conferring with subspecialty consultants as needed.

6. Function as the multi-specialty team leader by coordinating timing and sequencing of operative interventions of the chest, abdomen, head, and orthopedic considerations.

7. Function with faculty in planning for disasters by performing the following:

    a. Instruct ACLS, ATLS, and FCCS courses

    b. Assist in the training of emergency medical service (EMS) personnel

    c. Deliver community service lectures to citizens' groups

8. Demonstrate technical capability in advanced trauma care in the emergency department, intensive care units, and operating rooms.

9. Manage emergency services for an elderly patient, maximizing communication channels regarding:

    a. History

    b. Baseline cognitive and functional status

    c. Presence of advance directives

    d. Extent of work-up required

Practice-Based Learning and Improvement that involves investigation and evaluation of their own patient care, appraisal and assimilation of scientific evidence, and improvements in patient care.

INFORMATION TECHNOLOGY AND POPULATION COMPARISONS
REFERENCES

Abrams JH, Cerra FB. Essentials of Critical Care: Clinical Cases and Practical Solutions. St. Louis : Quality Medical Publishing, Inc., 1993.

Abrams JH, Cerra FB. Essentials of Surgical Critical Care. St. Louis : Quality Medical Publishing, Inc., 1993.

Bongard FS, Sue DY. Current Critical Care Diagnosis and Treatment. Norwalk CT : Appleton and Lange, 1994.

Civetta JM, Taylor RW, Kirby RR. Critical Care (3rd ed). Philadelphia : Lippincott-Raven Co., 1997.

Cobbs EL, Duthie EH, Jr, Murphy JB (eds), Geriatrics Review Syllabus: A Core Curriculum in Geriatric Medicine (4th ed). Dubuque IA : Kendall/Hunt Publishing Company, 1999.

Committee on Trauma, American College of Surgeons. Resources for Optimal Care of the Injured Patient, 1999.

Deitch Edwin (ed). Tools of the Trade and Rules of the Road: A Surgical Guide. Philadelphia : Lippincott Raven, 1997. (Chapt 25 Intubation, Chapt 26 Vascular Access).

Hall JB, Schmidt GA, Wood LDH. Principles of Critical Care (2nd ed). New York : McGraw-Hill, 1998;1-1767.

Knudson MM. Definitive care phase: geriatric trauma. In: Greenfield LJ, Mulholland M, Oldham KT, Zelenock GB, Lillemoe KD (eds), Surgery: Scientific Principles and Practice (2nd ed). Philadelphia : Lippincott-Raven, 1997;386-390.

Sanders AB, Witzke DB, Jones JS, et al. Principles of care and application of the geriatric emergency care model. In: Sanders AB (ed), Emergency Care of the Elder Person. St. Louis : Beverly Cracom Publications, 1996;59-93.

Tintinalli JE, Ruiz E, Krome RL, American College of Emergency Physicians. Emergency Medicine: A Comprehensive Study Guide (4th ed). New York : McGraw-Hill, 1996;1-1555.

SECTION 12.2   DIAGNOSTIC AND THERAPEUTIC RADIOLOGY

UNIT OBJECTIVES:

Demonstrate the appropriate, efficient, and economic use of radiologic resources for the clinical management of surgical procedures.

Demonstrate basic knowledge regarding the indications, contraindications, and possible adverse effects of diagnostic radiologic techniques.

Demonstrate knowledge and application of the use of radioisotopes and ionizing radiation in the management of vascular and non-vascular disease.

Utilize radiologic consultation to enhance the diagnostic evaluation and therapeutic options of complex surgical patients.

Medical Knowledge about established and evolving biomedical, clinical, and cognate (e.g. epidemiological and social-behavioral) sciences and the application of this knowledge to patient care.

Section One: Background

1.   Discuss the four basic densities and their radiologic/ pathologic correlations.

2.   Demonstrate an understanding of the fundamental physics and potential hazards of the following imaging techniques:

      a.   X-irradiation, including plain radiographic films, mammography, fluoroscopy, angiography, and computed axial tomography (CAT)

      b.   Ultrasound

      c.   Nuclear medicine

      d.   Magnetic resonance imaging (MRI)

      e.   Positron emission tomography (PET)

3.   Discuss the specific patient preparations for the aforementioned radiological studies, including oral intake restrictions and bowel preparative regimens.

Section Two: Diagnostic Studies

1. Discuss the following typical plain radiographs utilized to evaluate blunt and penetrating trauma, and identify cardinal features of commonly injured organs:

   a. Spine radiographs

   b. Chest radiographs

   c. Kidney-ureter-bladder radiographs

   d. Pelvis radiographs

2. Develop a strong foundation in the interpretation of chest radiographs, particularly involving a consistent, systematic, and reproducible approach to their interpretation.

3. Recognize radiologic findings that may be associated with age-related normal variations and degenerative processes.

4. Identify practical adjustments that may be necessary for the radiographic examination of the geriatric patient, considering:

   a. Physical and/or behavioral patient conditions that may limit or modify the procedure

   b. Stressful rigors of some radiographic examinations

   c. Influence of patient anxiety

   d. Patient positioning issues which may lead to suboptimal imaging, such as immobilization devices

5. Summarize the components of an acute abdominal series in the evaluation of a potentially acute surgical abdomen. Be prepared to identify typical radiographic abnormalities and their implications, including pneumoperitoneum and calcification.

6. Select the appropriate preoperative studies utilized to diagnose surgical pathology occurring in the following organ systems:

   a. Central nervous system

   b. Thorax

   c. Cardiovascular system

   d. Peripheral vascular system

   e. Gastrointestinal system

   f. Genitourinary system

g.   Retroperitoneum

h.   Musculoskeletal system

i.   Vascular

j.   Breast

7.   Recognize the potential applications and limitations of the following common imaging modalities utilized to diagnose surgical lesions:

     a.   Computed axial tomography

     b.   Ultrasound

     c.   Magnetic resonance imaging

     d.   Nuclear Medicine

8.   Given a specific clinical condition, identify the most efficacious imaging stratagem to confirm or dismiss the working diagnosis.

9.   Formulate a therapeutic plan based on variable imaging outcomes, being cognizant of:

     a.   Atypical manifestation of common disease

     b.   Realistic limitations of the radiologic study

     c.   Discrepancies in clinical and radiographic findings

10.   Analyze the applications and limitations of commonly utilized radioisotopic studies, including:

     a.   Bleeding scans

     b.   Thyroid and parathyroid imaging

     c.   Ventilation/perfusion scans

11.   Utilize the radiologist as a consultant to:

     a.   Review studies

     b.   Recommend the most appropriate or additional studies

     c.   Provide diagnostic intervention

     d.   Provide therapeutic intervention

Section Three: Therapeutic Radiology

1. Discuss the use of radioisotopes in the treatment of appropriate conditions, including:

    a. Endocrine disorders   b. Oncologic disorders

2. Assess the potential utility, limitations, and complications of interventional radiological procedures in various clinical settings.

3. Discuss the technical approaches and limitations of fine-needle and needle-core biopsies of masses performed using radiologic guidance.

4. Summarize the indications, limitations, and risks of interventional procedures for peripheral ding angioplasty, stents, and thrombolytic therapy.

Patient Care that is compassionate, appropriate, and effective for the treatment of health problems and the promotion of health.

Junior Level:

1. Demonstrate a practical knowledge of basic radiographic interpretation

2. Identify appropriate imaging modalities given various clinical situations.

3. Recognize and communicate potential patient-specific conditions, including allergic, which may impact on the safety and efficacy of radiographic evaluation.

4. Obtain appropriate preparatory studies for selected radiographic procedures.

Senior Level:

1. Supervise and/or request pertinent radiographic investigations in diagnostic evaluation.

2. Teach junior-level residents radiologic principles and pitfalls.

3. Identify the utility of adjunct imaging modalities to better define surgical conditions.

4. Recognize interventional radiological procedures that may provide definitive or complementary treatment of surgical conditions.

5. Initiate radiologic consultation on complex cases to avoid potential delay in diagnosis.

Practice-Based Learning and Improvement that involves investigation and evaluation of their own patient care, appraisal and assimilation of scientific evidence, and improvements in patient care.

INFORMATION TECHNOLOGY AND POPULATION COMPARISONS
REFERENCES

Brant W, Helms C. *Fundamentals of Diagnostic Radiology*. Baltimore: Williams & Wilkins Co., 1998;1-1460.

Daffner RH. *Clinical Radiology: The Essentials* (2nd ed). Baltimore: Williams & Wilkins, 1999;1-590.

Grainger R, Allison DJ. *Grainger and Allison's Diagnostic Radiology*. New York: Churchill Livingston, Inc., 2001.

Kadell BM, Zimmerman PT, Lu DS. Radiology of the abdomen. In: Zinner MJ, Schwartz SI, Ellis H (eds), *Maingot's Abdominal Operations* (10th ed). CT: Appleton & Lange 1997;3-116. Putman CE, Ravin CE. *Textbook of Diagnostic Imaging* (2nd ed). Philadelphia: WB Saunders Co., 1994.

Rheinhold RB, Doherty FJ, Mele FM, et al. Selected technologies and general surgery. In: O'Leary JP (ed), *The Physiologic Basis of Surgery* (2nd ed). Baltimore: Williams and Wilkins, 1996;618-644.

Silverman FN, Kuhn JP, Caffey J. *Caffey's Pediatric X-ray Diagnosis: An Integrated Imaging Approach* (9th ed). St. Louis: Mosby Year Book, Inc., 1993.

http://www.rsna.org

SECTION 12.3   PHARMACOTHERAPEUTICS

UNIT OBJECTIVES:

Demonstrate an understanding of general pharmacologic principles and knowledge of specific pharmacotherapeutic classes of drugs.

Apply this knowledge to effectively prescribe and monitor medications in the surgical patient.

Medical Knowledge about established and evolving biomedical, clinical, and cognate (e.g. epidemiological and social-behavioral) sciences and the application of this knowledge to patient care.

Junior Level:

1.   Describe general pharmacokinetic principles, including:

    a.   Absorption   c.   Metabolism

    b.   Distribution   d.   Elimination

2.   Describe how aging affects the following pharmacokinetic parameters:

    a.   Absorption   c.   Metabolism

    b.   Distribution   d.   Elimination

3.   Define pharmacodynamics, and explain its place in therapeutics.

4.   Identify clinically significant drug interactions, including:

    a.   Drug-drug interactions   b.   Drug-nutrient interactions

5.   Identify which medications are pharmacodynamically altered in elderly people.

6.   Identify adverse reactions to medications from clinical and laboratory observations.

7.   Describe the various pharmacological effects of giving medications via different routes of administration, including:

    a.   Oral   e   Rectal

    b.   Parenteral   f.   Inhalation

    c.   Topical   g.   Sublingual

    d.   Intrathecal

8. Discuss the association between increasing age and the occurrence of adverse medication reactions.

9. Identify five medication classes which are common causes of adverse medication reactions in elderly people.

10. Describe the essential components of an inpatient drug order and an outpatient prescription, including:

    a. Date/time   d. Schedule

    b. Drug name   e. Route of administration

    c. Strength   f. Refills or duration of therapy

11. List three reasons for reduced medication compliance in elderly people.

12. Identify the following medications for which an antidote exists, and describe how the antidote should be administered:

    a. Narcotic analgesics   d. Digoxin

    b. Benzodiazepines   e. Warfarin

    c. Heparin

13. Relate the key components of a drug and allergy patient history.

14. Explain the pharmacologic profile and clinical use of the following core groups of medications:

    a. Analgesics and anesthetics

    b. Antibiotics

    c. Cancer chemotherapeutic agents

    d. Cardiovascular drugs

    e. Modulators of the immune response

    f. Hormones

    g. Modulators of coagulation

    h. Modulators of wound healing

    i. Neuropsychiatric medications

    j. Gastrointestinal drugs

    k. Anti-inflammatory medications

l.   Respiratory agents

m.   Skeletal muscle relaxants

n.   Blood derivatives

15.   Analyze the methods for effective medication monitoring.

16.   Become familiar with and utilize a variety of terms with older patients that may be used synonymously with <u>pain</u>, such as:

a.	Burning	d.	Soreness
b.	Discomfort	e.	Heaviness
c.	Aching	f.	Tightness

17.   Discuss the potential side effects associated with the medication groups listed in #14 above, and identify treatment choices for these complications.

18.   Identify indications for use of the following classes of medications in emergency or critical care:

a.	Inotropes	e.	Antihypertensives
b.	Pressors	f.	Volume expanders
c.	Diuretics	g.	Neuromuscular blocking agents
d.	Antiarrhythmics	h.	Analgesics

19.   Explain the principles of perioperative drug use, including antimicrobial agents.

20.   Summarize the management of pain through the use of appropriate pharmacologic analgesia.

21.   Summarize the prophylactic and therapeutic use of anticoagulants in the surgical patient.

<u>Senior Level</u>:

1.   Formulate pharmacotherapeutic-dosing strategies in patients with altered pharmacokinetics such as:

a.	Hepatic dysfunction	d.	Ascites
b.	Kidney dysfunction	e.	Short bowel

c. Cardiovascular dysfunction   f. Advanced age

2. Utilize serum concentration monitoring to modify dosage regimens of medications with
    narrow therapeutic indices such as:
    a. Aminoglycosides
    b. Theophylline
    c. Vancomycin
    d. Phenytoin
    e. Digoxin
    f. Cyclosporine

3. Design, evaluate, and modify pharmacotherapeutic strategies to treat patients in complex
    clinical situations, including:
    a. Multiple diseases   c. Intensive care setting
    b. Multiple medications   d. Polypharmacy in the elderly

Patient Care that is compassionate, appropriate, and effective for the treatment of health
problems and the promotion of health.

Junior Level:

1. Take and record an appropriate drug and allergy history.
2. Write appropriate inpatient medication orders and outpatient prescriptions, under
    supervision.
3. Monitor the pharmacologic preparation of a patient for surgery.
4. Monitor the pharmacotherapeutic effects of medications.
5. Prescribe medications for patients without altered pharmacokinetic parameters.
6. Prescribe medications such as inotropes, pressors, diuretics, antiarrhythmics, and
    antihypertensives in emergency and critical care situations.
7. Prescribe medications pre- and post- operatively to prevent surgical complications,
    including infection, thromboembolic events, and stress related occurrences.

477

8. Prescribe and monitor appropriate analgesic therapy based on an assessment of a patient's pain.

9. Prescribe appropriate antimicrobial therapy for given surgical infections, and monitor the effectiveness of such therapy.

10. Appropriately prescribe and monitor the effects of anticoagulant therapy in surgical patients with thromboembolic disease.

11. Apply microbiology and antimicrobial knowledge in selecting appropriate therapeutic or empiric antibiotic coverage for a suspected infection.

Senior Level:

1. Manage patients in complex clinical pharmacotherapeutic situations.

2. Monitor and adjust the dose of medications (described as groupings in #14 of the first section) for patients with altered pharmacokinetics.

3. Monitor and alter the dose of selected medications based on serum concentrations.

4. Appropriately prescribe the following medications in the geriatric patient:

    a. Antihypertensives   d. Anticoagulants

    b. Digoxin   e. Analgesics

    c. Benzodiazepines   f. Antimicrobials

5. Monitor and alter the dose of medications listed above in the elderly patient.

Practice-Based Learning and Improvement that involves investigation and evaluation of their own patient care, appraisal and assimilation of scientific evidence, and improvements in patient care.

INFORMATION TECHNOLOGY AND POPULATION COMPARISONS REFERENCES

Abrams WB, Beers MH, Berkow R (eds). Clinical pharmacology. *The Merck Manual of Geriatrics* (2nd ed). Whitehouse Station, NJ: Merck Research Laboratories, Merck & Co., Inc., 1995;255-275.

AGS (American Geriatrics Society) Panel on Chronic Pain in Older Persons. The management of chronic pain in older persons. *J Am Geriatr Soc* 1998;46(5):635-651.

Backes WL, Moerschabaecher JM, Principles of pharmacology. In: O'Leary JP (ed), *The Physiologic Basis of Surgery* (2nd ed). Baltimore: Williams and Wilkins, 1996;228-246.

Chernow B, Brater DC. *The Pharmacologic Approach to the Critically Ill Patient* (3rd ed). Baltimore: Williams & Wilkins, 1994.

Cobbs EL, Duthie EH, Jr, Murphy JB (eds), Pharmacology and appropriate prescribing. *Geriatrics Review Syllabus: A Core Curriculum in Geriatric Medicine* (4th ed). Dubuque IA: Kendall/Hunt Publishing Company, 1999.

Dalen JE, Hirsch J (eds). Third ACCP consensus conference on antithrombotic therapy. *Chest* 1995;108:2255-5225.

De Piro JT, Talbert RL, Hayes PE, et al (eds). *Pharmacotherapy: A Pathophysiologic Approach* (3rd ed). New York: Elsevier Science Publishing Co., 1997.

Evans R, Ireland G, Morley J, Sheahan S. Pharmacology and aging. In: Sanders AB (ed), *Emergency Care of the Elder Person*. St. Louis: Beverly Cracom Publications, 1996;29-41.

Hammerlein A, Derendorf H, Lowenthal DT. Pharmacodynamic changes in the elderly: clinical implications. *Clin Pharmacokinetics* 1998;35:49-64.

Hanlon JT, Schmader KE, Ruby CM, et al. Suboptimal prescribing in older patients and outpatients. *J Am Geriatr Soc* 2001;49:200-209.

Lamy P, Wiser TH. Pharmacotherapeutic considerations in the elderly surgical patient. In: Katlic MR (ed), *Geriatric Surgery: Comprehensive Care of the Elderly Patient*. Baltimore: Urban & Schwarzenberg, 1990;209-239.

Prisant LM, Moser M. Hypertension in the elderly: can we improve results of therapy? *Arch Int Med* 2000;160:283-289.

Rosenthal RA, Andersen DK. Physiologic considerations in the elderly surgical patient. In: Miller TA (ed). *Modern Surgical Care: Physiologic Foundations and Clinical Applications* (2nd ed). St. Louis: Quality Medical Publishing, Inc., 1998;1362-1384.

Shrimp LA. Safety issues in the pharmacologic management of chronic pain in the elderly. *Pharmacotherapy* 1998;18:1313-1322.

Worden JP, Jr. Geriatric pharmacotherapy. *Curr Surg* 1996;53(9):522-526.

SECTION 12.4   ANESTHESIOLOGY

<u>UNIT OBJECTIVES:</u>

Demonstrate an understanding of the pathophysiology of pain and its management.

Demonstrate an understanding of the pharmacology and principles of regional and general anesthesia in analgesia.

Demonstrate the ability to use these principles in the management of surgical patients.

Recognize the condition of malignant hyperthermia and its treatment.

Medical Knowledge about established and evolving biomedical, clinical, and cognate (e.g. epidemiological and social-behavioral) sciences and the application of this knowledge to patient care.

1.   Discuss the rationale governing the use of local, regional, and general anesthesia, including the following concepts:

    a.   Careful cardiovascular, respiratory, and neurologic monitoring is the mainstay of safe anesthesia

    b.   No specific anesthetic is inherently safer than any other; and as such, risk assessment must be considered in each case

    c.   Regional anesthesia may provide some advantages, including:

        (1)   Decreased blood loss

        (2)   Improved perioperative graft patency in vascular reconstruction

        (3)   Reduced incidence of venous thrombosis

    d.   Combined regional and general techniques may improve outcomes in selected patient populations:

        (1)   Significant cardiovascular disease and major abdominal or thoracic surgery

        (2)   Severe pulmonary disease and major abdominal or thoracic surgery

    e.   Preemptive analgesia, such as the use of epidural anesthesia, enhances perioperative comfort

2.   Summarize the essential elements of the pre-anesthesia assessment, including:

a. Targeted history and physical examination (review of systems, emphasizing cardiovascular and pulmonary disease)

    (1) Effects of chronic medications (anticoagulants, insulin, and antiarrhythmics)

    (2) Effects of preoperative medications (narcotics, anxiolytics, and atropine)

    (3) Effects of postoperative medications (including antihypertensives and antiemetics)

b. Anatomic and physiologic variables germane to anesthetic success:

    (1) Airway anatomy, including the Mallampati classification.

        (a). Class 1: Visualization of all oro- and hypo- pharyngeal structures

        (b). Class 2: Anterior and posterior tonsillar pillars are obscured by tongue

        (c). Class 3: Soft palate and base of uvula are visible

        (d). Class 4: Only the soft palate is visualized

        (e). Increasing Mallampati score is associated with the reduced likelihood of successful direct laryngoscopic intubation.

            (1) Skeletal deformities

            (2) Neuromuscular diseases

            (3) Aspiration risk (pregnancy, scleroderma, hiatal hernia)

c. Assigned Anesthesia Society of America class and physical status:

    (1) Class 1: No organic disease

    (2) Class 2: Mild to moderate systemic disease

    (3) Class 3: Severe systemic disorders

    (4) Class 4: Severe systemic disturbance; life threatening

    (5) Class 5: Patient is moribund with little chance of survival

    (6) Class E: Patient requires an emergency procedure

3. Outline the major characteristics of the pharmacokinetics and pharmacodynamics of anesthetic agents (local, volatile, opioid), considering:

a. Lipid solubility

b. Protein binding

c. Partition coefficients

4.   Summarize the use and monitoring of drugs for sedation and analgesia to include:

    a.   Minimum anesthetic monitoring (pulse oximetry, electrocardiogram, blood pressure)

    b.   Advantages of scheduled postoperative analgesia versus intermittent dosing

    c.   Indications for patient-controlled anesthesia (PCA)

    d.   Importance of periodic assessment to determine:

        (1)   Level of consciousness

        (2)   Pulmonary status in sedated patients

5.   Summarize the principles of administration for and compare the effectiveness of the following methods of anesthesia:

    a.   General   c.   Regional

    b.   Spinal   d.   Local

6.   Describe the potential benefits of regional and local anesthesia, including:

    a.   Decreased respiratory depression

    b.   Diminished systemic effects (liver and renal toxicity)

    c.   Decreased direct cardiac depression

7.   Outline the potential complications associated with the use of regional anesthesia, including:

    a.   Spinal anesthetics (headache, cerebrospinal fluid leak, meningitis)

    b.   Regional nerve blocks (perineural hematomas)

8.   Discuss the indications for the use of muscle relaxants.

9.   Analyze anesthetic monitoring techniques, to include:

    a.   Swan-Ganz catheters

    b.   Arterial lines

    c.   Transvenous pacemakers

    d.   End-tidal carbon dioxide monitoring

    e.   Temperature monitoring

f.   Transesophageal echocardiography

10.   Describe the techniques and potential complications of managing an airway, including endotracheal and nasotracheal intubation.

11.   Describe and explain the most common immediate postoperative anesthetic issues:

        a.   Airway stability

        b.   Ventilation and oxygenation

        c.   Pain control

        d.   Nausea and vomiting

        e.   Temperature regulation

        f.   Hemodynamic stability

12.   Analyze therapeutic options for patients with chronic pain.

13.   Recognize the condition of malignant hypothermia and its management:

        a.   Incidence in general population (1:10,000)

        b.   Autosomal inheritance with variable penetrance

        c.   Pathophysiology of defective sarcoplasmic reticulum and secondary diminished reuptake of myoplasmic calcium leading to increased aerobic metabolism of skeletal muscle

        d.   Inducing medications, including inhaled anesthetics and succinylcholine

        e.   Hallmarks of hypermetabolism, skeletal muscle rigidity, and increased temperature

        f.   Therapy includes the discontinuance of anesthetic agents, dantrolene administration, and fluid resuscitation with proper physiologic monitoring.

Patient Care that is compassionate, appropriate, and effective for the treatment of health problems and the promotion of health.

<u>Junior Level:</u>

1.   Manage the airway in adults and children, employing appropriate:

a. Physical maneuvers

b. Oral/nasal support devices

c. Suctioning techniques to maintain clear airway

2. Perform nasal and oral intubation.

3. Recognize the stages of general anesthesia and their implications, particularly in regard to airway management.

4. Recognize and treat the signs and symptoms of complications due to anesthetic agents such as:

a. Cardiovascular collapse
    c. Malignant hyperthermia

b. Acute metabolic disturbances

5. Perform preoperative assessment of patients.

6. Recognize risks and possible side effects of drugs used for pain control.

Senior Level:

1. Monitor patients under anesthesia, including the use of peripheral and pulmonary artery catheters.

2. Administer pre- and post- anesthesia care.

3. Apply appropriate monitoring devices.

4. Establish vascular access in a child and in an adult.

5. Manage the difficult airway, including the performance of both rigid and fiberoptic bronchoscopy.

6. Establish an emergent airway, utilizing percutaneous or surgical techniques.

Practice-Based Learning and Improvement that involves investigation and evaluation of their own patient care, appraisal and assimilation of scientific evidence, and improvements in patient care.

INFORMATION TECHNOLOGY AND POPULATION COMPARISONS REFERENCES

Artmann SL, Giezentanner AL, Katz J. Physiology of anesthesia and pain. In: Miller TA (ed). *Modern Surgical Care: Physiologic Foundations and Clinical Applications* (2nd ed). St. Louis: Quality Medical Publishing, Inc., 1998;250-273.

Hopkins PM. Malignant hyperthermia: advances in clinical management and diagnosis. *B J Anes* 2000;85(1):118-128.

Kehlet H. Multimodal approach to control postoperative pathophysiology and rehabilitation. *B J Anes* 1997;78(5):606-617.

McLeskey CH (ed). *Geriatric Anesthesiology*. Baltimore: Williams & Wilkins, 1997;1-703.

Rosenthal RA, Andersen DK. Physiologic considerations in the elderly surgical patient. In: Miller TA (ed). *Modern Surgical Care: Physiologic Foundations and Clinical Applications* (2nd ed). St. Louis: Quality Medical Publishing, Inc., 1998;1362-1384.

Rutter TW, Tremper KK. Anesthesiology and pain management. In: Greenfield LJ, Mulholland M, Oldham KT, Zelenock GB, Lillemoe KD (eds), *Surgery: Scientific Principles and Practice* (2nd ed). Philadelphia: Lippincott-Raven, 1997;438-454.

Smith BE. Anesthetic considerations in elderly patients. In: Adkins RB, Jr., Scott HW, Jr. (eds), *Surgical Care for the Elderly* (2nd ed). Philadelphia: Lippincott-Raven Publishers, 1998;51-76.

Thomas MA, Riopelle JM. Anesthesia. In: O'Leary JP (ed), *The Physiologic Basis of Surgery* (2nd ed). Baltimore: Williams and Wilkins, 1996;602-617.

Wallace A, Layug B, Tateo I, et al. Prophylactic Atenolol reduces postoperative myocardial ischemia. *Anesthesiology* 1998;88(1):7-17.

http://www.asahq.org

SECTION 12.4A   ANESTHESIA FOR THE ELDERLY PATIENT

Demonstrate an understanding of the physiological alterations of the aging process and the potential impact on anesthetic administration.

Recognize and manage postoperative altered mental status in the elderly.

Medical Knowledge about established and evolving biomedical, clinical, and cognate (e.g. epidemiological and social-behavioral) sciences and the application of this knowledge to patient care.

1. Summarize how the physiology of aging interacts with the effects of anesthesia, with particular attention to:

    a. How high sympathetic tone, loss of beta-receptor responsiveness, and volume sensitivity to both hypovolemia and hypervolemia make blood pressure inherently unstable.

    b. How increased chest wall stiffness, increased lung compliance, and increased brain sensitivity to sedative/ analgesics increase the likelihood of hypoxia, atelectasis, and pneumonia.

2. Summarize the pharmacokinetic and pharmacodynamic principles underlying the effective use of anesthetic agents, particularly how aging often leads to increased sensitivity and prolonged duration of drug effects.

3. Understand how the anesthesiologist approaches patient evaluation and the optimization of patient condition in preparation for surgery.

4. Recognize those issues important to an elderly patient when faced with the decision to have surgery, and be able to determine when mental impairment does or does not preclude the patient from providing informed consent.

5. Understand how the elderly patients are predisposed to hypothermia and how hypothermia adversely affects the risk of infection and cardiac morbidity.

6. Be familiar with the causes, diagnosis, and management of postoperative delirium.

7. Explain the principles and techniques of preemptive analgesia, including non-steroidal analgesics and peripheral nerve and field blocks.

488

8. Analyze and compare the hemodynamic effects, benefits, risks, and contraindications for the following advanced techniques of postoperative pain control:

   a. Epidural infusions of local anesthetics and/or opioids.

   b. Continuous nerve blocks

   c. Intrapleural and extrapleural catheters

Patient Care that is compassionate, appropriate, and effective for the treatment of health problems and the promotion of health.

Junior and Senior Levels:

1. Assess the risk surrounding the stress of the proposed surgery relative to the benefit of the surgery, with the perspective of the physiological reserve of the patient, and be able to adjust the scope of the proposed surgery accordingly.

2. Appropriately select medications and adjust dosages for the elderly patient.

3. Recognize postoperative delirium and be able to diagnose and treat reversible causes.

4. Perform common field and nerve blocks for postoperative analgesia.

5. Establish effective dialogue with anesthesia and internal medicine colleagues for the comprehensive care of complicated patients.

INFORMATION TECHNOLOGY AND POPULATION COMPARISONS REFERENCES

Del Guercio LRM, Cohn JD. Monitoring operative risk in the elderly. *JAMA* 1980;243:1350-1355.

Executive summary of the ACC/AHA task force report: guidelines for perioperative cardiovascular evaluation for noncardiac surgery. *Anesth Analg* 1996;82:854-860.

Frank SM, Fleisher LA, Breslow MJ, et al. Perioperative maintenance of normothermia reduces the incidence of morbid cardiac events. *JAMA* 1997;277:1127-1134.

Kaiser AM, Zollinger A, DeLorenzi D, et al. Prospective, randomized comparison of extrapleural versus epidural analgesia for postthoracotomy pain. *Ann Thorac Surg* 1998;66:367-372.

Liu S, Carpenter RL, Neal JM. Epidural anesthesia and analgesia—their role in postoperative outcome. *Anesthesiology* 1995;85:1474-1506.

Mangano D. Effect of atenolol on mortality and cardiovascular morbidity after noncardiac surgery. *N Engl J Med* 1996;335:1713-1720.

McLeskey CH (ed). *Geriatric Anesthesiology*. Baltimore: Williams & Wilkins, 1997;1-703.

Rooke GA, Freund Pr, Jacobson AF. Hemodynamic response and change in organ blood volume during spinal anesthesia in elderly men with cardiac disease. *Anesth Analg* 1997;85:99-105. Syllabus on Geriatric Anesthesiology. ASA website (http://www.asahq.org), in Professional Information.

Tverskoy M, Cozacov C, Ayache M, et al. Postoperative pain after inguinal herniorrhaphy with different types of anesthesia. *Anesth Analg* 1990;70:29-35.

Vandermeulen EP, Van Aken H, Vermylen J. Anticoagulants and spinal-epidural anesthesia. *Anesth Analg* 1994;79:1165-1177.

SECTION 12.5   INTERNAL MEDICINE

UNIT OBJECTIVES:

Describe approaches to maximize communication when medical consultations are requested on surgical patients.

Summarize the principles of effective surgical consultation on medical patients.

Describe methods for preoperative assessment of perioperative cardiac risk in noncardiac surgery.

Describe the methods for preoperative assessment of pulmonary risk factors.

Discuss the perioperative management of common medical disorders.

Explain the risks of surgery in geriatric patients with respect to age and age-related changes in cardiovascular and pulmonary physiology, response to pharmacologic therapy, and response to surgical stress.

Medical Knowledge about established and evolving biomedical, clinical, and cognate (e.g. epidemiological and social-behavioral) sciences and the application of this knowledge to patient care.

1.   Discuss principles for effective communication when requesting a medical consultation, to include:

a.   Indications for requesting a pre- or post- operative medical evaluation on a surgical patient

b.   Clear articulation of reason(s) for requesting consultation

c.   Direct communication with the consultant whenever possible

d.   Medical records that provide meaningful clinical information from the history, physical examination, and laboratory

e.   Clarification of the role you wish the consultant to assume

2.   Describe effective communication with the patient's primary care provider when the patient is diagnosed with a surgical problem, to include:

a.   Maintaining a collaborative approach to management

b.   Enlisting the primary care provider in preoperative and postoperative care

      c.   Obtaining medical and psychosocial information about the patient, including other illnesses, social stressors and supports, patient preferences regarding end-of-life care.

3.   Discuss key components of a general surgical consultation performed on a medical patient with emphasis on:

      a.   Clarifying reasons for the consultation request and urgency

      b.   Assessing need for further laboratory or radiologic studies

      c.   Direct communication to responsible caregivers

      d.   Need for timely follow-up when definitive action is delayed

      e.   Importance of prompt communication with the primary care provider after performing a surgical procedure

4.   Explain preoperative assessment of cardiovascular risk in noncardiac surgery:

      a.   Review rationale for preoperative risk stratification and commonly used clinical risk assessment scales (Goldman criteria, Detsky criteria)

      b.   Clinical risk factors for perioperative cardiovascular events

      c.   Indications for preoperative stress ECG, exercise or pharmacologic stress test with nuclear perfusion imaging, stress echocardiography, ambulatory ECG monitoring, or coronary angiography

      d.   Methods to reduce risk of perioperative cardiovascular events such as beta-blockers in elderly patients

      e.   Common presentations of perioperative cardiovascular events such as angina, myocardial infarction (MI), arrhythmias, and congestive heart failure (CHF)

5.   Explain preoperative assessment of pulmonary risk factors for perioperative morbidity and mortality:

      a.   History of cigarette smoking, exercise capacity, COPD, asthma

      b.   Clinical evaluation using physical examination and observation of the patient walking

      c.   Indications for preoperative pulmonary function tests and their interpretation

    d.   Predictors of difficulty weaning after general anesthesia

    e.   Pre- and post- operative measures that can reduce risk of pulmonary complications

    f.   Perioperative management of bronchospasm

6.   Discuss measures to reduce risk for perioperative deep venous thrombosis and pulmonary emboli:

    a.   Stratification of risk for perioperative venous thrombosis based on patient characteristics and type of surgery (high, medium, low)

    b.   Choice of deep venous thrombosis (DVT) prophylaxis based on risk stratification

    c.   Indications for Coumadin, subcutaneous low dose heparin, subcutaneous low molecular weight heparin, pneumatic compression devices, early mobilization

    d.   Clinical and laboratory methods for diagnosing DVT and pulmonary embolus (PE) based on pretest likelihood

7.   Describe assessment and management of hypertension in the perioperative period:

    a.   Definitions of hypertensive urgency, emergency, and malignant hypertension.

    b.   Impact of hypertension on operative risk, including assessment of end-organ damage

    c.   Perioperative management of hypertension, including pharmacologic management in patients who have restricted oral intake

    d.   Management of hypertension in geriatric patients

    e.   Indications for seeking medical consultation in the hypertensive patient

8.   Describe the perioperative assessment and management of the diabetic patient:

    a.   Determination of glycemic control by glycosylated hemoglobin level

    b.   Assessment for ketoacidosis and/or hyperosmolar state

    c.   Appreciate presentation of diabetes in the elderly

    d.   Describe methods for intraoperative and perioperative management in Type I and II diabetes

e.   Describe formulas for determining insulin dosage during and after surgery in insulin-requiring patients

f.   Discuss indications for sliding scale insulin treatment

g.   Appreciate common side effects of oral hypoglycemic agents

h.   Describe emergent management of hypoglycemia

i.   Discuss indications for medical consultation in the diabetic patient

9.   Discuss the perioperative assessment and management of other common endocrinology problems, including:

a.   Hypothyroidism and hyperthyroidism

b.   Hypoparathyroidism and hyperparathyroidism

10.   Describe assessment and management of common electrolyte disturbances:

a.   Hypo- and hyper- natremia

b.   Hypo- and hyper- kalemia

c.   Divalent homeostasis

11.   Discuss approach to the patient with jaundice:

a.   Interpretation of liver function tests and imaging studies to distinguish hepatocellular disease from biliary obstruction (intrahepatic and extrahepatic)

b.   Causes of postoperative jaundice

c.   Presentation of viral hepatitis (acute and chronic)

d.   Impact of liver disease on drug metabolism

12.   Discuss approach to the surgical patient with renal failure

a.   Describe clinical and laboratory assessment of renal function

b.   Distinguish acute renal failure from chronic renal failure

c.   Segregate causes of acute renal failure into prerenal, intrarenal, and postrenal (obstructive)

d.   Describe clinical signs and symptoms of uremia

e.   Discuss differential diagnosis of postoperative acute renal failure

f.   List indications for acute hemodialysis and hemofiltration

g.   Describe medical management of acute renal failure

h.   Appreciate impact of renal failure on drug excretion

i.   List medications that can cause acute renal failure

13.   Describe indications for subacute bacterial endocarditis (SBE) prophylaxis based on type of valvular problem and type of procedure.

14.   Describe preoperative assessment and management of a patient with a coagulopathy.

15.   Describe how to assess and manage postoperative fever.

16.   Describe surgical risks in the obese patient.

17.   Recognize unique features of the geriatric surgical patient:

     a.   Impact of age on operative morbidity and mortality

     b.   Age-related changes in cardiovascular and pulmonary physiology

     c.   Pharmacologic alterations with aging and polypharmacy

     d.   Risk factors for postoperative delirium and its management

     e.   Cardiovascular risk assessment and use of beta-blockers to reduce risk of perioperative ischemic events

     f.   Skin care

     g.   Nutritional assessment and correction of nutritional deficiencies

     h.   Diminished special senses such as hearing and eyesight

     i.   Ethical issues such as informed consent in the demented patient, advanced directives, do-not-resuscitate (DNR), end-of-life care, communicating with families

     j.   Assessment for post-surgical care, including home nursing and nursing home placement

     k.   Importance of the care team in managing elderly patients

Patient Care that is compassionate, appropriate, and effective for the treatment of health problems and the promotion of health.

1. Diagnose and manage surgical patients with concomitant acute and/or chronic medical illnesses.

2. Properly perform perioperative evaluation of the surgical patient with:

   a. Moderate to high cardiovascular and respiratory risk

   b. Immunosuppressed state

   c. Significant psychiatric problem

3. Perform a general surgery consultation to a medical service patient.

Practice-Based Learning and Improvement that involves investigation and evaluation of their own patient care, appraisal and assimilation of scientific evidence, and improvements in patient care.

INFORMATION TECHNOLOGY AND POPULATION COMPARISONS REFERENCES

Berman AR. Pulmonary embolism in the elderly. *Clin Geriatric Med* 2001;17(1):107-130.

Caputo GM, Gross RJ. Medical consultation on surgical services: an annotated bibliography. *Ann Intern Med* 1993;118:290-297.

Clark E. Preoperative assessment: primary care work-up to identify surgical risks. *Geriatrics* 2001;56(7):36-40.

Drugs in the perioperative period: 1-Stopping or continuing drugs around surgery. *Drug Ther Bull* 1999;37(8):62-64.

Duncan G, Card FI. Collaboration between geriatricians and general surgeons. *Health Bull* 1992;50(21):163-167.

Ferguson MK. Preoperative assessment of pulmonary risk. *Chest* 1999;115(5 Suppl):58S-63S.

Gilbert K, Larocque BJ, Patrick LT. Prospective evaluation of cardiac risk indices for patients undergoing noncardiac surgery. *Ann Intern Med* 2000;133(5):356-359.

Gross RJ, Caputo GM (eds). *Kammerer and Gross' Medical Consultation: the Internist on Surgical, Obstetric, and Psychiatric Services* (3rd ed). Baltimore: Williams & Wilkins. 1998.

Haas S. Prevention of venous thromboembolism: recommendations based on the International Consensus and the American College of Chest Physicians Sixth Consensus Conference on Antithrombotic Therapy. *Clin Appl Thromb Hemost* 2001;7(3):171-177.

Hazzard WR, Blass JP, Ettinger WH, Jr., et al. (eds). *Principles of Geriatric Medicine and Gerontology* (4th ed). New York: McGraw-Hill, 1998;1-4440.

Kearon C, Hirsh J. Management of anticoagulation before and after elective surgery. *N Engl J Med* 1997;336(2):1506-1511.

King MS. Preoperative evaluation. *Am Fam Physician* 2000;62(2):387-396.

Mangano D, Layug EL, Wallace A, Tateo I. Effect of atenolol on mortality and cardiovascular morbidity after noncardiac surgery. *N Engl J Med* 1996;335:1713-1720.

Park KW. Critical review of the ACC/AHA algorithm for stratifying cardiac patients for noncardiac surgery. *Int Anesthesiol Clin* 2001;39(4):81-92.

Proctor MC, Greenfield LJ. Thromboprophylaxis in an academic medical center. *Cardiovasc Surg* 2001 9(5):426-430.

Vogt AW, Henson LC. Unindicated preoperative testing: ASA physical status and financial implications. *J Clin Anesthesia* 1997;9(6):437-441.

Wolfsthal S. *Medical Perioperative Management*. Norwalk CT: Appleton and Lange, 1990.

SECTION 12.6   PSYCHIATRY

<u>UNIT OBJECTIVES:</u>

Demonstrate an understanding of psychiatric principles in the management of surgical patients.

Demonstrate the ability to apply appropriate psychiatric principles in the management of surgical patients.

Medical Knowledge about established and evolving biomedical, clinical, and cognate (e.g. epidemiological and social-behavioral) sciences and the application of this knowledge to patient care.

Review diagnosis of psychiatric illness pertinent to surgical patients:

1.   Describe the signs and symptoms of psychiatric disorders of significance to the general medical management of surgical patients, including:

    a.   Disorders diagnosed in childhood

    b.   Schizophrenia and psychotic disorders

    c.   Cognitive disorders

    d.   Mood disorders

    e.   Anxiety-related disorders

    f.   Eating disorders

    g.   Substance-related disorders

    h.   Personality disorders

2.   Outline the medical treatment of psychiatric disorders, and describe their pharmacologic side effects:

    a.   Antilytics

        (1)   Central nervous system (CNS)

        (2)   Depression

        (3)   Addiction/tolerance

    b.   Antipsychotic medications, including: (side effects, including

        (1)   Sedation   (4)   Extrapyramidal symptoms

        (2)   Hypotension   (5)   Lower seizure threshold

          (3)   Anticholinergic effects

    c.   Antidepressants, including: (side effects, including sedation

          (1)   Sedation

          (2)   Anticholinergic effects

          (3)   Monoamine oxidase inhibitors (MAOI)

          (4)   Food and drug interactions, including anesthesia conduction

    d.   Mood stabilizers

          (1)   Lithium (side effects, including tremor, gastrointestinal

               (a) Tremor

               (b) Gastrointestinal disturbances

               (c) Renal effects

          (2)   Carbamazepine (side effects, including leukopenia,

               (a) Leukopenia

               (b) Agranulocytosis

               (c) Aplastic anemia

    e.   Hypnotics

3.   Understand the etiology and treatment options for acute mental status changes that can follow surgery, including:

    a.   Somnolence   d.   Agitation

    b.   Confusion   e.   Convulsions

    c.   Disorientation   f.   Hallucinations

4.   Summarize common psychiatric reactions to surgical treatments and procedures, including:

    a.   "ICU psychosis"   d.   Anxiety reaction

    b.   Delirium   e.   Acute drug withdrawal

    c.   Depression   f.   "Sundowning"

5.   Identify and assess characteristics of the suicidal patient:

    a.   Identifying signs

        (1)   Drug overdose

        (2)   Self-inflicted injuries

  b.   Predisposing conditions

        (1)   Depression

        (2)   Alcoholism

        (3)   Personality disorders

        (4)   Addiction

        (5)   Schizophrenia

        (6)   Manic-depressive psychosis

  c.   Risk Factors

        (1)   History of suicide attempts

        (2)   Advanced age

        (3)   Recent loss

        (4)   Chronic illness

6.   Recognize the need for the prescription of suicide precautions.

7.   Recognize the management of patients with altered mental status.

8.   Understand general principles of drug and/or alcohol withdrawal and their impact on surgical patients.

9.   Discuss the epidemiology of mental health problems in elderly patients, including:

  a.   Normal changes of aging

        (1)   Reaction time

        (2)   Precision-requiring activities

        (3)   Risk taking

  b.   Medications

  c.   Psychiatric problems as primary or secondary diagnosis for nursing home residents

  d.   Organic disorders (Alzheimer's disease)

  e.   Primary and secondary depressions, including pseudodementia and sleep disorders

  f.   Interactions between mental and physical health

g.   Alcohol abuse

10.   Identify factors unique to elderly persons that predispose to delirium.

11.   Describe approaches to supporting the dying patient:

a.   Pain management/comfort measures

b.   Communication skills with patient and family

c.   Coping skills, patient support systems, and family dynamics

d.   Limiting/withdrawing support

(1)   "Do not resuscitate" orders

(2)   Living will

(3)   Health care proxy

(4)   Persistent vegetative state

(5)   Irreversible coma

(6)   Role of ethics consultation

(7)   Competency determination

(8)   Documentation

(9)   Potential organ donation

e.   Review the definitions of death

12.   Understand the role of the psychiatric consult team.

13.   Review the effect of psychiatric illness on surgical care and the effect of surgery on psychiatric illness:

a.   Identify common psychiatric reactions to surgical treatments/procedures (see objective #4 and #5 above).

b.   Outline procedures utilized to assess competency in the hospitalized patient.

c.   Describe the signs and symptomatology of child, partner, or elder abuse and the institutional and legal procedures for reporting suspected abuse cases.

d.   Formulate appropriate responses for managing disruptive patients, including agitated patients, malingerers, and sociopaths.

14.   Implement initial psychiatric treatment and access referral systems for ongoing psychiatric evaluation and care:

    a.   Specify the considerations for management of surgical patients with complex psychiatric illness.

    b.   Outline plans for follow-up care and referrals for surgical patients with psychiatric problems.

    c.   Determine the special psychiatric issues associated with the management of:

        (1)   Burn patients (burn delirium, pain management, deformity)

        (2)   Transplant patients

        (3)   Cancer patients

        (4)   Head and spinal cord injury patients

Patient Care that is compassionate, appropriate, and effective for the treatment of health problems and the promotion of health.

1.   Apply knowledge of the impact of psychiatric illness to the management of surgical patients:

    a.   Incorporate the review of psychiatric symptomatology in the evaluation of surgical patients.

    b.   Obtain a psychiatric drug profile.

    c.   Monitor use of psychiatric medications

    d.   Assess pain and prescribe appropriate medication.

    e.   Manage minor psychiatric problems in postoperative patients.

2.   Apply knowledge of the initial management of psychiatric problems to surgical patients:

    a.   Manage disorientation and anxiety in intensive care patients.

    b.   Assess suicidal potential, request psychiatric consultation, and institute suicide precautions.

    c.   Inform families of patient deaths, request autopsies, and organ donation.

    d.   Consider recommendations from psychiatric consultations.

    e.   Record signs and symptoms of abuse and initiate required reports.

f.   Evaluate the effect of disruptive behavior and deliberate non-compliance on surgical outcomes.

3.   Facilitate a team approach to surgical patients with psychiatric problems and assure follow-up as needed:

a.   Manage the surgical care of patients with complex psychiatric illness.

b.   Monitor the psychiatric treatment of general surgical patients.

c.   Arrange for appropriate follow-up care and/or referral of patients with complex psychiatric illness.

d.   Assist with competency determinations in appropriate cases.

e.   Manage patients with special psychiatric concerns such as:

(1)   Trauma

(2)   Burns

(3)   Transplant

(4)   Malignancy

(5)   Head and spinal cord injury

Practice-Based Learning and Improvement that involves investigation and evaluation of their own patient care, appraisal and assimilation of scientific evidence, and improvements in patient care.

INFORMATION TECHNOLOGY AND POPULATION COMPARISONS REFERENCES

American Psychiatric Association. *Diagnostic and Statistical Manual of Mental Disorders* (4th ed). Washington DC: APA, 1994.

Arana GW, Rosenbaum JF. *Handbook of Psychiatric Drug Therapy* (4th ed). Philadelphia: Lippincott Williams and Wilkins, 2000;1-272.

Beers MH, Berkow R (eds). Section 3, Surgery and rehabilitation; Section 4, Psychiatric disorders. *The Merck Manual of Geriatrics* (3rd ed). Whitehouse Station, NJ: Merck Research Laboratories, 2000.

Chang PH, Steinberg MB. Alcohol withdrawal. *Med Clin N Amer* 2001;85(5):1191-1212.

Cobbs EL, Duthie EH, Jr, Murphy JB (eds), Geriatric psychiatry. *Geriatrics Review Syllabus: A Core Curriculum in Geriatric Medicine* (4th ed). Dubuque IA: Kendall/Hunt Publishing Company, 1999; 167-198.

Cohen D, Paveza GJ, Gorelick PB. Psychiatric changes. In: Katlic MR (ed), *Geriatric Surgery: Comprehensive Care of the Elderly Patient*. Baltimore: Urban & Schwarzenberg, 1990;165-172.

Ferrara PC, Chan L. Initial management of the patient with altered mental status. *Am Fam Physician* 1997;55(5):1773-1780.

Kalbfleisch M. Altered mental status. In: Sanders AB (ed), *Emergency Care of the Elder Person*. St. Louis: Beverly Cracom Publications, 1996;119-142.

Luce JM, Alpers A. End-of-life care: what do the American courts say? *Critical Care Med* 2001;29(2 Suppl):N40-45.

Margolin RA, Kwentus JA. Neuropsychiatric aspects of surgery. In: Adkins RB, Jr., Scott HW, Jr. (eds), *Surgical Care for the Elderly* (2nd ed). Philadelphia: Lippincott-Raven Publishers, 1998;131-150.

Mega MS. Differential diagnosis of dementia: clinical examination and laboratory assessment. *Clin Cornerstone* 2001;3(4):1-14.

Miller SS, Marin DB. Assessing capacity. *Emerg Med Clin N Amer* 2000;18(2):233-242.

Olmeda R, Hoffman RS. Withdrawal syndromes. *Emerg Med Clin N Amer* 2000;18(2):273-288.

Pollack ME, Billick SB. Competency to consent to treatment. *Psychiatr Q* 1999;70(4):303-311.

Pousada L, Fryer DM. Cerebrovascular accident. In: Sanders AB (ed), *Emergency Care of the Elder Person*. St. Louis: Beverly Cracom Publications, 1996;263-277.

Quinn DI, Wodak A, Day RO. Pharmacokinetic and pharmacodynamic principles of illicit drug use and treatment of illicit drug users. *Clin Pharmacokinet* 1997;33(5):344-400.

Smith RD, Tiel R, Johnson RJ. Basic neuroscience. In: O'Leary JP (ed). *The Physiologic Basis of Surgery* (2nd ed). Baltimore: Williams and Wilkins, 1996;522-560.

Tombaugh TN, McIntyre NJ. The Mini-Mental State Examination: a comprehensive review. *J Am Geriatr Soc* 1992;40:922-935.

http://www.psych.org

CHAPTER 13

Interpersonal and Communication

13.1.   ANATOMY

13.2   PHYSIOLOGY

Skills that result in effective information exchange and teaming with patients, their families, and other health professionals.

SECTION 13.1: ANATOMY

UNIT OBJECTIVES:

Demonstrate knowledge of anatomy that is pertinent to the practice of surgery.

Apply knowledge of anatomy to the diagnosis and treatment of patients, both in and out of the operating room.

Junior Level:

1. Outline the general concepts of anatomy and its subdivisions, including:

   a. Gross anatomy

   b. Cellular and subcellular anatomy

   c. Molecular biology

2. Compare the organization, characteristics, and functions of the tissues and their components within each organ system, including:

   a. Skin

   b. Circulatory system

   c. Nervous system

   d. Musculoskeletal system

   e. Respiratory system

   f. Digestive system

   g. Urinary system

   h. Reproductive system

   i. Organs of special sense

3. Review, identify, and delineate the vulnerable anatomical structures encountered in common general surgical operations such as:

   a. Venous and arterial access in infants

   b. Catheterization

   c. Colonoscopy

   d. Cricothyrotomy

   e. Mastectomy

   f. Inguinal hernia repair

   g. Cholecystectomy

   h. Cardiac procedures

   i. Aortic aneurysm repair

   j. Insertion of Swan-Ganz catheter

k.   Insertion of chest tubes

l.   Application of leg cast

m.   Appendectomy

n.   Burr holes

o.   Vagotomy and pyloroplasty

p.   Colectomy

q.   Renal transplant

r.   Thyroidectomy

s.   Resection of the liver

t.   Urinary procedures

4.   Recognize those anatomic structures commonly encountered in other surgical subspecialties, such as:

a.   Orthopedics   d.   Gynecology

b.   Otolaryngology   e.   Urology

c.   Neurosurgery

5.   Discuss the differences in visualization of organ structures by various technologies, such as:

a.   Routine radiograms

b.   Contrast studies

c.   Computed axial tomography (CAT) scans

d.   Ultrasound

e.   Magnetic resonance imaging (MRI) scans

f.   Angiograms

g.   Positron emission tomography (PET) scans

6.   List and access the source materials for anatomic references, guides for exposure, and the anatomic aspects of common general surgical procedures.

7.   Describe the anatomic aspects of conception, human development, normal embryology, and common developmental anomalies encountered in general surgery, such as:

a. Pelvic inflammatory disease

b. Appendicitis in pregnancy

c. Omphalomesenteric remnants

d. Diaphragmatic hernia

e. VATER syndrome

f. Tracheoesophageal fistula

g. Biliary atresia

h. Malrotation

i. Gastroschisis

j. Urachal cyst

k. Imperforate anus

l. Trisomy 18

m. Tetralogy of Fallot

n. Atrioseptal defect

8. Differentiate between the following anatomic terms:

a.	Topographic anatomy	f.	Ventral
b.	Radiographic anatomy	g.	Median plane
c.	Supination	h.	Midsagittal plane
d.	Pronation	i.	Coronal plane
e.	Dorsal		

9. Describe the anatomic changes due to aging on a gross, cellular, and molecular level with special emphasis on the following organs: eyes, bone, brain, GI tract, lungs, kidneys, reproductive system, and vascular system.

Senior Level:

1. Summarize the embryologic explanations for the common major birth anomalies.

2. Define and describe the anatomic aspects of even the most complex general surgical operations such as:

a. Repair of an abdominoperineal aneurysm

b. Whipple procedure

c. Pneumonectomy

d. Abdominoperineal resection

e. Liver resection

f. Liver transplantation

g. Bilateral radical neck dissection

h. Gastric bypass

3. Interpret various imaging technologies to derive anatomic information. Integrate knowledge of anatomy into the following:

a. The diagnosis of general surgical disease

b. Explanations to patients and families regarding:

   (1) Embryologic causes of disease

   (2) Planning of surgical procedures

   (3) Progress of disease

   (4) Explanation of complications

INFORMATION TECHNOLOGY AND POPULATION COMPARISONS
REFERENCES

Adkins RB, Jr., Marshall BA. Anatomic and physiologic aspects of aging. In: Adkins RB, Jr., Scott HW, Jr. (eds), Surgical Care for the Elderly (2nd ed). Philadelphia: Lippincott-Raven Publishers, 1998;11-24.

Jahnigen DW, Schrier RW. Geriatric Medicine (2nd ed). Cambridge MA: Blackwell-Science, 1996;1-867.

Netter FH, Jr. Atlas of Human Anatomy (2nd ed). East Hanover NJ: Novartis, 1997.

Pemberton LB, Colborn GL, Skandalakis JE. Workbook of Surgical Anatomy, New York: McGraw-Hill, Inc., Health Professions Division (A PreTest Publication), 1991.

Pokorny WJ, Rothenberg SS, Brandt ML. Growth and development. In: O'Leary JP (ed), The Physiologic Basis of Surgery (2nd ed). Baltimore: Williams and Wilkins, 1996;43-74.

Scott-Conner C, Dawson DL. Operative Anatomy. Philadelphia: JB Lippincott Company, 1993.

Skandalakis LJ, Rowe JS, Jr., Gray SW, et al. Surgical embryology and anatomy of the pancreas. Surg Cl of N Amer 1993;73(4):661-697.

Skandalakis JE, Skandalakis PN, Skandalakis LJ. Surgical Anatomy and Technique: A Pocket Manual. New York: Springer-Verlag 1995;1-674.

Wood WC, Skandalakis JE (eds). Anatomic Basis of Tumor Surgery. St. Louis: Quality Medical Publishing, Inc., 1999.

http://www.vesalius.com

Interpersonal and Communication Skills that result in effective information exchange and teaming with patients, their families, and other health professionals.

Patient and family communications, communication with associates, teamwork, counseling

Communicator

1. Effective doctor/patient communication

2. Establish a doctor/patient relationship characterized by understanding, trust, respect, empathy and confidentiality

3. Gather information about patient's beliefs, concerns and expectations about the illness and considers the influence of factors such as patient's age, gender, ethnic, cultural and socio-economic background and spiritual values on that illness

4. Deliver information to the patient and family in a humane manner and in a way that is understandable, encourages discussion and promotes patient's participation in decision making to the degree that they wish

5. Understand and demonstrate the importance of co-operation with other healthcare professionals involved in the care, such that the roles of these professionals are delineated and consistent messages are delivered to the patient and their families.

6. Demonstrate skills in working with others who present significant communication challenges such as anger or confusion, or an ethno-cultural background different from the patient's own.

SECTION 13.2   PHYSIOLOGY

UNIT OBJECTIVES:

Demonstrate knowledge of normal and disturbed human physiology causing surgical diseases.

Demonstrate knowledge of the effects of age, as reflected in the newborn, infants, children, and the older patients on the physiologic functions of the major organ systems.

Apply physiological knowledge to the clinical and operative management of surgical diseases.

1.   Describe concepts of normal physiology, including:

   a.   Fundamental processes of cell differentiation and growth

   b.   Endocrine and autocrine control of genetics and development

   c.   Normal pregnancy, embryology, and parturition

   d.   Concept of homeostasis and cellular mediators

   e.   Biochemistry of normal nutrition and metabolism

   f.   Fluid mechanics and dynamics

   g.   Hemostasis, coagulation, thrombogenesis, fibrinosis

   h.   Excretory and regulatory renal function

   i.   Biomechanics of normal respiration and gaseous exchange

   j.   Wound healing and inflammatory response

   k.   Oncogenesis

   l.   Neuroendocrine control of development of secondary sexual characteristics, breasts

   m.   Neurophysiology of pain

   n.   Response to sepsis

   o.   The immune response

   p.   Cellular division, telomeres, apoptosis

2.   In each of the above systems, identify physiologic variations in geriatric, pediatric, immunosuppressed, and pregnant patients.

3.   Indicate the normal values of commonly applied clinical tests.

4.   Describe the applications of physiologic principles to surgical monitoring and therapy, including the following approaches:

a.   Application of Swan-Ganz catheters

b.   Ventilator management

c.   Renal function studies

d.   Noninvasive vascular testing

e.   Interpretation of results of the common metabolic panel blood tests

f.   Interpretation of electrocardiogram (EKG), cardiac echograms and other cardiac function studies

g.   Interpretation of a nutritional profile

h.   Endocrine function studies

5.   Describe how aging affects the tests listed in the section immediately above.

6.   Describe the abnormal physiology of complex diseases or entities such as:

a.	Cardiac failure		f.	Intestinal obstruction
b.	Renal failure		g.	Malnutrition
c.	Pulmonary failure		h.	Cardiopulmonary bypass
d.	Immunosuppression		i.	Advanced age
e.	Malignancy			

7.   Analyze the aspects of aging within each organ system that can alter the surgeon's approach to care of the elderly patient, to include consideration of:

a.   Genetic factors (e.g., alterations in DNA synthesis and chromosomal functioning)

b.   Cumulative cellular damage (e.g., changes from free radicals and radiation)

c.   Errors in protein synthesis

d.   Alterations in the immune system

e.   Effects of endogenous steroid hormones

f.   The cross-linkage theory (resulting in loss of elasticity, increased tissue brittleness)

g.   Apoptosis

h.   Telomere function

8.   Interpret laboratory tests and clinical findings based upon physiologic concepts.

9. Manage patients with surgical illnesses and/or major physiologic disruptions such as:

   a. Liver failure

   b. Malnutrition

   c. Renal failure/bowel obstruction

   d. Hemorrhage

   e. Cardiopulmonary failure

   f. Electrolyte imbalance

   g. Endocrine disorders such as multiple endocrine neoplasia (MEN)

   h. Sepsis

   i. Shock

   j. Immunosuppression

   k. Diabetes

   l. Advanced age

10. Adapt treatment plans to reflect physiologic variations in pediatric, geriatric, and pregnant patients.

11.. Utilize clinical findings, laboratory tests, and hemodynamic measurements to alter patient physiology.

12. Adjust treatment plans in response to abnormal physiologic values.

13. Identify and formulate treatment plans for improved nutrition.

14. Interpret hemodynamic monitoring and adjust treatment to restore homeostasis:

   a. Insert and maintain arterial venous and central lines.

   b. Monitor catheters.

15. Solve problems interfering with normal hemostasis.

16. Analyze pulmonary function tests, solve problems causing abnormal respiration, and delineate weaning parameters.

INFORMATION TECHNOLOGY AND POPULATION COMPARISONS
REFERENCES

Adkins RB, Jr., Marshall BA. Anatomic and physiologic aspects of aging. In: Adkins RB, Jr., Scott HW., Jr. (eds), Surgical Care for the Elderly (2nd ed). Philadelphia: Lippincott-Raven Publishers, 1998;11-24.

Cobbs EL, Duthie EH, Jr, Murphy JB (eds). Biology of aging/age-related physiologic changes. Geriatrics Review Syllabus: A Core Curriculum in Geriatric Medicine (4th ed). Dubuque IA: Kendall/Hunt Publishing Company, 1999.

Evers BM, Townsend CM Jr, Thompson JC. Organ physiology of aging. In: Zenilman ME, Roslyn JJ (eds), Surgery in the elderly patient, Surg Cl of N Amer 1994;74(1):23-39.

Guyton AC, Hall JE, Human Physiology and Mechanisms of Disease (6th ed). Philadelphia: Saunders, 1997;1-737.

Jahnigen DW, Schrier RW. Geriatric Medicine (2nd ed). Cambridge MA: Blackwell-Science, 1996;1-867.

McLeskey CH (ed). Physiologic changes of aging. Geriatric Anesthesiology. Baltimore: Williams & Wilkins 1997;29-142.

Rosenthal RA, Andersen DK. Physiologic considerations in the elderly surgical patient. In: Miller TA (ed), Modern Surgical Care: Physiologic Foundations and Clinical Applications (2nd ed). St. Louis: Quality Medical Publishing, Inc., 1998;1362-1384.

Sanders AB. Physiology of aging. In: Sanders AB (ed), Emergency Care of the Elder Person. St. Louis: Beverly Cracom Publications, 1996;11-28.
Schiller HJ, Kort KC, Sillin LF. Physiologic principles in preparing patients for surgery. In: Miller TA (ed), Modern Surgical Care: Physiologic Foundations and Clinical Applications (2nd ed). St. Louis: Quality Medical Publishing, Inc., 1998;293-317.

Schwesinger WH, Moyer MP. Cell biology. In: O'Leary JP (ed), The Physiologic Basis of Surgery (2nd ed). Baltimore: Williams and Wilkins, 1996;1-42.

Zenilman ME. Preoperative assessment of the elderly. In: Cameron JL (ed), Current Surgical Therapy (6th ed). St. Louis: Mosby, 1998;1070-1075.

CHAPTER 14

Professionalism

14.1   ETHICAL AND LEGAL PRACTICE

14.2   PRACTICE MANAGEMENT

14.3   PALLIATIVE CARE

Professionalism as manifested through a commitment to carrying out professional responsibilities, adherence to ethical principles, and sensitivity to a diverse patient population

SECTION 14.1.   ETHICAL AND LEGAL ISSUES IN SURGICAL PRACTICE

UNIT OBJECTIVES:

Demonstrate knowledge of basic ethical and legal principles applicable to the practice of medicine.

Demonstrate the ability to recognize ethical and legal issues that arise in the practice of surgery.

Demonstrate the ability to employ strategies for effectively managing ethical and legal issues associated with the practice of surgery.

Medical Knowledge about established and evolving biomedical, clinical, and cognate (e.g. epidemiological and social-behavioral) sciences and the application of this knowledge to patient care.

Conditions, treatments, outcomes, new advances

Section One: Ethical, and legal issues associated with the practice of medicine

1.   a.   Define the following terms, and analyze their application to the practice of surgery:

   b.   Abortion

   c.   Advance Directives

      (1)   Patient Self-Determination Act

      (2)   Living Will (your state requirements)

      (3)   Durable Power of Attorney for Health Care

      (4)   Right to Die concept

   d.   Authoritarianism (importance of patient choices)

   e.   Autonomy

      (1)   As 'capacity for self-determination'

      (2)   As 'right to self-determination'

   f.   Beneficence

   g.   Bioethics

   h.   Casuistry (based on the study of case histories)

   i.   Causation

   j.   Civil law

k. Codes of ethics

l. Competence

m. Confidentiality

n. Continuity of care

o. Cost of care

p. Cost-benefit analysis

q. Cost-containment, including use of clinical pathways

r. Access to health care

s. Rights to health care

t. Covenant

u. Criminal law

w. Death (including various legal definitions)

x. Deontological ethics

y. 'Do Not Resuscitate' decisions

z. Duty

    (1) As the analysis of human behavior according to given principles, values, virtues, and/or according to specific methods of reasoning

    (2) As the rules or patterns of behavior expected within certain groups (e.g., professions, religious communities) or by virtue of holding a specific role

aa. Eugenics

bb. Euthanasia

cc. "Futile" treatment

dd. Hospital Ethics Committee

ee. Impaired physician

ff. Informed consent

gg. Institutional Review Board

hh. Justice

    (1) As 'distributive'

    (2) As 'retributive'

    (3) As 'commutative' (justice in transactions)

ii. Liability (including forms and limits of coverage)

jj.   Malpractice

kk.   Managed care

ll.   Medical ethics

mm.   Morality

nn.   Natural law

oo.   Natural rights

pp.   Negligence

qq.   Omission (morally not performing an act or not performing a moral act)

rr.   Palliative care

ss.   Paternalism (relation with patients)

tt.   Peer review

uu.   Physician-assisted suicide

ww.   Pragmatism

xx.   Prima facie duty

yy.   Principles

zz.   Privacy

aaa.   Quality assurance (and associated concepts such as Continuous Quality Improvement)

bbb.   Quality of life

ccc.   Research on human and animal subjects

ddd.   Right

    (1)   As a 'negative right'

    (2)   As a 'positive right'

eee.   Rule

fff.   Situation ethics

ggg.   Social contract

hhh.   Standard of care

iii.   Surrogate decision-maker (proxy)

jjj.   Teleological ethics

kkk.   Tort

lll.   Truthfulness

mmm.   Utilitarianism

nnn.   Utilization review (and related concepts)

ooo.   Values (patient defines benefit and quality)

ppp.   Virtue ethics

qqq.   Withdrawal or withholding treatment

2.   Identify and evaluate similarities and differences between the ethical and the technical aspects of clinical decision making.

3.   Specify the ethical and legal values and principles associated with the profession of surgery and clinical surgical decision-making.

4.   Discuss ethical and legal considerations for the development and use of new technologies in human subjects, including stem cell research, cloning, and gene therapy.

5.   Assess the professional and institutional resources and methods for managing ethical and legal issues including the management of conflict.

Section Two: The physician-patient relationship

6.   Analyze and explain the ethical and legal characteristics of the physician-patient relationship, including:

a.   Establishing the relationship

b.   Maintaining the relationship, including continuity of care

c.   Observing a patient's right to privacy and the confidentiality of clinical information

d.   Severing the relationship; patient abandonment

7.   Predict possible implications of 'managed care' on the traditional physician-patient relationship.

Section Three: The medical record

8.   Analyze the ethical and legal considerations of the medical record by performing these tasks:

a.   Describe the essential components of a medical record that meet both clinical and legal requirements.

b.   Describe the role of the inpatient/outpatient medical record and its use as:

    (1)   An accurate and complete account of the surgical management of a patient

    (2)   A legal document

c.   Specify the legal implications of altering or destroying medical records.

d.   Identify the proper method of making corrections or additions to the medical record.

Section Four: Informed consent

9.   Analyze the concept of informed consent by performing these tasks:

a.   Define competence, and discuss its application in obtaining informed consent.

b.   Determine how to ensure that patient consent to treatment is given voluntarily.

c.   Describe your institutional requirements for informed consent.

d.   Review the concept that physicians disclose all risks that would be considered material to the competent person (Canterbury v. Spence).

e.   Discuss the role of second opinion in surgical decision-making.

f.   Recommend a response to patient's refusal of recommended treatment.

g.   Discuss the ethical and legal issues associated with the performance of prophylactic surgery.

h.   Define the physician's responsibilities in the performance of experimental procedures.

i.   Define the ethical and legal obligations to inform patients of a physician's HIV status.

10.   Analyze patient advance directives, including:

a.   Identify federal, state, institutional, and individual responsibilities under the Patient Self-Determination Act.

b.   Review statutory requirements for legally valid advance directives.

c.   Compare and contrast living wills versus durable powers of attorney

11. Summarize ethical and legal issues associated with death and dying, considering:

   a. "Do Not Resuscitate" orders

   b. Discontinuing or foregoing treatment

   c. Withholding or withdrawing life-prolonging medical treatment

   d. Nutrition and hydration

   e. Euthanasia

   f. Physician-assisted suicide

   g. Determination of death

Section Five: Professional responsibility

12. Formulate an appropriate approach to the management of:

   a. The impaired physician

   b. Physician error

      (1) Own error   (2) Another's error

13. Explain the ethical and legal implications of refusing requested medical treatment under the following circumstances:

   a. Where treatment would be futile

   b. Where medical treatment poses risks to the physicians or others

   c. Where the physician opposes the treatment for moral reasons

   d. Where the physician opposes treatment for economic reasons

14. Identify the physician's ethical obligation to participate in:

   a. Medical review of individual physician/surgeon activities

   b. General evaluation of surgical therapies

15. Discuss the following aspects of medical staff appointment and disciplinary decisions:

   a. Role of economic credentialing

   b. Utilization review

   c. Implications of the American's with Disabilities Act

16.	Review the confidentiality of medical peer review records and proceedings.

17.	Discuss the responsibilities of the profession to provide access to health care.

18.	Discuss political and social activism in the profession regarding:

    a.	Membership and participation in professional associations

    b.	Communication with legislators

    c.	Community activism and education

    d.	Participation in physician "union" activities

Section Six: Professional licensure and certification

19.	Describe the processes and identify the agencies associated with:

    a.	Residency program accreditation

    b.	Physician/surgeon certification

    c.	Licensure

    d.	Credentialing

20.	Assess the value of recertification.

Section Seven: Professional liability

21.	Analyze the characteristics and issues involved in the current malpractice climate by performing the following tasks:

    a.	Characterize the relationships between the legal and medical professions and the insurance industry in resolution of malpractice claims.

    b.	Discuss the function and process of litigation in resolving malpractice claims.

    c.	Summarize the issues and goals involved in legislative reform of the civil justice system in the area of professional liability.

22.	Compare various types of professional liability insurance with regard to forms of coverage, limits of coverage, availability, and cost.

23.	Outline the process of a medical liability action and the role of each of the following in the process:

a.	Subpoena	d.	Settlement
b.	Discovery	e.	Directed verdict
c.	Deposition	f.	Appeal

24. Outline the process of a medical malpractice trial.

25. Describe criteria for the entry of legal actions into the National Practitioner Data Bank.

26. Estimate the significance of the following variables:

   a. Potential litigious situations

   b. Malpractice avoidance/practice management techniques

   c. Corporate negligence or negligent credentialing

   d. Spoliation of evidence

27. Review the general rules for:

   a. Professional liability insurance carrier involvement

   b. Attorney selection

   c. Preparation of defense

   d. Role and selection of expert witnesses

28. Discuss the role, practices, and procedures of the following in reducing professional liability:

   a. Risk management

   b. Quality assurance

29. Review the legal aspects of ex parte contacts with attorneys representing physicians in malpractice actions.

Practice-Based Learning and Improvement that involves investigation and evaluation of their own patient care, appraisal and assimilation of scientific evidence, and improvements in patient care.

1. Illustrate various moral concepts using examples from health care, especially those cases that have set a legal precedent or significantly influenced medical ethics (e.g., Roe v. Wade, Quinlan, Bouvia, Cruzan, Sakiewicz, Tuskegee Syphilis Study).

2. Describe the pluralistic nature of the United States and the role of health care as a 'public arena.'

3. Determine the course of action to be followed in the event of a malpractice claim, including interaction with plaintiffs, lawyers, and insurance companies.

4. Outline the appropriate steps to take when one suspects that a colleague is impaired.

5. Identify the professional liability concerns of other members of the healthcare team, including nurses, pharmacists, dieticians, and other medical specialists.

6. Obtain proxy consent in appropriate cases, including those involving minors.

7. Demonstrate proper methods of correcting medical records.

8. Participate in discussions and decisions regarding the discontinuation or foregoing of treatment.

9. Ascertain patient and family wishes regarding discontinuation or foregoing treatment.

10. Write orders for treatment limitation in appropriate cases.

11. Participate in the identification and resolution of cases involving surgical error.

12. Determine the degree of personal involvement in professional liability issues.

13. Formulate a plan for involvement in the political and legislative arenas regarding civil justice reform of professional liability litigation.

14. Determine a personal plan for achieving recognition and certification in surgery or its subspecialties.

15. Participate in surgical case review activities.

16. Participate in utilization review activities.

17. Review options for reform of the U.S. healthcare system, and identify possible consequences of reform proposals for surgical practice, patient access to care, and the cost of health care.

INFORMATION TECHNOLOGY AND POPULATION COMPARISONS
REFERENCES

Abrams WB, Beers MH, Berkow R (eds). Quality of life issues. Care of the dying patient. Legal issues. Ethical issues. Elder abuse and neglect. The Merck Manual of Geriatrics (2nd ed).

Whitehouse Station, NJ: Merck Research Laboratories, Merck & Co., Inc., 1995;235-238; 238-249; 1379-1391; 1392-1399; 1408-1416.

Achenbaum WA. From generation to generation: why US health care reform is so difficult in the twentieth century. In: Callahan D, Meulen RHJ, Topinkova E (eds), A World Growing Old: The Coming Health Care Challenges. Washington DC: Georgetown University Press, 1995;137-147.

American College of Surgeons Regents Committee on Ethics. http://www.facs.org/about/committees/ethics/index.html.

American College of Surgeons Professional Liability Program. http://www.facs.org/dept/hpa/proliab/index.html

American Medical Association. Code of Medical Ethics: Current Opinions with Annotations. Chicago: AMA, 1998.

Angelos P. Annotated bibliography of ethics in surgery. J Am Coll Surg 1999;188(5):538-544.

Angelos P, DaRosa DA, Derossis AM, Kim B. Medical ethics curriculum for surgical residents: results of a pilot project. Surgery 1999;126:701-707.

Atchley RC. The longevity revolution. In: Seltzer MM (ed), The Impact of Increased Life Expectancy: Beyond the Gray Horizon, New York, NY: Springer Publishing Company; 1995:33-50.

Benson J, Britten N. How much truth and to whom? Respecting the autonomy of cancer patients—ethical theory and the patient's view. BMJ 1996;313:729-731.

Binstock RH. Dementia and Aging; Ethics, Values, and Policy Choices. Baltimore: The Johns Hopkins University Press, 1992;1-184.

Binstock RH, Post SG (eds). Too Old for Health Care? Controversies in Medicine, Law, Economics, and Ethics. Baltimore: The Johns Hopkins University Press, 1991;1-209.

Brock DW, Wartman SA. When competent patients make irrational choices. N Engl J Med 1990;322:1595-1599.

Clarke DE, Goldstein MK, Raffin TA. Ethical dilemmas in the critically ill elderly. Clin Geriatr Med 1994;10:91-101.

Cobbs EL, Duthie EH, Jr, Murphy JB (eds), Ethical and legal issues. Geriatrics Review Syllabus: A Core Curriculum in Geriatric Medicine (4th ed). Dubuque IA: Kendall/Hunt Publishing Company, 1999.

Da Rosa DA, Angelos P. Teaching ethics to surgical residents: a starter package. Focus on Surg Ed 1999;16(3):16-17.

Department of Professional Liability of the American College of Obstetricians and Gynecologists. Litigation Assistant. Bull Am Coll Surg 1987;72(5):1-18.

Dingell JD. Misconduct in medical research. N Engl J Med 1993;328(22):1610-1615.

Drickamer M. Ethics in clinical practice. In: Rosenthal RA, Zenilman ME, Katlic MR. Principles and Practice of Geriatric Surgery. New York City, NY: Springer, 2001;195-201.

Emmanuel EJ, Emmanuel LL. Four models of the physician patient relationship. JAMA 1992;267:2221-2226.

Fleetwood J, Gracely E, Vaught W, et al. Medical EthEx online: a computer-based learning program in medical ethics and communication skills. Tch and Learn in Med 2000;12(2):96-104.

Hafferty FW, Franks R. The hidden curriculum, ethics, teaching, and the structure of medical education. Acad Med 1994;69(11):861-871.

Hakim RB, Teno JM, Harrell FE, Jr, et al. Factors associated with do-not-resuscitate orders: patients' preferences, prognoses, and physicians' judgments. Ann Int Med 1996;125:284-293.

Hepburn K, Reed R. Ethical and clinical issues with Native-American elders: end-of-life decision making. Cl in Geriatr Med 1995;11(1):97-111.

Hudson RB (ed). The Future of Age-Based Public Policy. Baltimore: The Johns Hopkins University Press, 1997;1-384.

Katlic MR. Surgery in centenarians. In: Rosenthal RA, Zenilman ME, Katlic MR. Principles and Practice of Geriatric Surgery. New York City, NY: Springer, 2001;211-218.

Kramer AM. Health care for elderly persons—myths and realities. N Engl J Med 1995;332:1027-1029.

Longino CF, Jr., Murphy JW. Paradigm strain: the old age challenge to the biomedical model. In: Seltzer MM (ed), The Impact of Increased Life Expectancy: Beyond the Gray Horizon, New York, NY: Springer Publishing Company; 1995:193-212.

McCullough LB, Jones JW, Brody BA (eds). Surgical Ethics. New York: Oxford University Press, 1998.

Moody HR. Ethics in an Aging Society. Baltimore: The Johns Hopkins University Press, 1992;1-288.

Mouton CP, Johnson MS, Cole DR. Ethical considerations with African-American elders. Cl in Geriatr Med 1995;11(1):113-129.

Nora PF (ed). Professional Liability/Risk Management: A Manual for Surgeons (2nd ed). Chicago: American College of Surgeons, 1997.

Reich WT (ed). Encyclopedia of Bioethics. New York: Macmillan, 1995.

Roberts M. Should surgery be rationed for the elderly on cost-effectiveness data? In: Rosenthal RA, Zenilman ME, Katlic MR. Principles and Practice of Geriatric Surgery. New York City, NY: Springer, 2001;111-117.

Rowe JW. Health care myths at the end of life. Bull Am Coll Surg 1996;81:11-18.

Sass H-M, Veatch RM, Kimura R. Advance Directives and Surrogate Decision Making in Health Care: US, Germany, and Japan. Baltimore: The Johns Hopkins University Press, 1998;1-311.

Shenk D, Keith J. Culture as constraint and potential for a long-lived society. In: Seltzer MM (ed), The Impact of Increased Life Expectancy: Beyond the Gray Horizon, New York, NY: Springer Publishing Company; 1995:87-108.

Sugarman J, McCrory DC, Hubal RC. Getting meaningful informed consent from older adults: a structured literature review of empirical research. J Amer Geriatr Soc 1998;46(4):517-524.

Thomasma DC. The ethical challenge of providing health care for the elderly. Camb Q Healthc Ethics 1995;148-162.

Zenilman ME. Surgery in the frail elderly: nursing home patients. In: Rosenthal RA, Zenilman ME, Katlic MR. Principles and Practice of Geriatric Surgery. New York City, NY: Springer, 2001;202-210.

Systems-Based Practice, as manifested by actions that demonstrate an awareness of and responsiveness to the larger context and system of health care and the ability to effectively call on system resources to provide care that is of optimal value.

Focus on standards of practice, delivery differences, access to care differences, cost issues, assess system problems, cooperation with hospital services, advocacy, and technology

Medical expert

1. Elicit a history that is relevant, concise, accurate and appropriate to the patient's problem
2. Demonstrate effective consultation skills in presenting well documented assessments and recommendations in written and/or verbal form in response to a request from another healthcare provider
3. Demonstrate the attitudes and the skills necessary to retrieve and implement the information necessary to provide healthcare services to patients in meeting the needs and expectations of the community
4. Demonstrate insight into his/her limitations by self-assessment
5. Demonstrate medical expertise in situations other than those involving direct patient care
6. Elicit a history that is relevant, concise, accurate and appropriate to the patient's problem

Discipline-Based Objectives

1. Display attitudes commonly accepted as essential to professionalism
2. Use appropriate strategies to maintain and advance professional competence
3. Continually evaluate one's abilities, knowledge and skills and know one's limitations of professional competence

Personal Professional Boundary Objectives

1. Adopt specific strategies to heighten personal and professional awareness and explore and resolve interpersonal difficulties in professional relationships
2. Consciously strive to balance personal and professional roles and responsibilities and to demonstrate ways of attempting to resolve conflicts and role strain

Objectives related to Ethics and Professional Bodies

1. Know and understand the professional, legal and ethical codes of the General Medical Council and any other codes to which the physician is bound

2. Recognize, analyze and attempt to resolve in clinical practice ethical issues such as truth telling, consent, advanced directives, confidentiality, end-of-life care, conflict of interest, resource allocation, research ethics etc.

3. Understand and be able to apply relevant legislation that relates to the health care system in order to guide one's clinical practice

4. Recognize, analyze and know how to deal with unprofessional behaviors in clinical practice, taking into account local and national regulations

SECTION 14.3   PRACTICE MANAGEMENT

UNIT OBJECTIVES:

Demonstrate knowledge of the principles of management associated with a surgical career.

Demonstrate the ability to apply sound management principles in establishing and managing a surgical practice that is clinically efficient, financially sound, and ethically correct.

Medical Knowledge about established and evolving biomedical, clinical, and cognate (e.g. epidemiological and social-behavioral) sciences and the application of this knowledge to patient care.

Junior Level:

1. Analyze the surgeon's responsibilities to society as they are associated with the management of a surgical practice.

2. Summarize the responsibilities and obligations of a surgeon regarding his/her social leadership in the community and health care facilities.

3. Analyze how the health care delivery system affects the socioeconomic wellbeing of the local community and nation.

4 Discuss the characteristics and relationships of the multiple components of the health care delivery system, including:

    a. Treatment facilities such as hospitals, long-term care facilities, community clinics

    b. Health care legislation currently in effect

    c. Management/provision of health care, including third party payment systems:

        (1) Medicare and Medicaid requirements

        (2) Employer-provided health insurance

        (3) Private health insurance

        (4) Responding to insurance denials

        (5) Dealing with gatekeepers

        (6) Case management (Large Case Management) procedures

        (7) Closed panel managed care plans

d. Diagnosis and processing codes; use of Fee Allowance Schedule

e. Physician practice organizations

f. Medical equipment and pharmaceutical manufacturing, sales, and distribution

5. Assess the cost-containment responsibilities of a physician in the ordering of diagnostic and therapeutic measures, to include consideration of effectiveness and efficiency.

6. Demonstrate familiarity with the political, economic, and social changes and trends likely to affect future surgical practice.

7. Discuss the characteristics and importance of effective interpersonal communication with colleagues, consultants, clinical and administrative support personnel, and patients.

8. Describe approaches about how to involve the patient's family and spiritual counselor in clinical decisions and discussions.

9. List the institutional and social service agencies in your community, and describe their role in the surgical management of patients and in assisting families.

10. Summarize the career options available at the conclusion of the residency, including:

a. General surgery practice (private practice or academic)

b. Fellowship in subspecialty

c. Other choices (e.g., research, entrepreneurial business, administration)

11. Discuss the types and characteristics, potential and shortcomings of organizational structures that affect the practice and fiscal aspects of surgical practice, including:

a. Solo practice

b. Group practice

    (1) Partnership

    (2) Professional Association

    (3) Corporation

    (4) Group practice without walls (GPWW)

c. Academic practice

d. Health Maintenance Organization (HMO)

    (1) Preferred Provider Organization (PPO)

    (2) Independent Practice Association (IPA)

        (3)   Staff model (to employ providers directly)

   e.   Exclusive Provider Organization (EPO)

   f.   Federal

        (1)   Medicare

        (2)   Medicaid

        (3)   Title XX of the Social Security Act

        (4)   Older Americans Act

        (5)   Veterans Administration

12.   Summarize significant aspects of the following critical issues as they relate to surgical practice management:

   a.   Legislative/regulatory requirements

        (1)   Americans with Disabilities Act (ADA)

        (2)   Clinical Laboratory Improvement Amendments (CLIA)

   b.   Federal/professional regulatory institutions

        (1)   Health Care Financing Administration (HCFA)

        (2)   Joint Commission for the Accreditation of Healthcare Organizations

        (3)   Occupational Safety and Health Administration (OSHA)

   c.   Societal expectations

        (1)   Affirmative action

        (2)   Equal opportunity

        (3)   Sexual harassment

13.   Describe patient eligibility variability through the Medicare program, financed through HCFA, for coverage of:

   a.   Elderly

   b.   Disabled persons receiving Social Security

   c.   Persons with end-stage renal disease

   d.   Certain federal employees

14.   Define the range of current coverage and aspects of implementation for the following:

a. Medicare Part A and Part B

b. Diagnosis-related groups (DRG's)

c. Medigap

15. Describe the range of support available for home and community-based care for the elderly.

16. Demonstrate a working knowledge of the organization, content, and analysis of the outpatient record.

17. Demonstrate a working knowledge of International Classification of Diseases (ICD) and Current Procedural Terminology (CPT) coding and data analysis.

18. Outline a plan for evaluating personal and professional considerations in making a career choice.

19. Recognize the importance of spouse and family involvement in making career choices, including choice of geographic location.

Senior Level:

1. Select a specific planning methodology to be used in career decisions.

2. Review the availability, requirements, and application procedures for post-residency fellowships under consideration.

3. Review and critique the following issues as they relate to a planned surgical practice:

a. Health care delivery systems, including managed care

b. Health care economics

c. Political and legislative processes in health care

4. Obtain demographic studies of potential practice locations to include population and medical demographics.

5. Outline the essential characteristics of the business side of medical practice, including:

a. Content and interpretation of financial reports

b. Management of human resources

      c.   Facilities design and management, including site selection and equipment requirements

      d.   Accounting procedures such as billing and collections

6.   Analyze the financial issues associated with the selection of the career options under consideration.

7.   Describe and evaluate the essential components of the following topics associated with the management of a planned surgical practice:

      a.   Financial management and accounting

      b.   Coding, billing, and collections

      c.   Selection and management of facilities, including real property and equipment

      d.   Human resources management

      e.   Marketing and planning

      f.   Data management using computer technology

      g.   Contractual and legal issues

      h.   Quality assurance

      i.   Risk management (professional and employer)

      j.   Cost-containment

8.   Describe the content, managed care relationships, interpretation, and utilization of the following financial documents:

      a.   Balance sheet

      b.   Income and expense statement

      c.   Accounts payable and receivable

      d.   Collection analysis

9.   Determine the insurance requirements related to the planned surgical practice, including:

      a.   Casualty, fire, and theft

      b.   Liability/malpractice

      c.   Personal health and disability

d. Personal life

10. Outline quality assurance activities required in surgical practice, including:

   a. Clinical record adequacy and accuracy

   b. Risk management

   c. Documentation of morbidity and mortality

   d. Periodic review of morbidity and mortality

   e. Appropriate provision of second opinion

11. Formulate plans to acquire and maintain managerial skills appropriate for the practice.

Practice-Based Learning and Improvement that involves investigation and evaluation of their own patient care, appraisal and assimilation of scientific evidence, and improvements in patient care.

<u>Junior Level</u>:

1. Discuss post-residency career options with:

   a. Faculty

   b. Other residents

   c. Family

2. Locate sources for review of:

   a. Social, legal, and ethical issues associated with post-residency career decisions

   b. Health care economics and structure

3. Begin to accumulate information about surgical practice opportunities, including type of practice and location.

4. Accumulate information about pertinent fellowship opportunities.

5. Explore other post-residency career choices.

6.   Assess own interpersonal skills and their impact on career choice.

7.   Develop and implement strategies for improving interpersonal communications skills.

8.   Select and implement a logical plan for making decisions about a post-residency career. Include a timetable and milestones.

9.   Involve appropriate family members in career planning.

10.   Accumulate a notebook with basic laws covering office management (e.g., CLIA)

11.   Maintain accurate and current documentation of patient care experiences while in training, utilizing the appropriate software package for ACGME-RRC documentation and American Board of Surgery application completion. Determine and follow a plan of action for meeting required case number minimums.

12.   Develop a personal resume/curriculum vitae and collection file for updating scholarly accomplishments and other credentials appropriate for preparing professional announcements.

13.   Locate sources for review of the physician's role in cost-containment.

Senior Level:

1.   Obtain specific information about post-residency fellowships including availability, requirements, and application procedures.

2.   Gather information about specific types of surgical practice of personal interest.

3.   Analyze current medical and population demographics associated with the types and locations of surgical practice being considered.

4.   Prepare a detailed financial plan for each selected career option. Include repayment of educational loans in the plan.

5.   Select type of surgical practice to pursue.

6.   Review practice facility requirements, including:

    a.   Location, including proximity to hospital, consultants, diagnostic services

    b.   Space, including floor plan, patient flow, waiting room capacity

    c.   Patient access, including parking

    d.   Equipment

7.   Develop a business plan for surgical practice.

8.   Develop an accounting system for surgical practice.

9.   Determine requirements and select systems to manage:

    a.   Clinical records

    b.   Finance, accounting, billing, and collection

    c.   Schedules and appointments

10.   Complete a financial plan for the proposed surgical practice to include:

    a.   Start up costs

    b.   Revenue generation including fee schedules

    c.   Practice expenses

    d.   Insurance requirements and costs

    e.   Human resources compensation and costs

    f.   Income projections

    g.   Equipment costs, including maintenance

11.   Determine human resource requirements, including recruiting and training.

12.   Prepare professional job descriptions for all personnel requirements.

13.   Construct a basic plan for fair and appropriate personnel mentoring and evaluation.

14.   Complete licensure and registration requirements for your chosen location.

15.   Complete applications for hospital staff membership and clinical privileges.

16.   Develop a marketing strategy for the chosen community.

17.   Formulate a plan for personal and practice promotion to include:

    a.   Active participation in medical staff affairs

    b.   Attendance at appropriate hospital and medical staff committee meetings and meetings of local medical societies

    c.   Participation in medical education programs for:

        (1)   Medical staff

        (2)   Residents and medical students

        (3)   Nursing and hospital ancillary staff

        (4)   Public

    d.   Participation in emergency call as appropriate

e. Involvement in clinical and/or basic science research

f. Participation in community social, cultural, and service activities

g. Being available, dependable and visible

18. Formulate plans to maintain clinical skills appropriate for practice through continuing medical education (CME) activities:

a. Preparation for recertification

b. CEM documentation for re-licensure

19. Prepare materials for Website formulation appropriate for dispensing information for patients and colleagues in surgery and other disciplines.

Practice-Based Learning and Improvement that involves investigation and evaluation of their own patient care, appraisal and assimilation of scientific evidence, and improvements in patient care.

INFORMATION TECHNOLOGY AND POPULATION COMPARISONS

REFERENCES

Abrams WB, Beers MH, Berkow R (eds). Health insurance. The Merck Manual of Geriatrics (2nd ed). Whitehouse Station, NJ: Merck Research Laboratories, Merck & Co., Inc., 1995;1440-1448.

Brummel-Smith KV (ed). Essential components of geriatric care provided through health maintenance organizations. J Amer Geriatr Soc 1997;46:303-308.

Callahan D, Meulen RHJ, Topinkova E (eds). A World Growing Old: The Coming Health Care Challenges. Washington DC: Georgetown University Press, 1995.

Carrico CJ. Scudder oration on trauma; in search of a voice. Bull Amer Coll Surg 1999;84(5):14-22.

Cobbs EL, Duthie EH, Jr, Murphy JB (eds), Geriatrics Review Syllabus: A Core Curriculum in Geriatric Medicine (4th ed). Dubuque IA: Kendall/Hunt Publishing Company, 1999.

Dunkle RE, Lynch S. Social work: more of the same or something new? In: Seltzer MM (ed), The Impact of Increased Life Expectancy: Beyond the Gray Horizon, New York, NY: Springer Publishing Company; 1995:131-147.

Friedsam HJ. Long-term care in the very long term. In: Seltzer MM (ed), The Impact of Increased Life Expectancy: Beyond the Gray Horizon, New York, NY: Springer Publishing Company; 1995:165-188.

Kongstvedt PR (ed). Essentials of Managed Health Care. Gaithersburg MD: Aspen Publishers, Inc., 1995;1-309.

Longino CF, Jr., Murphy JW. Paradigm strain: the old age challenge to the biomedical model. In: Seltzer MM (ed), The Impact of Increased Life Expectancy: Beyond the Gray Horizon, New York, NY: Springer Publishing Company; 1995:193-212.

Patterson DJ. Indexing Managed Care: Benchmarking Strategies for Assessing Managed Care Penetration in Your Market. New York: McGraw-Hill, 1997.

Pawlson LG, Infeld DL, Lastinger DM. The health care system. In: Ham RJ, Sloan PD (eds), Primary Care Geriatrics: A Case-Based Approach (3rd ed). St. Louis: Mosby, 1997;70-81.

Rosenthal RA, Andersen DK. Physiologic considerations in the elderly surgical patient. In: Miller TA (ed), Modern Surgical Care: Physiologic Foundations and Clinical Applications (2nd ed). St. Louis: Quality Medical Publishing, Inc., 1998;1362-1384.

Walt AJ. Can cost containment be learned in a surgical residency? Bull Am Coll Surg 1994;79(9):8-12.

SECTION 14.3   PALLIATIVE CARE

UNIT OBJECTIVES:

Outline resources available to patients at end of life, both locally and nationally.

Demonstrate an understanding of the differences between curative and palliative patient care models.

Integrate patient care, considering life-prolongation and palliation.

Utilize effective principles of communication, bioethical concepts, and practical bedside care in working with patients, families, and other health care providers.

Evaluate differential goals of treatment options/palliative care options available for geriatric patients.

Learn and apply the principles of palliative care for patients with advanced illness and those at the end of life

Principles of organ donation: Knowledge of the principles of organ donation.

Medical Knowledge about established and evolving biomedical, clinical, and cognate (e.g. epidemiological and social-behavioral) sciences and the application of this knowledge to patient care.

Conditions, treatments, outcomes, new advances

1.   Discuss the evolution of palliative care. Utilize the following terms in your discussion of the evolution: to alleviate, to mitigate, to lessen pain, and to give temporary relief.

2.   Discuss the principles and rationale for the goal of palliative care as achieving the best quality of life for patients and their families, utilizing the following core principles:

a.   Respect the dignity of patient and caregivers.

b.   Be sensitive to and respectful of the wishes of patient and family.

c.   Use the most appropriate measures that are consistent with patient choices.

d.   Ensure alleviation of pain and management of other physical symptoms.

e.   Recognize, assess, and address psychologic, social, and spiritual and religious problems.

f.   Ensure appropriate continuity of care by the patient's primary and specialist physicians.

g.   Provide access to any therapy that may realistically be expected to improve the patient's quality of life.

h.   Provide access to appropriate palliative care and hospice care.

i.   Respect the patient's right to refuse treatment.

j.   Recognize the physician's responsibility to forgo treatments that are futile.

3.   Summarize and give examples of how to comply with patient and family expectations in the five domains of quality end of life care from the patient's perspective:

a.   Receiving adequate pain and symptom management

b.   Avoiding inappropriate prolongation of dying

c.   Achieving a sense of control

d.   Relieving burden

e.   Strengthening relationships with loved ones

4.   Outline considerations for determining measures of quality of life.

5.   Illustrate how one would go about assessing quality of life for:

a.   Patient   b.   Caregivers

6.   Explain the significance and interrelationship between these two basic clinical tasks as they relate to palliative care:

a.   Communication skills

b.   Symptom control/management

7.   Analyze the significance of and mechanisms for implementing a team approach for caring for the patient with advanced illnesses include consideration of:

a.   Other physicians

b.   Nursing staff

c.   Other health care team members

8.   Analyze and discuss the significance of the "active, optimistic, interventionist" tradition of surgery for cure as compared with the needs of the patient who is "beyond cure" regarding these issues:

   a.   Time to pursue various treatments

   b.   Realistic vs. unrealistic goal accomplishment

   c.   Use of these verbs: cut, sew, resect vs. bypass, stabilize, decompress

9.   The literature indicates that the most prominent concern voiced by patients facing life-limiting disease is of pain and poorly controlled symptoms.   Evaluate the surgeon's professional and ethical obligation in dealing with this patient concern. Discuss this issue, considering:

   a.   The surgeon has the patient's comfort as priority

   b.   Every resource is accessed to attain patient comfort

10.   Care of the terminally ill

   a.   Analgesia

      (1)   Antiemetics

      (2)   Laxatives

11.   Circumstances in which consideration of organ donation is appropriate

12.   Principles of brain death

13.   Understanding the role of the coroner and the certification of death

Practice-Based Learning and Improvement that involves investigation and evaluation of their own patient care, appraisal and assimilation of scientific evidence, and improvements in patient care.

1.   Complete an evaluation and treatment plan for a patient who is at the end of life and for whom integration of life-prolongation and palliation are important considerations. Consider the following:

a.   Patient risks

b.   Treatment options

c.   Patient goals and values

2.   Utilize the principles of appropriate palliative care to counsel patients and their families about surgical and medical procedures to be employed, including obtaining informed consent after discussing the risks, benefits, and alternatives to the procedure.

3.   Demonstrate communication skills in end of life care through establishing interpersonal relationships with patients while discussing problems with them.

4.   Establish collegiality with non-surgical partners in patient care, especially regarding the spiritual care of the patient.

5.   Utilize professional resources such as Websites to assist and improve patients' palliative care.

6.   Perform selected palliative general surgical procedures such as:

a.   Drainage of effusions (ascites, pleural, pericardial)

b.   Intervention for obstructions (respiratory, gastrointestinal, urologic, vascular)

c.   Control of pain

d.   Palliative tumor resection

e.   Supportive intervention (tissue sampling, vascular access, enteral feeding tubes)

Attitudes:

1.   Recognize the concerns of patients and their families regarding their fear of uncontrolled pain.

2.   Respond positively and actively to the efforts of other members of the healthcare team for the total care of the patient, including consideration of:

a.   Non-medical consequences of treatment

b.   Quality of life issues

c.   Spiritual needs of patient and caregivers

d.   Interpersonal relationships

Practice-Based Learning and Improvement that involves investigation and evaluation of their own patient care, appraisal and assimilation of scientific evidence, and improvements in patient care.

INFORMATION TECHNOLOGY AND POPULATION COMPARISONS

REFERENCES

Abrams WB, Beers MH, Berkow R. History and physical examination. Comprehensive geriatric assessment. Establishing therapeutic objectives: quality of life issues. Surgery: preoperative evaluation and intraoperative and postoperative care. In: Abrams WB, Beers MH, Berkow R (eds), The Merck Manual of Geriatrics (2nd ed). Whitehouse Station, NJ: Merck Research Laboratories, Merck & Co., Inc., 1995;205-224; 224-235; 235-238; 321-345.

Angelos P. Palliative philosophy: the ethical underpinning. In: Dunn GP, (ed). The surgeon and palliative care. Surg Oncol Cl January, 2001;10:1:31-38.

American College of Surgeons: Principles guiding care at the end of life. Bulletin of the American College of Surgeons 1998:83:46.

Annas GJ. Informed consent, cancer, and truth in prognosis. N Engl J Med 1994;330:223-225.

Argent J, Faulkner A, Jones A, O'Keefe C. Communication skills in palliative care: development and modification of a rating scale. Med Educ 1994;28:559-565.

Bruera E, Beattie-Palmer LN. Pharmacologic management of nonpain symptoms in surgical patients. In: Dunn GP, (ed). The surgeon and palliative care. Surg Oncol Cl January, 2001;10:1:89-108.

Buckman R. Communication in palliative care: a practical guide. In: Doyle D, Hanks GWC, MacDonald N (eds). Oxford Textbook of Palliative Medicine. Oxford, United Kingdom: Oxford University Press: 1998:141-159.

Buckman R. How to Break Bad News: A Guide for Healthcare Professionals. Baltimore: The Johns Hopkins University Press: 1992.

Carron A, Lynn J, Kenney P. End of life care in medical textbooks. Ann Intern Med 1999;130:82-6.

Civetta JM. Critical palliative care: intensive care redefined. In: Dunn GP, (ed). The surgeon and palliative care. Surg Oncol Cl January, 2001;10:1:137-160.

Doyle D, Hanks GWC, MacDonald N (eds). Oxford Textbook of Palliative Medicine (2nd ed). Oxford, United Kingdom: Oxford University Press: 1998:141-159.

Dunn GP. The surgeon and palliative care: an evolving perspective. In: Dunn GP, (ed). The surgeon and palliative care. Surg Oncol Cl January, 2001;10:1:7-24.

Dunn GP, (ed). The surgeon and palliative care. Surg Oncol Cl January, 2001;10:1:242pp.

Friedsam HJ. Long-term care in the very long term. In: Seltzer MM (ed), The Impact of Increased Life Expectancy: Beyond the Gray Horizon, New York, NY: Springer Publishing Company; 1995:165-188.

Milch RA. The surgeon-patient relationship in advanced illness. In: Dunn GP, (ed). The surgeon and palliative care. Surg Oncol Cl January, 2001;10:1:25-30.

Parker RA. Caring for patients at the end of life: reflections after 12 years of practice. Ann Intern Med 2002;136(1):72-75.

Quill TE, Arnold RM, Platt F. "I wish things were different": expressing wishes in response to loss, futility, and unrealistic hopes. Ann Intern Med 2001;135(7):551-555.

Ray JB. Pharmacologic management of pain: the surgeon's responsibility. In: Dunn GP, (ed). The surgeon and palliative care. Surg Oncol Cl January, 2001;10:1:71-88.

Singer PA, Martin DK, Kelner M. Quality of life issues: patients' perspectives. JAMA 1999;281:163-8.

The SUPPORT Principal Investigators. A controlled trial to improve care for seriously ill hospitalized patients. JAMA 1995;274:1591-8.

Weissman DE, Ambuel B. Improving End-Of-Life Care. A Resource Guide for Physician Education. (2nd ed). Milwaukee: Medical College of Wisconsin Research Foundation; 2000.

Wrede-Seaman L. Symptom Management Algorithms. A Handbook for Palliative Care (2nd ed). Yakima WA: Intellicard;1999.

Wylie N, Mast T, Kennerly J. Sharing the Final Journey: Walking with the Dying. Huntsport, Nova Scotia: Robert Pope Foundations, 1996;176 pp.

Web resources
      a.   American Academy of Hospice and Palliative Medicine (AAHPM)
                http://www.aahpm.org
      b.   American Academy of Pain Management http://www.aapainmanage.org
      c.   American Academy of Pain Medicine http://www.painmed.org
      d.   International Association of the Study of Pain
                (IASP) http://www.pslgroup.com/dg/1ff02.html
      e.   Last Acts http://www.lastacts.org

Systems-Based Practice, as manifested by actions that demonstrate an awareness of and responsiveness to the larger context and system of health care and the ability to effectively call on system resources to provide care that is of optimal value.

Focus on standards of practice, delivery differences, access to care differences, cost issues, assess system problems, cooperation with hospital services, advocacy, and technology

Collaborator

1. Describe roles, expertise and limitations of all members of an interdisciplinary team required to achieve a goal related to patient care, a research problem, an educational activity or an administrative responsibility

2. Develop a care plan for a patient they have assessed, including investigation, treatment and continuing care, in collaboration with members of an interdisciplinary team

3. Participate in an interdisciplinary team meeting, demonstrating the ability to accept, consider and respect the opinion of others team members, while contributing specialty-specific expertise him/herself

4. Describe how healthcare governance influences patient care, research and educational activities at a local, regional and national level

5. Communicate with members of an interdisciplinary team in the resolution of conflicts, provision of feedback, and where appropriate, be able to assume a leadership role

Manager

1. Understand how to function effectively in a healthcare organization from an individual clinical practice to organizations at the local regional and national level

2. Understands the structure, financing, and operation of the NHS and its facilities, function effectively within it and be capable of playing an active role in its change

3. Ability to access and apply a broad base of information to the care of patients in community care, hospital and other healthcare settings

4. Make clinical decisions and judgments based upon sound evidence for the benefit of individuals and the population served. This allows for an advocacy role primarily for the

individual but in the context of societal needs when monitoring and allocating needed resources

5. Understand population based approaches to healthcare services and their implication for medical practice

6. Participate in planning, budgeting, evaluation and outcome of a patient care program

7. Be able to work effectively as a member of a team or a partnership and to accomplish tasks whether one is a team leader or a team member

Health Advocate

Demonstrate an understanding of determinants of health and public policy in relation to:

1. Individual patients by identifying the patient's status with respect to one or more determinants of health (i.e. unemployment);

2. adapting the assessment and management accordingly (i.e. the medical history to the patients social circumstances); and

3. assessing the patient's ability to access various services in the health and social system

4. Demonstrate an understanding of public health policy by describing how public policy is developed; identifying current policies that affect health, either positively or negatively (i.e. communicable diseases, tobacco, substance abuse); and citing examples of how policy was changed as a result of actions by physicians

5. Demonstrate an understanding of determinants of health and public policy in relation to: *Practice populations* by work with specialty society and other organizations in identifying current "at risk" groups within a given specialty practice and applying the available knowledge about prevention to "at risk" groups within the practice; and contributing "group data" for better understanding of health problems within the population

6. *General Population* by describing in broad terms the key issues currently under debate regarding changes in the National Health System, indicating how these might affect societal health care outcomes and advocating to decrease the burden of illness (at a community or societal level) of a condition or problem relevant to his/her specialty

society, community based advocacy group, or other public education bodies, or private organizations

7. *Individual patients* by identifying the patient's status with respect to one or more determinants of health (i.e. unemployment); adapting the assessment and management accordingly (i.e. the medical history to the patients social circumstances); and assessing the patient's ability to access various services in the health and social system

CHAPTER 15

Systems-Based Practice

15.1   RESEARCH AND STATISTICS

15.2   EPIDEMOLOGY

System based practice as manifested by actions that demonstrate an awareness of and responsiveness to the larger context and system of health care and the ability to effectively call on system resources to provide care that is of optimal value.

SECTION 15.1: RESEARCH AND BIOSTATISTICAL METHODS

UNIT OBJECTIVES:

Demonstrate an understanding of research principles and their application to the practice of general surgery.

Demonstrate knowledge about the use and application of study designs and statistical methods.

Demonstrate knowledge of the role of clinical databases in clinical research and patient care.

Demonstrate knowledge of the principles underlying evidence-based surgery.

Demonstrate the ability to critically evaluate the information provided by drug companies and medical instrument and equipment manufacturers.

Medical Knowledge about established and evolving biomedical, clinical, and cognate (e.g. epidemiological and social-behavioral) sciences and the application of this knowledge to patient care.

1.   Differentiate between the following study designs:
    a.   Descriptive or case-series
    b.   Case control (retrospective)
    c.   Cross-sectional (prevalence)
    d.   Cohort (prospective/incidence)
    e.   Clinical trial
    f.   Sequential (repeated measures)
    g.   Crossover

2.   Discuss the following concepts related to study design:
    a.   Internal versus external validity (generalizability)
    b.   Major threats to internal and external validity
    c.   Randomization, random selection, random assignment
    d.   Inclusion versus exclusion criteria
    e.   Blinding, blocking, stratification
    f.   Number needed to treat

g.   "Intention to Treat" principle

3.   Explain the differences between the following scales of measurement:

    a.   Nominal   c.   Interval

    b.   Ordinal   d.   Ratio

4.   Distinguish between the following techniques/methods for exploring and presenting data:

    a.   Frequency distribution   d.   Histogram

    b.   Bar chart   e.   Frequency polygon

    c.   Contingency table   f.   Scatterplot

5.   Distinguish between the following statistics used to summarize or describe data:

    a.   Mean, mode, median

    b.   Range, standard deviation

    c.   Percentile, interquartile range

    d.   Proportion, ratio, rate

6.   Interpret the following vital statistics rates:

    a.   Mortality, morbidity, cause-specific mortality rates

    b.   Prevalence, incidence

    c.   Adjusted rates

7.   Distinguish between the following measures of relationship between two variables:

    a.   Pearson correlation coefficient

    b.   Coefficient of determination

    c.   Spearman rank correlation

    d.   Relative risk, odds ratio

8.   Interpret the following terms and concepts related to drawing inferences from research data:

    a.   Population versus sample

b.   Population distribution, sampling distribution, standard normal distribution

c.   Standard error versus standard deviation

d.   Hypothesis testing, null and alternative (research) hypothesis

e.   Parametric versus nonparametric tests

f.   Confidence intervals, confidence limits

g.   One-tailed versus two-tailed tests

h.   Level of significance, alpha level, P value

i.   Type I error, type II error, power

9.   Identify the following tests of significance and concepts related to the comparison of means:

   a.   Independent and paired t-test (parametric tests)

   b.   Wilcoxon rank-sum test (also called the Mann-Whitney U or the Mann-Whitney-Wilcoxon rank-sum test) (nonparametric test)

   c.   Wilcoxon signed-ranks test (nonparametric test)

   d.   One-way analysis of variance (ANOVA)

   e.   Two-way ANOVA

   f.   Repeated measures ANOVA

   g.   Statistical interaction

   h.   Planned comparisons

   i.   Posterior or post hoc comparisons such as the Turkey, Schaffer, Newman-Keels, Bonferroni, and Dunnett procedures

10.   Identify the following tests of significance and concepts related to the comparison of proportions:

   a.   Z-approximation test

   b.   Chi-square test

   c.   McNemar test for comparing proportions in paired groups

   d.   Sample size and strength of association in the interpretation of the chi-square statistic

   e.   Fisher's Exact Test

11. Identify the following tests of significance and concepts related to investigating the relationship between two or more variables:

    a.   t-test for testing the significance of the correlation

    b.   Fisher's Z transformation

    c.   Confidence intervals for the relative risk and odds ratio

    d.   Simple and multiple linear regression

    e.   Standard error of estimate

    f.   Confidence bands for a regression line

    g.   Comparing two regression lines

    h.   Testing the significance of the regression line and the regression coefficients

    i.   Stepwise multiple regression

    j.   Logistic regression

12. Identify the following concepts related to the analysis of survival data:

    a.   Actuarial or life table analysis versus Kaplan-Meier

    b.   Comparing two survival curves using the Gehan or generalized Wilcoxon test, the log rank test, and the Mantel-Haenszel chi-square test

    c.   Censored observations

    d.   Cox regression

13. Interpret the following concepts related to evaluating diagnostic tests and procedures:

    a.   Sensitivity and specificity

    b.   Gold standard

    c.   Predictive value of a positive or negative test

    d.   Index of suspicion or prior probability

    e.   Likelihood ratio method

14. Discuss the following procedures, principles, and concepts related to the ethics of medical research:

    a.   The Declaration of Helsinki (see Troidl reference)

b. Informed consent

c. Institutional review boards and animal use review committees

d. Ethical use of animals in research

e. Confidentially and anonymity concerns

f. Truth and accuracy in the publication of research results

15. Explain the following procedures and concepts related to clinical databases:

a. Role of clinical databases in clinical research and outcomes research

b. Database terminology such as field, record, query, report generation, ASCII file, computer file, and merging

c. Data coding, data entry, and data verification

d. Use of standardized databases such as hospital tumor registries or state trauma registries

e. Database development

16. Discuss the following principles, methods, and concepts related to evidence-based surgery:

a. Basic skills needed to critically evaluate the published evidence:

(1) Defining the clinical question

(2) Translating the question into searchable keywords

(3) Conducting the search

(4) Selecting the best articles

b. Users' guides for selecting and evaluating articles about therapy, diagnosis, harm, and prognosis

c. Selection and evaluation of integrative articles such as review articles, meta-analyses, practice guidelines, and decision analyses

d. Use of administrative databases to link patient outcomes to costs related to producing these outcomes

e. Use of patient-reported outcome measures as another method for evaluating the success of surgical treatments

Practice-Based Learning and Improvement that involves investigation and evaluation of their own patient care, appraisal and assimilation of scientific evidence, and improvements in patient care.

1.   Critically evaluate the published evidence for a surgical therapy using a computer search engine such as MEDLINE, using the users' guide for evaluating therapy articles, and summarizing your findings in writing, to include your recommendation for surgical practice.

2.   Write a summary of the literature review, including a synthesis of the major findings and a recommendation for surgical practice.

3.   Develop and implement a computer-based clinical database using a software package such as EXCEL, ACCESS, SPSS, SAS, FileMaker, or other commercially available software.

4.   Identify and prepare a case study suitable for presentation or publication.

5.   Design and conduct a surgical research study, utilizing the following activities:

    a.   Select/search for a researchable project, involving an attending or other clinician-mentor

    b.   Search and review the literature

    c.   Formulate hypotheses

    d.   Identify key variables (both predictor and outcome), decide on the optimal level of measurement, create operational definitions, and assess reliability

    e.   Develop a research design

    f.   Identify population and study sample

    g.   Develop sample selection procedures

    h.   Select or develop measures

    i.   Develop study protocol and prepare institutional review board (IRB) proposal

    j.   Collect and analyze data

    k.   Interpret results

    l.   Identify various journal formats and related instructions to authors

    m.   Write paper

n.   Review techniques for optimal presentation of papers and posters, including related media

o.   Convert paper into an appropriate presentation

p.   Deliver the presentation

INFORMATION TECHNOLOGY AND POPULATION COMPARISONS REFERENCES

Black J, Troidl H, et al. Surgical Research (3rd ed). New York: Springer-Verlag, Inc., 1997.

Davis AT. Biostatistics. In: O'Leary JP, Capote LR (eds), The Physiologic Basis of Surgery (3rd ed). Philadelphia: Lippincott Williams and Wilkins, 2002.

Dawson B, Trapp RG. Basic and Clinical Biostatistics (3rd ed). New York: McGraw-Hill, 2000.

Glaser AN. High-Yield Biostatistics (2nd ed).Philadelphia: Lippincott Williams & Wilkins, 2001.

Gordon T, Cameron JL. Evidence-Based Surgery. Hamilton, Ontario: BC Decker, Inc., Publisher, 2000.

Hulley S, Cummings S, et al. Designing Clinical Research: An Epidemiologic Approach (2nd ed). Philadelphia: Lippincott Williams & Wilkins, 2000.

Huth EJ. Writing and Publishing in Medicine (3rd ed). Philadelphia: Lippincott Williams & Wilkins, 1998.

Kahn JP, Mastroianni AC, Sugarman J. Beyond Consent: Seeking Justice in Research. New York: Oxford University Press, 1998.

SECTION 15.2: CLINICAL EPIDEMIOLOGY AND OUTCOMES RESEARCH
PART A: CLINICAL EPIDEMIOLOGY
UNIT OBJECTIVE:

Medical Knowledge about established and evolving biomedical, clinical, and cognate (e.g. epidemiological and social-behavioral) sciences and the application of this knowledge to patient care.

1. Explain the discipline of clinical epidemiology to include the study of groups of people and the background evidence needed for clinical decisions in patient care.

2. List the clinical events of primary interest in clinical epidemiology, including: death, disease, disability, discomfort, and dissatisfaction.

3. Distinguish mass screening from case finding.

4. Discuss the following criteria used to determine for which diseases people should be screened:

    a.   Sensitivity

    b.   Specificity

    c.   Positive predictive value; negative predictive value

    d.   Number of false positives

    e.   Test factors (e.g., simplicity, cost, safety, patient acceptability)

5. For a given disease/condition, compare the advantages and disadvantages of applying multiple diagnostic tests all at once versus consecutively.

6. Discuss clinical decision analysis, including:

    a.   Defining the problem, alternative actions, and possible outcomes

    b.   Developing a decision tree to assign probabilities for each outcome

    c.   Assigning a value or utility for each outcome

7. Differentiate risk factors from prognostic factors for a given disease/condition (e.g., for acute myocardial infarction, older age and male gender are both risk factors and prognostic factors, whereas hypertension is a risk factor but hypotension is a prognostic factor).

8. Discuss the following five <u>rates</u> commonly used to predict prognosis:

a.	Five-year survival	d.	Remission
b.	Case-fatality	e.	Recurrence
c.	Response		

9. Identify locations of potential bias in randomized, controlled clinical trials, including:

   a. Patient selection

   b. Patient allocation to study groups

   c. Patient compliance

   d. Definition of outcomes

   e. Generalizability of results

10. Distinguish between clinical significance and statistical significance.

11. Analyze the following situations in which a physician's personal experience is insufficient to establish a relationship between a disease and its cause. Personal experience is insufficient when:

   a. The disease is common

   b. The disease has multiple causes

   c. The disease has a low incidence

   d. The disease has a long latency period

12. For non-experimental studies, define the following criteria for determining cause and effect:

   a. Temporality

   b. Strength of the measure of association

   c. Presence of a dose/response relationship

   d. Consistency of results

   e. Biological plausibility

   f. Specificity of effect

Practice-Based Learning and Improvement that involves investigation and evaluation of their own patient care, appraisal and assimilation of scientific evidence, and improvements in patient care.

1. Recognize when to apply a specific screening test in a case finding situation.

2. Apply clinical decision analysis to the treatment of a given patient with a given disease.

3. Estimate risk of disease development for a given patient given a history of exposure to specific risk factors.

4. Decide whether a given association is one of cause and effect.

PART B: OUTCOMES RESEARCH

Medical Knowledge about established and evolving biomedical, clinical, and cognate (e.g. epidemiological and social-behavioral) sciences and the application of this knowledge to patient care.

1. Explain the traditional negative clinical outcomes for a given surgical procedure, including death, disease, disability, and complications.

2. Discuss the modern clinical outcomes for a given surgical procedure, including discomfort, dissatisfaction, quality of life, and cost-effectiveness.

3. Identify the most frequently occurring negative outcome(s) of a given surgical procedure, (e.g., thrombosis following arterial venous prosthetic shunt formation).

4. Compare the following different ways of measuring outcomes for a given surgical procedure:

    a. Chart reviews

    b. Clinical evaluations

    c. Questionnaires

5. Discuss each of the following steps in conducting prospective outcomes research:

    a. Hypothesis formation

    b. Computerized literature search

    c. Selection of a study design

    d.   Estimation of sample size

    e.   Specification of inclusion and exclusion criteria

    f.   Allocation of patients to groups

    g.   Evaluating outcome(s)

    h.   Analyzing data

6. Provide examples of potentially confounding patient variables, including age, sex, race, income, education, occupation, religion, marital status, residence, nationality, disease stage, comorbidities, and complications.

7. Provide examples of potentially confounding treatment variables, including extent of surgery, timing of surgery, anesthetic technique, postsurgical nursing care, drug therapy, chemotherapy, radiotherapy, physical therapy, and nutritional therapy.

8. Describe the following common problems in collecting useful outcomes data:

    a.   Inadequate sample size

    b.   Inaccurate characterization of patient population

    c.   Inappropriate comparison group

    d.   Uncontrolled patient variables

    e.   Uncontrolled treatment variables

    f.   Patient noncompliance

Practice-Based Learning and Improvement that involves investigation and evaluation of their own patient care, appraisal and assimilation of scientific evidence, and improvements in patient care.

1. Demonstrate the ability to review the surgical literature critically.

2. Design a clinical outcomes research study.

INFORMATION TECHNOLOGY AND POPULATION COMPARISONS
REFERENCES

Aickin M. Causal Analysis in Biomedicine and Epidemiology: Based on Minimal Sufficient Causation. New York: Dekker Publications, Inc., 2002.

Blancett SS, Flarey DL. Health Care Outcomes: Collaborative, Path-Based Approaches. Frederick MD: Aspen Publishers, Inc., 1998;1-432.

Dawson-Saunders B, Trapp RG. Basic and Clinical Biostatistics (2nd ed). Norwalk CT: Appleton and Lange, 1994.

Fallon WF, Wears RL, Tepas JJ. Resident supervision in the operating room: does this impact on outcome? J Trauma 1993;35(4):556-561.

Fletcher RH, Fletcher SW, Wagner EH. Clinical Epidemiology: The Essentials (2nd ed). Baltimore: Williams & Wilkins, 1988.

Green ML. Graduate medical education training in clinical Epidemiology, critical appraisal, and evidence-based medicine: a critical review of curricula. Acad Med 1999;74(6):686-694.

Hennekens CH, Buring JE. Epidemiology in Medicine. Boston: Little, Brown, and Co., 1987.

Jenicek M. Clinical Case Reporting in Evidence-Based Medicine. Boston: Edward Arnold Co., 2001. Journal of Surgical Outcomes. Published by WB Saunders Co., First issue: November, 1998.

Kane RL. Understanding Health Care Outcomes Research. Frederick MD: Aspen Publishers, Inc., 1997;1-288.

McGuire HH, Horsley JS, Salter DR, Sobel M. Measuring and managing quality of surgery: statistical vs. incidental approaches. Arch Surg 1992;127:733-738.

Sackett DL, Haynes RB, Guyatt GH, Tugwell P. Clinical Epidemiology: A Basic Science for Clinical Medicine (2nd ed). Boston: Little, Brown, and Co., 1991.

Seltzer MM (ed). The Impact of Increased Life Expectancy: Beyond the Gray Horizon, New York, NY: Springer Publishing Company; 1995:1-237.

Sheps SB. Research methods for surgeons: an overview. J Invest Surg 1993;6:321-328.

Stewart M, Tudiver F, Bass MJ, et al. (eds). Tools for Primary Care Research. Newbury Park CA: Sage Publications, Inc., 1992.

Troidl H, Spitzer WO, McPeek B, et al. (eds). Principles and Practice of Research: Strategies for Surgical Investigators (2nd ed). New York: Springer-Verlag, Inc., 1991.

Wallace RB, Woolson RF (eds), The Epidemiologic Study of the Elderly. New York: Oxford University Press, 1992:1-387.

Wilkin D, Hallam L, Doggett M. Measures of Need and Outcome for Primary Health Care. Oxford: Oxford University Press, 1992.

EPILOGUE

"I have never let my schooling interfere with my education."

Mark Twain

SUCCESSES: PERFORMANCE

In surgical education, we seem to have been very successful in modeling residents. Their first choice of activities is to be in the operating room learning by observation and direction. They are eager to operate and become proficient in surgical skills and in performing successful operations. Unfortunately, this may only represent a third or less of what is important in providing quality surgical care[1].

Outside of the operating room, residents seem to learn best in environments with clear protocols and standards and with good clinician mentors. Residents learn the logistics of providing care relatively easily in this situation, but the critical decision making, practice based and system based management often falter.

"Study without desire spoils the memory, and it retains nothing that it takes in."
Leonardo Da Vinci

FAILURES: INTEGRATION

One of our biggest failures in applying educational approaches to surgery has been a lack integration of the curriculum into current work. Since the curriculum is only a "guide", it's successful integration into the curriculum is usually not measured and like most un-appraised activities, it is often unmanaged and its impact uncertain. This failure usually stems from a second problem, in that the residents and faculty do not "own" the curriculum. Usually the staff teaches from their practice, they do not feel an accountability to assure the residents successfully reach all the goals in the faculty's specialty area. The lack of appreciating the educational value of the curriculum is also why updating, refining and prioritizing the curriculum is considered such a heinous job. The resident's attitude toward using the curriculum usually represents the same type of distain.

"Intelligence plus character-that is the goal of true education."
Martin Luther King Jr.

INCLUSIONS: ASSESSMENT AND CULTURE

As this volume started, we noted the companion volume; "General Surgical Residency Assessment Program" would provide details on assessment tools and approach. Part of that volume is a focus on culture. A discriminator of quality in surgical training programs is the internal standards by which the residents perform and interact with each other, the staff and faculty. Our assessment in surgical education has been heavily weighted toward medical knowledge and skills attainment. There are those that believe that we can "train" residents on Interpersonal behaviors and Professionalism, but we cannot "educate" them because this relates to personal intrinsic values. Our failure to address this issue with surgical residents is evident by the fact that, in most surgical departments, interpersonal behavior and professionalism issues are more predominant with surgical faculty then those of competency.

A focus on a culture of integrity and professionalism may be the way to create an opportunity for the resident to examine their own personal value system and for change.

"You can never be overdressed or overeducated."
Oscar Wilde

OMISSIONS: BALANCE

As noted above, most surgical programs are successful at generating surgeons with competent surgical skills and that know how to follow treatment plans. Most trainees have a good fund of knowledge regarding evidence based medicine. Unfortunately, based on medical advances, this preparation is only adequate for a 5 or 10 year period. Additionally, the skill and application components of surgery is such a consuming aspect of the discipline that training, the "knowing how", overwhelms education, the "knowing why"[2]. Modeling dominates over independent behavior. Rules govern flexibility. This is most apparent in two areas; system management and quality improvement. At the time of its introduction, the ACGME competency of System based practice seemed both intrinsically obvious and valuable and simultaneously virtually undefined. There is a glaring void in systems management, the critical factor of "knowing why", which is required for successful implementation of training in this competency. Similarly, successful training in quality improvement tools and approaches is compromised without independent behavior and flexibility in the approach to medical managment.[3] The failure of so many medical institutions in their quality improvement programs may be seated in this lapse in true educational approaches.[4] A Surgical educational program should strain to balance training versus education.

"There's a difference between interest and commitment. When you're interested in doing something, you do it only when circumstance permit. When you're committed to something, you accept no excuses, only results."

Art Turock

EXECUTION: COMMITMENT

The volume on quality; Surgical Systems: Quality Management, ended with a quote from Donabedian on the basic truth on how to succeed in quality management.

"A genuine persistent, unshakable resolve to advance quality must come first. If that is present, almost any reasonable method for advancing quality will succeed. If the commitment to quality is absent, even the most sophisticated methods will fail."[5]

A. Donabedian

It is striking how this same sentiment applies to the resolve required for successful surgical educational programs. If there is a genuine commitment and concern for your surgical residents; teaching and improving their educational program becomes innate.

REFERENCES

1. Guru, V et al Relationship between preventability of death after coronary artery bypass surgery and all cause risk adjusted mortality rates. Circulation 2008;117:2969-2976.

2. Essenhigh, RH. A few thoughts on the difference between education and training. Letter to the editor; National Forum. Phi Kappa Phi Journal 2000:46.

3. Fabri PJ. Is there a difference between education and training? 2008 http://www.facs.org/education/rap/fabri0408.html.

4.   Vest JR, Gamm LD. A critical review of the research literature on Six Sigma, Lean and StuderGroup's Hardwiring Excellence in the United States: the need to demonstrate and communicate the effectiveness of transformation strategies in healthcare. Implementation Science 2009; 4:35(1-9)

5.   Donabedian, A. An introduction to Quality Assurance in Healthcare, Oxford Press, NY 2003.

www.ingramcontent.com/pod-product-compliance
Lightning Source LLC
Chambersburg PA
CBHW050644150426

42813CB00054B/1172